# SIMPLE LIVING

## in the 21st Century

**Robert Spaccarelli**

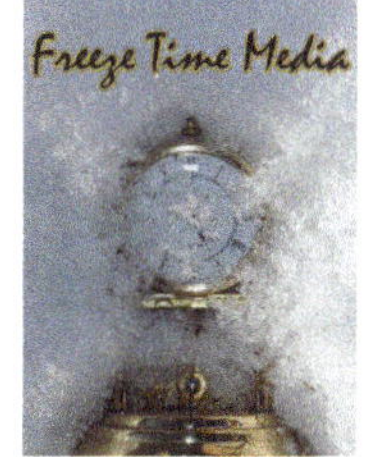

Simple Living in the 21st Century



www.robertspaccarelli.com

Freeze Time Media

ISBN-13: 978-1-946702-02-9

ISBN-10: 1-946702-02-1



Editor: JJ McKeever

Interior layout: Di Freeze

Cover: James McKeever III, Di Freeze

Unless otherwise noted, all images in this book were taken by Robert Spaccarelli.

# Praise for *Simple Living in the 21st Century*

Knowing Robert Spaccarelli is like living with a verbal encyclopedia. Robert first came into our lives and world when my wife and I were looking for an expert to control and manage the acreage around our beautiful barn in Putnam County. Robert brought with him so many talents in so many fields. I asked how honey was made. Within a week, we had a wild flower garden planted and six working beehives, which eventually supplied us with forty pounds of honey. Each year we have an abundance of the healthiest vegetables I've ever tasted.

Who needs to cook when Robert puts on his chef's apron? Every week he creates unbelievable luncheons of homegrown vegetables and freshly procured fish from special markets only he knows of. His main dish could easily earn three stars in a Michelin guidebook, and for dessert, we just reach over and pluck a dozen of his delicious figs from the trees he's stored over the winter months. Need to catch your own fish? Then follow Robert to the Adirondacks where his expertise will teach you to catch the biggest pike the lake has to offer. Robert is an all-round expert on — you name it, he'll be it.

So glad he's in our lives.

*Jim and Julie Dale*

I serendipitously met Robert Spaccarelli at a time when it became clear that transforming Grape Hollow Farm, a 47-acre property in Dutchess County, into a permaculture paradise required more than just a plan on paper. It required someone with his expertise and experience to maintain and grow an agriculturally productive ecosystem with the diversity, stability, and resilience of natural ecosystems.

Rob knows firsthand how to work with nature, rather than against it. Completely intuitive and self-taught, he's created and educated me on how to build beehives, bountiful gardens abundant in Jerusalem artichokes, kale, ground cherries, green peppers, tomatoes, eggplants, and a plethora of earth's treasures. He planted an orchard with 500 fruit trees, taught me how to tap trees and make maple syrup, and sourced apples for hard cider. In short, he's been an indispensable part of the growth and success of Grape Hollow Farm.

*Scott Berrie*

We lovingly refer to Robert as the Dr. Doolittle of plants.

Over the last six years, Rob has helped us transform our land into a magical organic garden and oasis for bees and butterflies. My favorite day of the week during the spring, summer, and fall is the day I spend with Rob in the garden learning the ins and outs of organic gardening and sharing the wonders of nature. Rob has taught us the fundamentals of gardening, the Zen patience one must have with mother nature, and the subtle hints that nature gives you to detect the presence of disease, predators, and new growth.

Throughout the season, we create a bounty of produce that we proudly enjoy and also freeze or can for the winter months. There's nothing like opening a hearty soup in mid-January that was created from the fruits of the summer garden!

Rob has helped us transform our front lawn into a walking oasis of native plants, fruits, and berries as we try to keep our bees and butterflies healthy and thriving.

If you're interested in sustainable living, a farm-to-table organic life, and watching your own bees pollinate the flowers on a tree that will shortly burst with fruit, this is a must-read book!!

*Melissa and Lewis Kohl*

*This book is dedicatd to my parents — Lucy and Victor Spaccarelli. They inspired me to be who I am today and all I accomplished. Mom was a wonderful cook and inspired my own love of cooking. She taught me a lot. Dad was an incredible gardener, stonemason, and bricklayer who built many buildings at Fordham University in the Bronx. He was a forager and could live off the land. Much of what they taught me led to this book. I know they would have gotten a kick out of it.*

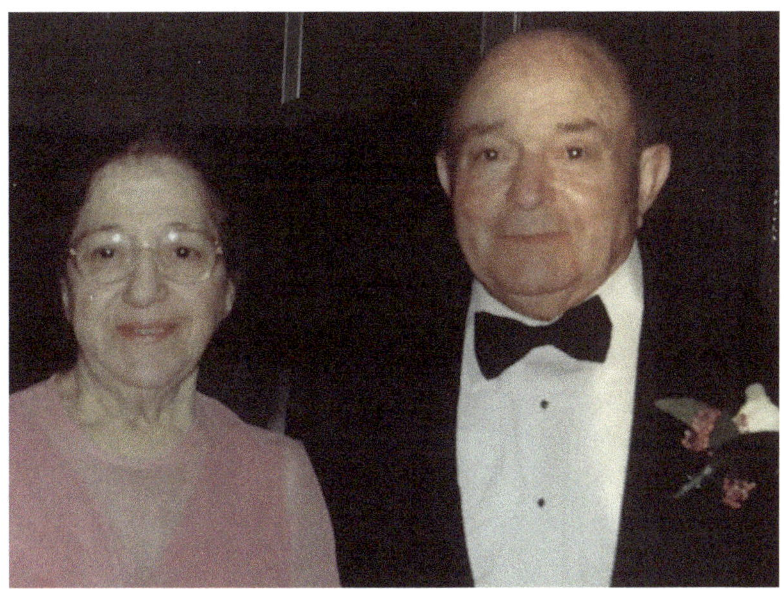

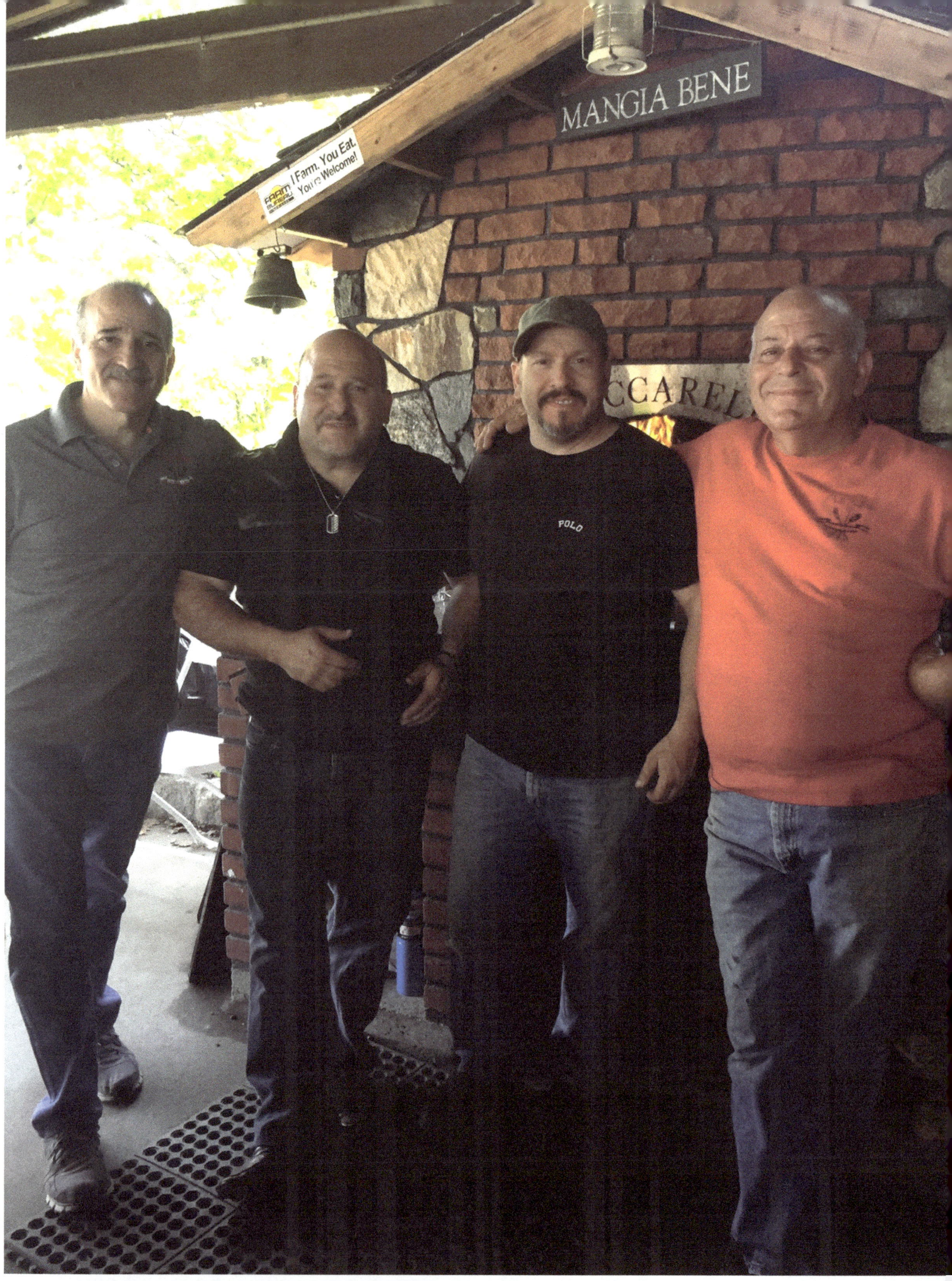
MANGIA BENE
I Farm. You Eat.
POLO

# Acknowledgments

I'd like to give a special thanks to the following people who made such an impact on my life, leading to the creation of this book:

My parents, Victor and Lucy, for showing me many things about the woods that I use to this day. Dad took me along as a child and taught me quite a bit. Mom was a very good cook and I learned many of her recipes.

A special thanks to my brother Victor. He's the one who took me to a fair when I was 10 years old, which got me hooked on beekeeping.

My brother Mike took me fishing as a young boy. He also built my beautiful home with his own hands.

My sister Phyllis for always being there for me.

My sister Jean for watching me as a child. She was my babysitter and looked after me for quite a while.

My brother John, who also took me in the woods and taught me a lot about mushrooms.

John Alfano, who introduced me to pike fishing on Bantam Lake in Connecticut. He is my best friend and always will be.

To my kids, Julian and Lucy. You have been an inspiration to me, and I see the apple hasn't fallen far from the tree. Julian is following in my footsteps with gardening, honey harvesting, and growing plants and fruit trees. He has also become a great fisherman. Lucy is a wonderful chef, baker, jelly and jam maker, and helps harvest the figs and make the chutney we all enjoy.

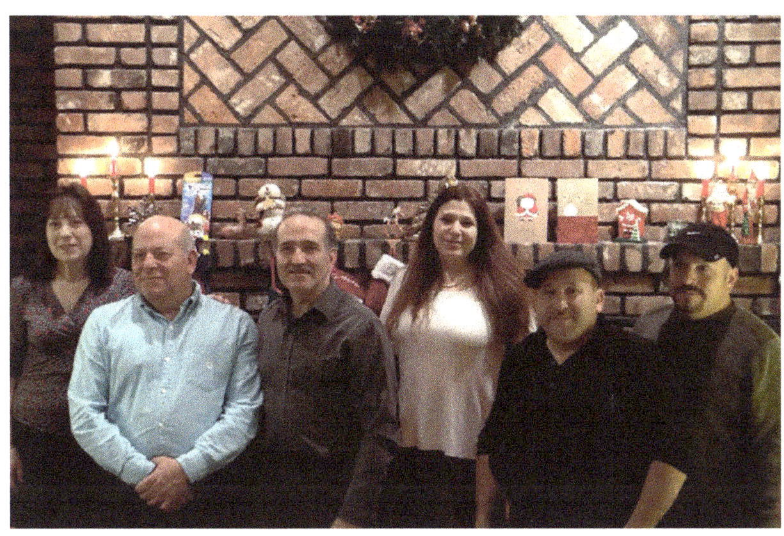

*Above: Jean, Victor, John, Phyllis, Mike, and Robert Spaccarelli.*

*Left: John, Mike, Robert, and Victor.*

# Contents

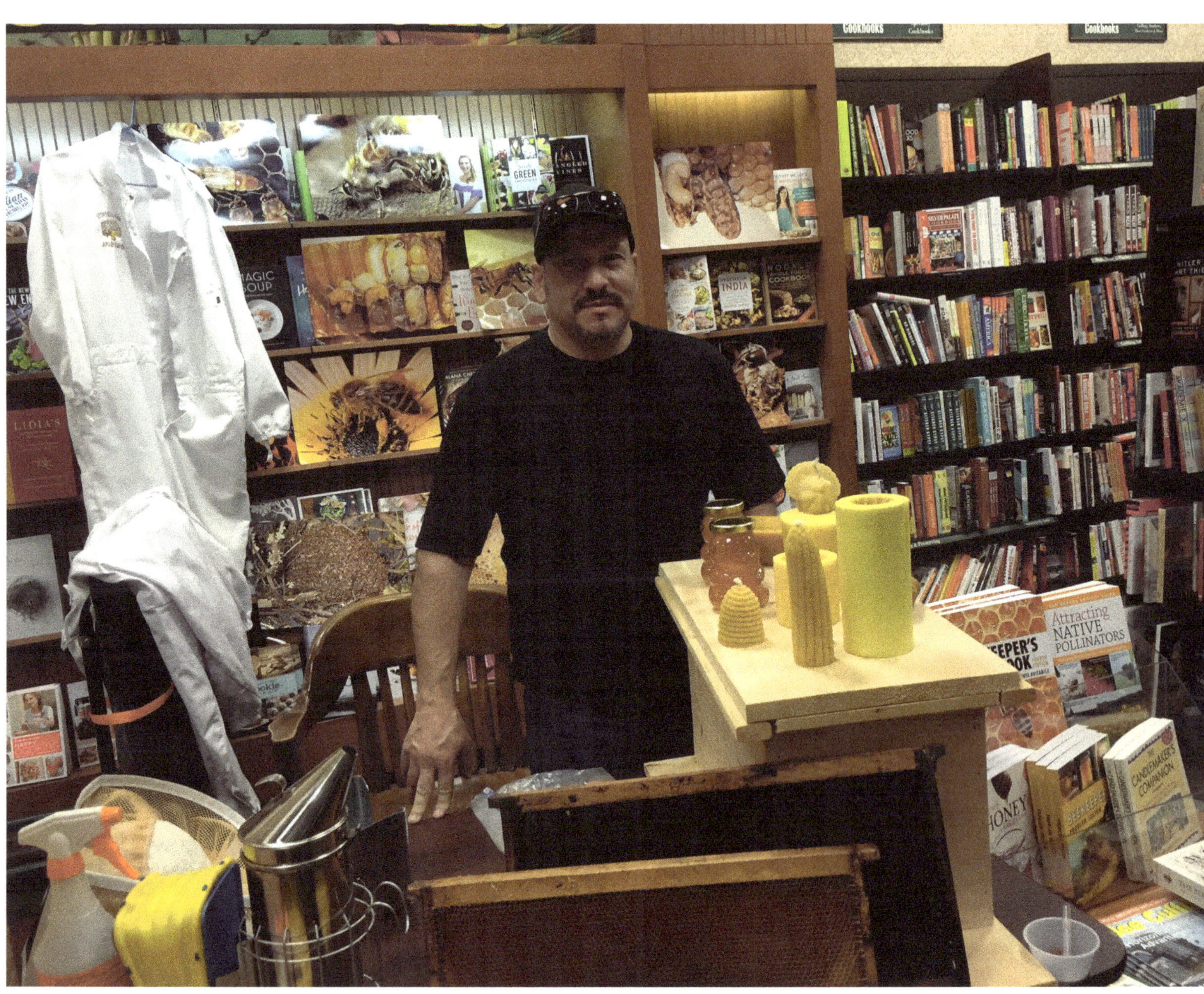


*Beekeeping speech at Barnes & Noble.*

# Introduction

I was born on August 4, 1969. I say that to put some things in perspective. I grew up at a time when the country was going through unprecedented technological advances. Computers went from big and expensive to one being in almost every home. Cars do everything except drive themselves — and that's even coming into existence. We have more computer power in our smartphones than all of NASA had when they put a man on the moon three weeks before I was born. Every year we witness more discoveries than happened in the entire preceding decade.

This book doesn't shortchange all the technological progress we've made just in my lifetime. In the grand scheme of things, all those things are just tools to make life easier to navigate. Yes, I can look up anything on my phone for immediate information, but who's to say that being able to do that is more important than the discovery of fire, or of the wheel! It's all relative depending on humankind's situation at the time of an invention.

However, there are things that men and women want to get back to that we've delegated to others. These are the building blocks of life, such as healthy eating, growing some of our own food, and learning more about nature, so we'd better understand it and incorporate it into our lives. While technology may be great, it really doesn't make life easier for many of us. Quite often, it seems to make things more hectic and frustrating. Many desire to live life more simply.

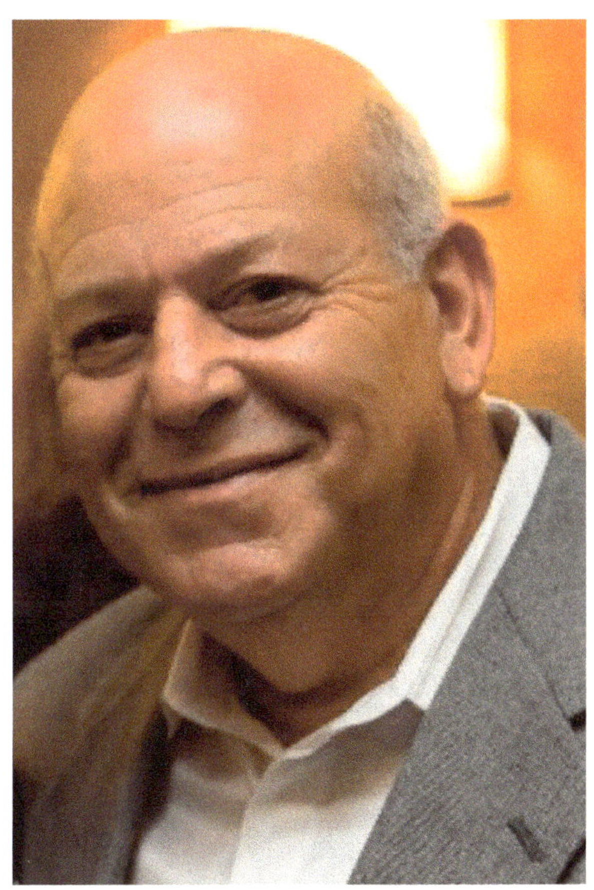

*My brother Victor indirectly got me involved in beekeeping.*

I believe I do that and I want to share with others some of the things I've learned. I'm a beekeeper, raise figs and vegetables, use nature's bounty to add to what my family eats, manage other people's farms, help homeowners create a sustainable landscape, and use my knowledge of wildlife and nature to be a practitioner of sustainable living in whatever way possible.

It isn't like I had an epiphany while I was an adult and decided to live my life this way. I've been like this since I was a boy. When I was 10, I didn't want a toy truck; I wanted seeds to plant and get them to grow! The fascination and wanting to learn more about the process of anything in nature has never left me.

Looking back, it isn't a surprise why I was that way. My parents were an inspiration. By profession, my father was a bricklayer and stonemason. He was also a gardener, searched for wild mushrooms, foraged in nature, and showed me how to hunt and fish. He and my mother were hard workers and passed on that quality to me and my five brothers and sisters.

Yes, there were six of us, with me as the youngest. The others are Victor, Phyllis, Jean, Michael, and Johnny.

My mom never minded me making greenhouses out of cellophane and cardboard to grow my seeds on the windowsill. Victor was the one who indirectly got me involved in beekeeping. When I was 10 years old, he took me to our local fair, the Yorktown Grange Fair. While there, he took me to meet Tom Rippilon, a beekeeper who had a stand at the fair where he was selling his honey and other products. Victor asked him if I could hang out there for a while selling honey with him, and Tom said sure. While I helped him with his honey, we talked about bees and honey. I was fascinated, and I was hooked.

Ever since then, I've been a beekeeper. The world of honeybees fascinates me. When I was a teenager, and the first video games came on the market, they weren't something that interested me. Learning more about bees and increasing my hives kept my attention. Honey is one of the most nutritious natural substances known to man with many healthy properties. It's also delicious and you can use it in many ways.

That's part of what I want to share with you in this book. I'm also very good at foraging for wild mushrooms and plants. For me, it's inspirational to find edible plants and share them with my family. To this day, I still go foraging for wild mushrooms in the places my father took me. I want to share with you some information we've lost over time as a culture, since people began buying their food at grocery stores. It doesn't take much to learn how to raise your own mushrooms, go out and forage for some, and collect edible plants.

My son, Julian, and daughter, Lucy, often accompany me on my foraging adventures in the spring. I started teaching them when they were little children. They're growing up knowing how to forage and grow their own veggies. I include them in all I do so they'll know in the future how to be sustainable, eat healthily, and share their knowledge with others.

Sharing with others prompted this book. Something deep inside of us yearns for a simple life more in tune with nature. There's a beauty in the land and vast resources available if you know where to look. I still enjoy catching salmon in September and smoking them. Most people don't realize how beautiful nature is and what it has to offer. Growing seeds, starting a garden, and then eating the fruits of your labor is satisfying. Many people would like to learn how to do this.

Some have hired me to help them. As an adult, I've taken all I've learned to another level. As I mentioned, I help people with their farms and teach them sustainable living. I go in and organize their landscaping. I utilize ground cover and bring in blueberries and strawberries. Not only do I show them how to dress up their land with plants like this, but now they're also producing food. Nothing is better than biting into a fresh strawberry. You know you used all natural material to help grow it. You find the taste of a fresh berry so much better than what you buy in a store that was probably grown in a greenhouse.

The knowledge of sustainable living is becoming lost. Other adults hire me to show them how it works or to bring it about on their property, so I know there's a desire to learn. The yearning for knowledge goes much younger than that, though. I go to elementary schools, resurrect their gardens, and teach the students about gardening.

I started helping at a local school where keeping up the gardens just wasn't in the budget anymore. The first school I went to had gardens completely overgrown with poison ivy and weeds. I ripped everything out of the beds and coaxed the soil back to life with nitrogen, compost, and manure. Then I had the kids bring in seeds and brought some plants from my greenhouse. Soon we had a bumper crop of various flowers and vegetables growing. What I was able to teach their kids touched the hearts of the parents. As they learn about growing veggies, they're also learning about eating healthier.

I want to help those looking for a little guidance in sustainable living or wanting more out of life. It isn't like what I do makes a person anti-technology. There's a place for everything. I use computers and smartphones. I also start new hives from my bees and make a mean fig chutney from my own fruit. I think trying to live simpler in the 21st century is achieving a better balance. Maybe you're on a computer all day for work. It doesn't mean that you couldn't get your hands dirty in your garden when you come home or harvest your own honey when it's time.

For this book, I'm mainly focusing on beekeeping, gardening, growing figs, wild mushrooms, fishing, and foraging. I'll also share some recipes because I'm a darn good chef with all these natural ingredients. It all comes from practical experience. I learned from success and failure. There's no reason you should make some of the mistakes I did!

I love that my children are growing up with an appreciation for living as we do as a family, and learning as we go. I want all my readers to leave this book with more knowledge, and the desire to put it to use.

Enjoy!

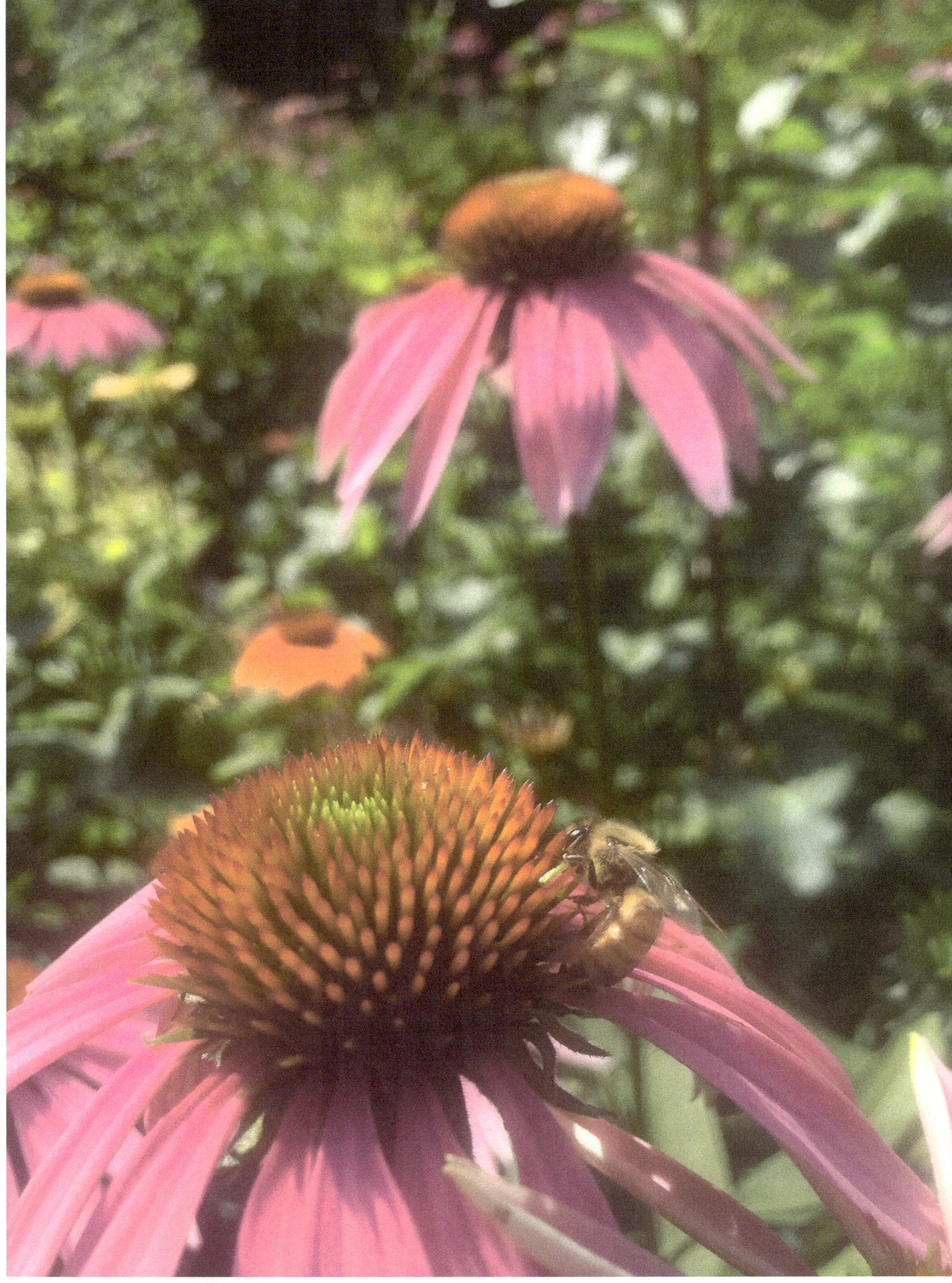

# Bees and Honey

*"The keeping of bees is like the direction of sunbeams."*

**— Henry David Thoreau**

Honey is a natural sugary food substance made and stored by certain social insects. The best known and the easiest of them to colonize is the honeybee. To give you the technical process of how a bee makes honey, the insect produces it from the sugary essence of plants that it gathers. Through regurgitation, applying enzymes, and causing water evaporation, a group of bees can produce a copious amount of honey. This is the science of it, and I'll go into much more detail further on in this section.

Bees have fascinated me since I was a boy and began to work with them. The popularity of beekeeping and the threats to honeybees were the initial driving force in writing this book. I encourage others to get involved in beekeeping for honey production or just to help with pollination because it will have positive ramifications in the world. That's no exaggeration!

The variety of honey that comes from honeybees is the most popular. It's produced and consumed worldwide. Fructose and glucose give honey its sweetness. Most microorganisms don't grow in honey, and it has the same relative sweetness as granulated sugar. I have a section later in the book with some of my recipes, but honey is a wonderful sugar replacement in cooking and baking.

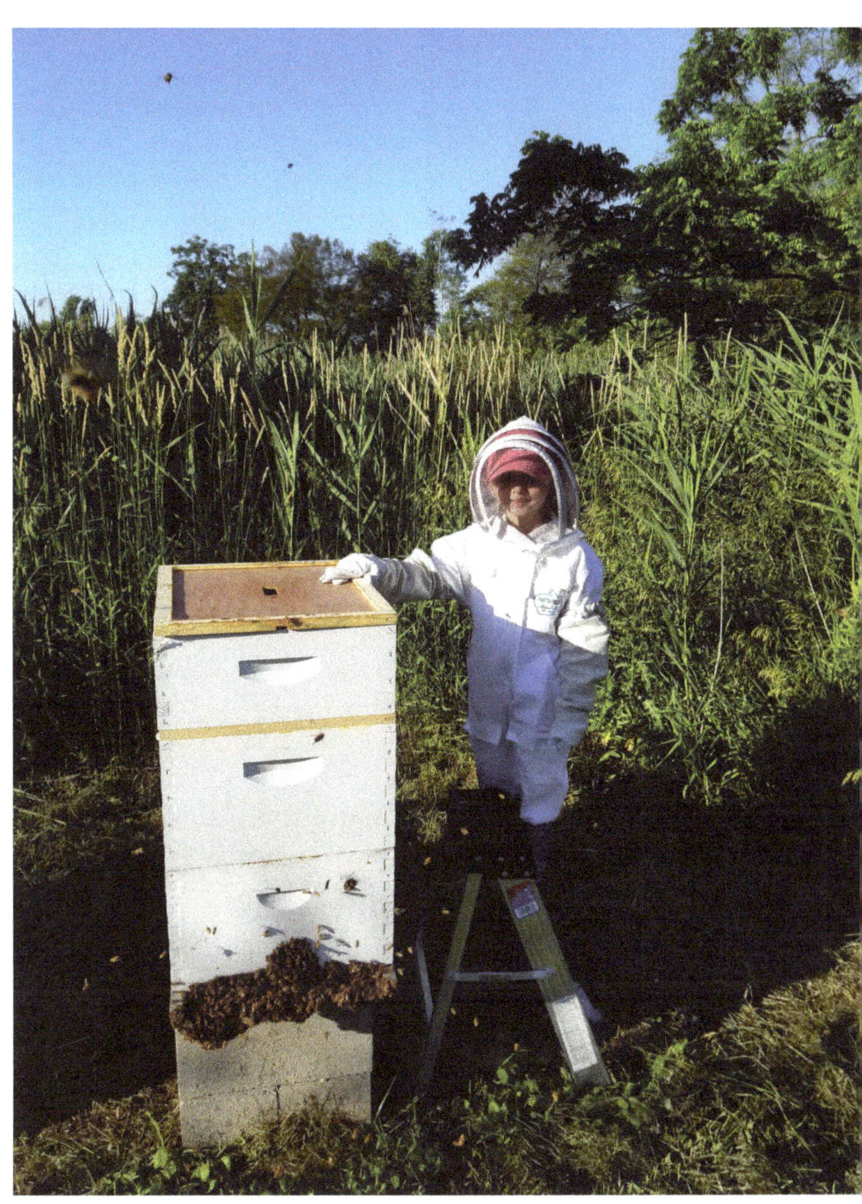

*Above: Like me, Olivia started beekeeping at an early age.*

*Left: Honeybee foraging nectar on echinacea.*

## *Honey in History*

Honey isn't some modern-day fad. I find the history of honey interesting. Here's a brief version of it, so you can appreciate your role in a long and needed industry.

The first ancient acknowledgment of honey is in a cave painting from Valencia, Spain. It shows humans searching for honey over 8,000 years ago. It depicts two figures gathering honey and honeycombs from a wild hive. The humans are lugging around baskets and gourds to collect the golden liquid. Furthermore, the painting shows a series of ropes or ladders the bee hunters used to approach the bees' nest. Experts in ancient civilizations speculate that people followed certain birds or animals attracted to honey to find the hives.

The country of Georgia holds the oldest honey remains that archaeologists have found. They discovered honey clinging to the surface of clay containers found in an ancient tomb. Dating on these items go back some 5,500 years ago. In a further study of tombs from that area and era, it appears that people buried several varieties of honey with the dead for their journey into the hereafter. Analysis of the different kinds of honey showed that they came from berry blossoms, linden, and various wildflowers.

The ancient Egyptians used honey in a great deal of cooking, including its use as a sweetener for cakes and biscuits. That's certainly something that hasn't changed for 3,000 years. Honey was also an ingredient they used for embalming the dead. Unlike cooking, honey isn't used much for that anymore! Min, the Egyptian fertility god of Egypt, received honey as an offering.

The roots of our own civilization, ancient Greece, produced great quantities of honey. Domestic beekeeping was very much in style 2,500 years ago in Greece. In fact, there were so many beehives around Athens that the government passed a law in 594 BC. It stated, "He who sets up hives of bees must put them 300 feet away from those already installed by another."

Archaeologists in Greece have unearthed hives from that ancient era. It appears that ancient Greek beekeepers were willing to move their hives over far distances to produce the most honey possible. It seems that they took advantage of different growing seasons for various flowers and fruits to maximize production.

As with Egypt, honey was a key sweetening ingredient in Greek and Roman food preparation in the absence of sugar. Many recipes mention the use of honey at the time, and the literary works of authors like Virgil, Homer, Cicero, and others talk about its uses.

As in Greek and Roman texts, there's also a rich trove of ancient texts from India like the Vedas and Ayurveda writings from 4,000 years ago that document the use of honey. Chinese history shows that beekeeping is so old in that area of the world that its origins are untraceable. Ancient scrolls mention beekeeping and how the type of wooden box used for storage was an important factor in its quality.

Before Europeans settled Central America, the Mayans also domestically produced honey. They colonized and gathered honey from the stingless bee for cooking purposes, and continue to do so today. The Mayan stingless bee was considered sacred.

## *Honey in Religion*

Speaking of sacred, you can find honey documented prevalently throughout many of the world's religions. Have you ever heard the saying that "Honey is the food of the gods?" In ancient Greece, the food of the twelve gods of Olympus and Zeus was honey in the form of nectar and ambrosia.

In Hinduism, honey, which they named Madhu, is one of the five elixirs of immortality or Panchamrita. In temples, priests poured honey over the deities in a ritual called Madhu Abhisheka. The Vedas and other ancient Indian literature mention the use of honey as a great medicinal and health food.

The Jewish tradition has honey as the symbol for their New Year, known as Rosh Hashanah. During the traditional meal commemorating the holiday, the Jewish people dip apple slices in honey and eat them to bring in a sweet new year. Many Rosh Hashanah greeting cards show honey and an apple, symbolizing the feast. In some synagogues, ushers give out small straws of honey to celebrate the New Year.

The Bible's Old Testament contains many references to honey. We read in the Book of Judges how Samson found a swarm of bees and honey in the carcass of a lion that helped him survive. Old Testament law encourages the Hebrew people to make offerings of honey in the temple to God. The Book of Leviticus says, "Every grain offering you bring to the Lord must be made without yeast, for you are not to burn any yeast or honey in a food offering presented to the Lord." (2:11). Jonathan finds himself in a confrontation with his father, King Saul, as related in the Book of Samuel. This occurred because Jonathan ate honey in defilement of a rash oath Saul made (14:24–47). Proverbs says, "Pleasant words are as a honeycomb, sweet to the soul, and health to the bones." The Promised Land is described in Exodus as a "land flowing with milk and honey."

In 2005, archeologists found an apiary dating from the 10th century B.C. in Tel Rehov, Israel. It contained 100 hives and estimates have it producing half a ton of honey annually! Pure honey is considered kosher, though produced by a flying insect, which is a non-kosher creature. In Jewish law, it's the only product of a non-kosher animal given kosher status.

The New Testament relates how John the Baptist survived for a long time on a diet consisting of locusts and wild honey while living in the wilderness. I always thought that proves anything tastes better with honey!

Buddhism tradition has honey playing a vital role during the festival of Madhu Purnima. Buddhists celebrate this holiday in India and Bangladesh. It commemorated the time Buddha made peace among his followers by leaving them. He retreated to the wilderness where it's said that a monkey brought Buddha honey to eat. On Madhu Purnima, Buddhists remember this occasion by giving honey to monks. Buddhist art frequently depicts the monkey's gift.

Islam has an entire chapter in the Quran called an-Nahl (the Bee). According to his teachings, Muhammad strongly recommended honey for healing purposes. In fact, honey's history as a health aid has been around for as long as people knew about the golden liquid.

## *Honey in Health*

Honey is nature's purest food. It contains 22 amino acids, 26 minerals, and is a powerful immune system booster. It contains up to 5,000 live enzymes. When looking at it for its health benefits, you want raw, unfiltered honey. Keep in mind that honey you buy from a supermarket is usually refined, filtered, and heated for easy marketing and bottling.

Raw honey comes directly from the hive. It's extracted through centrifugal force or crushed out of the comb. With the crushed method, you let the honey settle in a bucket and allow the wax and particles to float to the surface, which you can then scoop out. All the healing properties remain in the honey.

Civilizations have always believed honey has many practical health uses. People have used it as an ointment for rashes and burns. It's still used as a method to help soothe sore throats when other remedies aren't effective. In myths and folk medicine, honey has been used both orally and topically to treat various ailments including gastric disturbances, ulcers, skin wounds, and skin burns by ancient Greeks and Egyptians, and in Ayurveda and traditional Chinese medicine.

As a treatment for wounds and burns, honey may have antimicrobial properties, as first reported in 1892, and is useful as a safe, improvisational wound treatment. Consuming local raw honey is believed to help with seasonal allergies due to repeated exposure to the pollen in the area.

As for other health benefits, here's a synopsis gleaned from organic.net on the positive effects honey has on the human body:

**Sweetener:** Honey can be used as a sugar substitute in many drinks and foods. Since it's approximately 69 percent glucose and fructose, honey is better for your health and well-being as opposed to regular white sugar.

**Weight Control:** While honey does contain more calories than sugar, it helps with the breakdown of stored fat in your body. Simply mix the honey with warm water and drink it down. Combining lemon juice or cinnamon with honey also aids in losing weight.

**Energy Source:** According to the USDA, honey contains about 64 calories per tablespoon. Therefore, many people use it as a source of energy. On the other hand, one tablespoon of sugar will give you about 15 calories. Furthermore, even the most sensitive stomachs can easily convert the carbohydrates in honey into glucose, since it's very easy for the body to digest this pure, natural substance.

**Improving Athletic Performance:** Recent research has shown that honey is an excellent ergogenic aid and helps in boosting the performance of athletes. It's a great way to maintain blood sugar levels, muscle recuperation, and glycogen restoration after a workout, as well as regulating the amount of insulin in the body and energy expenditure.

**Source of Vitamins and Minerals:** It contains a variety of vitamins and minerals. The type of vitamins and minerals and their quantity depends on the type of flowers used for apiculture. Commonly, honey contains vitamin C, calcium, and iron. If you check the vitamin and mineral content in regular sugar from any other source, you'll find it to be completely absent or insignificant.

**Antibacterial and Antifungal Properties:** People often use it as a natural antiseptic in traditional medicines because of its antibacterial and antifungal properties.

**Antioxidants:** It contains nutraceuticals, which are very effective for the removal of free radicals from the body. As a result, our body immunity improves against many conditions, even potentially fatal ones like cancer or heart disease.

**Skin Care with Milk and Honey:** Milk and honey are often served together since both of these ingredients help in creating smooth, beautiful skin. Consuming this combination every morning is a common practice in many countries for this very reason.

**Honey in Wound Management:** Significant research is being carried out to study the benefits of honey in the treatment of wounds. The Nursing Standard explains some of these benefits in wound management in their documentation of its benefits.

Researchers continue to do a wide variety of studies on honey and its positive effect on people. It's a simple, but powerful natural substance. After all these years, we might have only scratched the surface of its uses. The wonderful thing is that it just tastes so good!

Realizing what honey is all about brings into focus just how amazing its production is — the result of a hard-working insect no bigger than the size of the tip of one of your fingers. As a group, bees are a complex community where every bee has a job to do, and the sustainability of the hive hinges on each bee performing to the best of its abilities. People could learn a lot about working together from observing this phenomenon.

*Summer wildflower honey on the left and fall Japanese knotweed honey on the right.*

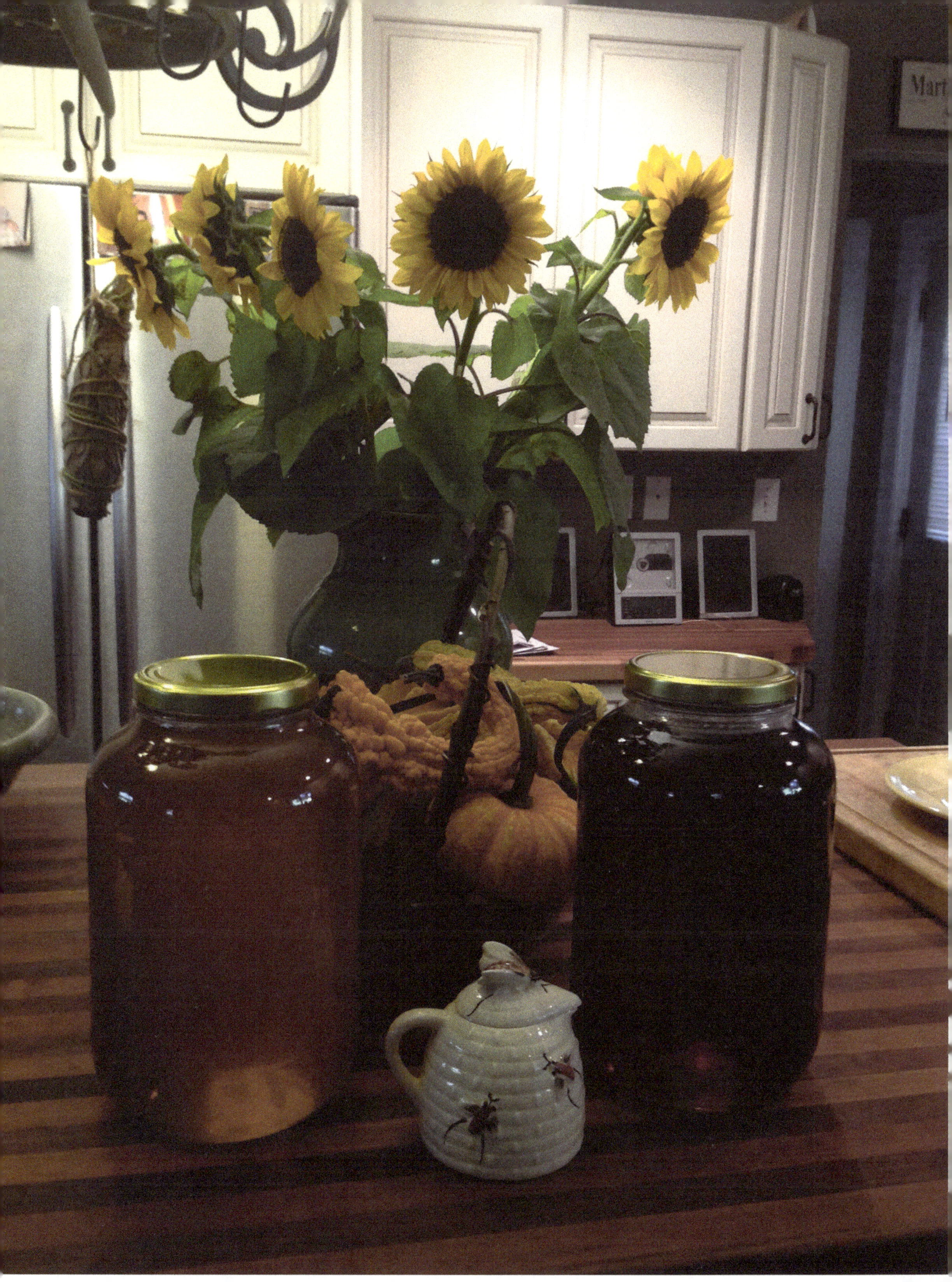

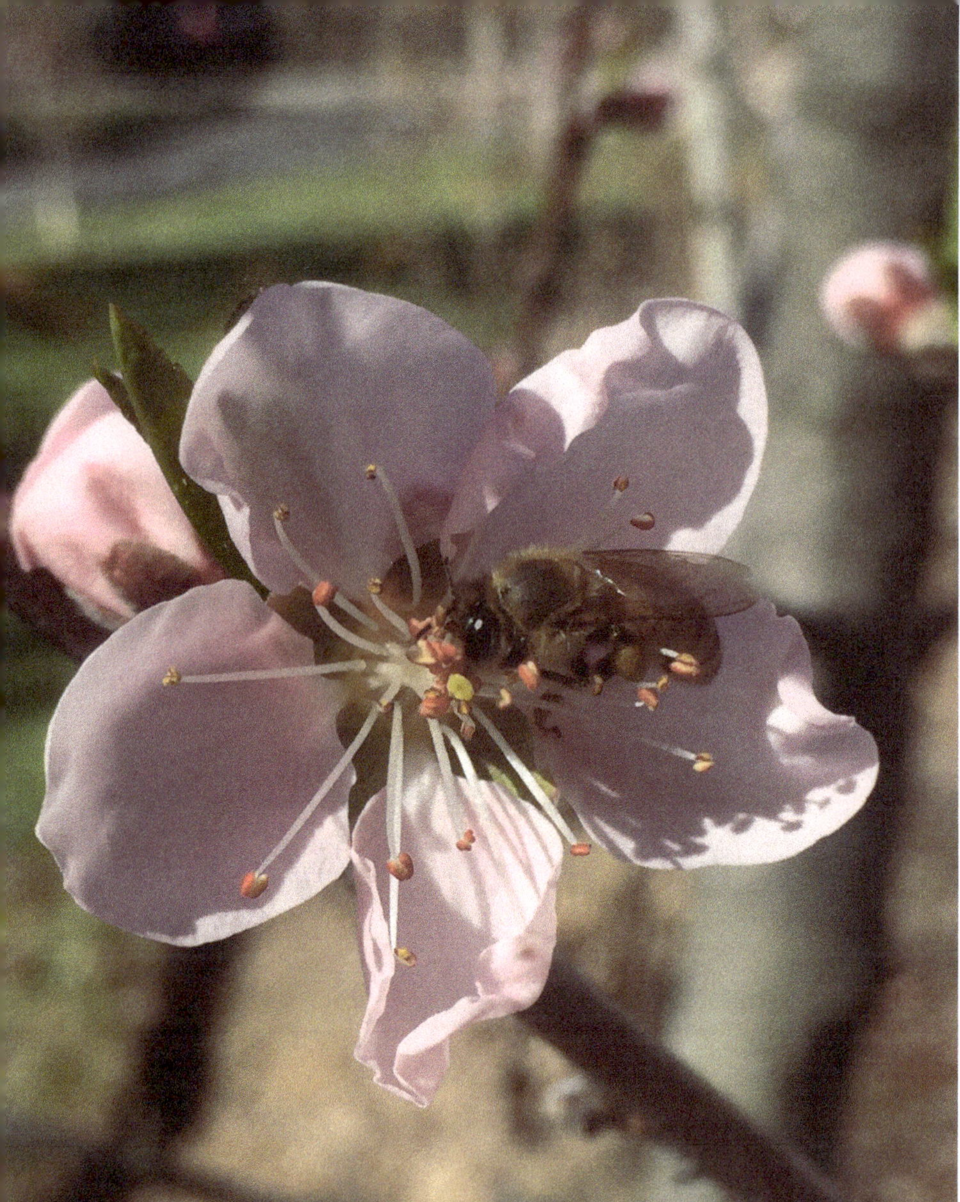

*Worker honeybee on a peach blossom.*

## The Honeybee

You can call a hive of bees a cluster. We call the clusters inside the hive a colony. When you see a picture of a mass of bees in their colony, it appears very confusing. In fact, honeybees are highly organized. This is even more awe-inspiring when you consider that a typical colony consists of 45,000 to 50,000 bees! A colony consists of just one queen and around 800 drones, which are the male bees. The rest are female workers.

Bees are very social for one important reason — a single bee cannot survive alone. They all work together and cooperate in doing their respective duties to organize the brood nest. For example, some jobs bees perform to maintain the life of the colony is to keep the larva at a proper temperature, fan nectar to evaporate water to produce honey, and collect pollen to feed brood developing larva. A colony of bees works together to ensure their survival.

The heart of the hive is the queen bee. She needs 16 days to emerge from her cell. She's the largest female of the hive. All the other worker bees are also females. The queen's job is to lay eggs all day to keep up the numbers of the colony.

The queen stays down in the hive in the brood chambers and raises the young. The other bees feed her royal jelly, which the worker bees secrete from their glands in the hypopharynx. This gives the queen the energy to lay thousands of eggs a day. She's a hard worker, and without her, the hive will go downhill. When her laying pattern develops a sparseness, it might be time to re-queen the hive. I share how to do this a little further along in this section. When you re-queen, the laying pattern will again become robust. Come spring, you will have a good brood cycle.

During honey production, the worker bees only live six to seven weeks. One of their jobs is to feed the queen bee. The only time the queen flies is in the spring to mate with a drone. In winter, workers live longer, usually around six months. This happens because their stored honey in the hive lessens from consumption. The honey left in the hive that they created over the summer months sustains them over the winter. They feed on the honey as they gather around the queen.

The only bee in the hive that doesn't play much of a role in the colony is the drone. The drone, one of the largest bees in the hive, doesn't have a stinger. They live off the nectar from the worker bees, and they just take up space in the hive during the summer months. Their critical role is in the spring when they vie to mate with the queen so that she lays up to 2,000 eggs a day.

The worker bees kick the drones out of the hive in the fall, and they then starve to death. New ones are born into the hive in the spring from new unfertile eggs laid by the queen. That way you have 200 to 300 drones in the colony during the busy season when the hive produces copious amounts of honey. As fall approaches and honey production begins to taper off and shut down, they're cast out so they won't take up space and eat food during the winter months. The colony won't allow it.

It takes twenty days for the worker honeybees to hatch from an egg laid by the queen. When worker bees hatch, they are known as nurse bees for their first week of life. They have a gland in their head known as the hypopharyngeal gland. After the first week, this gland starts to develop and produces royal jelly. They then feed this jelly to the larva along with bee bread, which is fermented pollen and nectar.

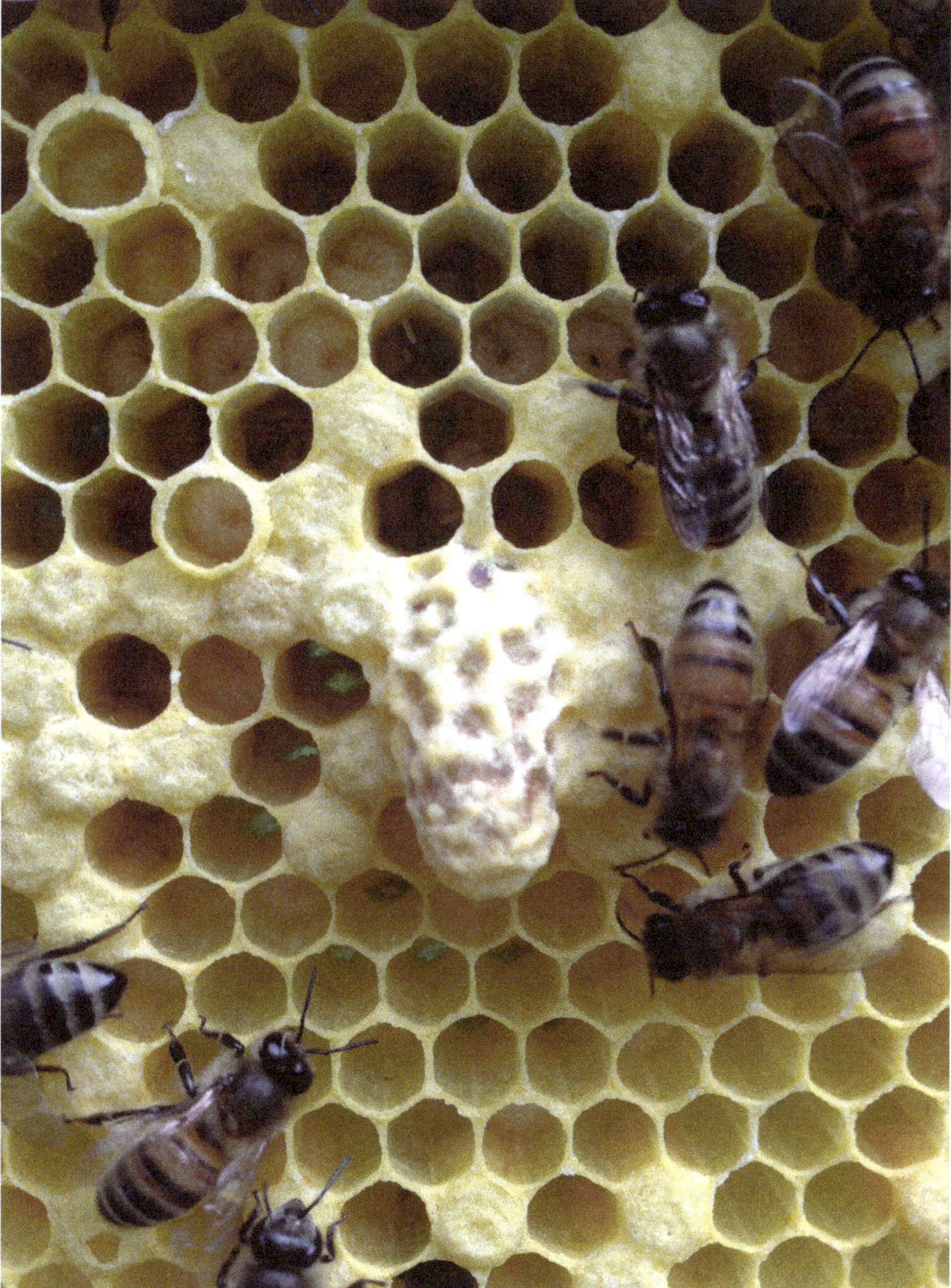

*Freshly made queen cell waiting to hatch.*

Once the bees develop in their cells, they go through their larva stage. This is where they wrap themselves with a cocoon, and then they pupate. After twenty days, they hatch. Their job in the colony is to learn the ropes of the hive. They tend and feed the other bees. First, they become acquainted with the other worker bees coming in. After a few weeks, they begin collecting pollen and nectar. When they bring the nectar back to the hive, they deposit it into the cells constructed in the colony. These cells start to fill with nectar. Once the cells are three-quarters of the way filled, the bees start fanning their wings rapidly, evaporating moisture from the nectar. This activity thickens it and before you know it — Eureka! You now have honey. Once the cell is 99 percent full, they start to build a thin layer of wax over the cell and cap it with capping wax. This preserves the honey for long periods of time over the winter months so the remaining bees in the colony can feed on it.

## *The Hive*

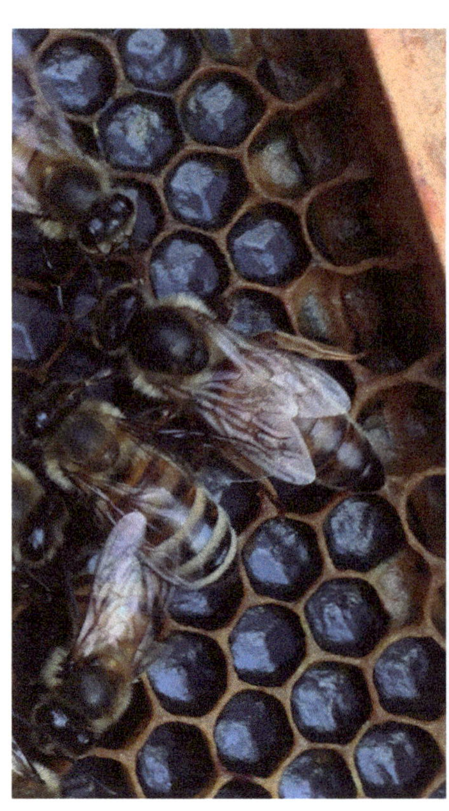

Swarming of the bees is a process the colony uses to regenerate. It's how they produce a new family. During the spring, you begin the time of mass brood production. This is when the "swarming" takes place. Queen cells form, and then the old queen flies off along with half of the colony. At this time, the old queen settles on a branch. It can be 20 feet or half a mile away from the previous colony. Once the rest of the bees that followed her settle on a branch, scout bees fly away to look for a new place to live. This is the time a beekeeper would love to locate a swarm. He or she is always on guard for this event when the swarming season approaches. It's the ideal way to start a hive.

Generally, in the Northeast, this happens around the last week of May and the first week of June. Once the swarm sends out the scout bees, they look for a hollow cavity, an old barn, or something conducive to starting a new hive. Wherever they decide to go, the swarm will follow them. If a beekeeper uses this opportunity to introduce them to a man-made hive, that will become their home.

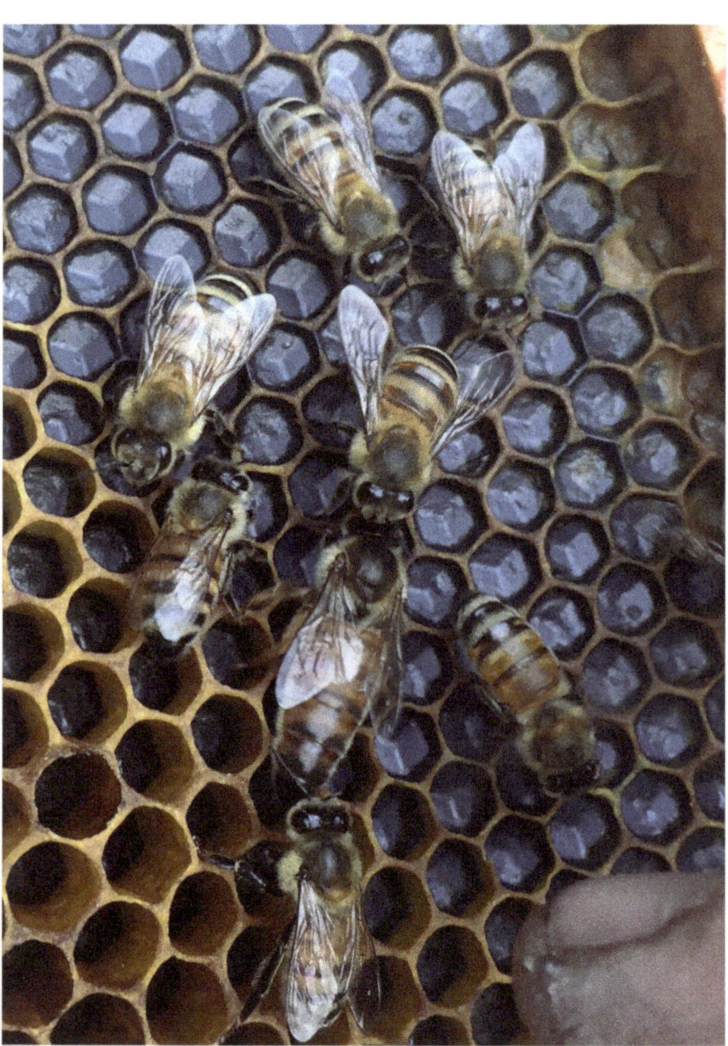

Once the swarm leaves the hive, the new queen that emerges will take the place of the former queen in the existing hive. It's only a matter of a few weeks before that old hive returns to full strength. This is when the new queen bee makes her only flight. It's a mating flight, and she flies straight up with several drones flying after her. The first drone that meets up with her will mate her for life. It's a very short life for the winning drone, as he falls to the ground and perishes once he and the queen complete mating. Now, the queen will return to the hive, and she begins her job of laying thousands of eggs a day to keep up with the demand of needing new workers to replenish the loss of those that die. Keep in mind that the worker bees only live for about six or seven weeks during the summer. Once the queen starts to lay eggs and the brood develops, they'll hatch out, and then begin collecting nectar and pollen from flowers to produce the honey to sustain themselves over the winter.

As a beekeeper, you can prevent these swarms from happening by removing the congestion of the colony before the swarming activity begins. You can split and increase your apiary by removing the cells and frames from the colony, and do your own split by introducing a new queen into the existing colony.

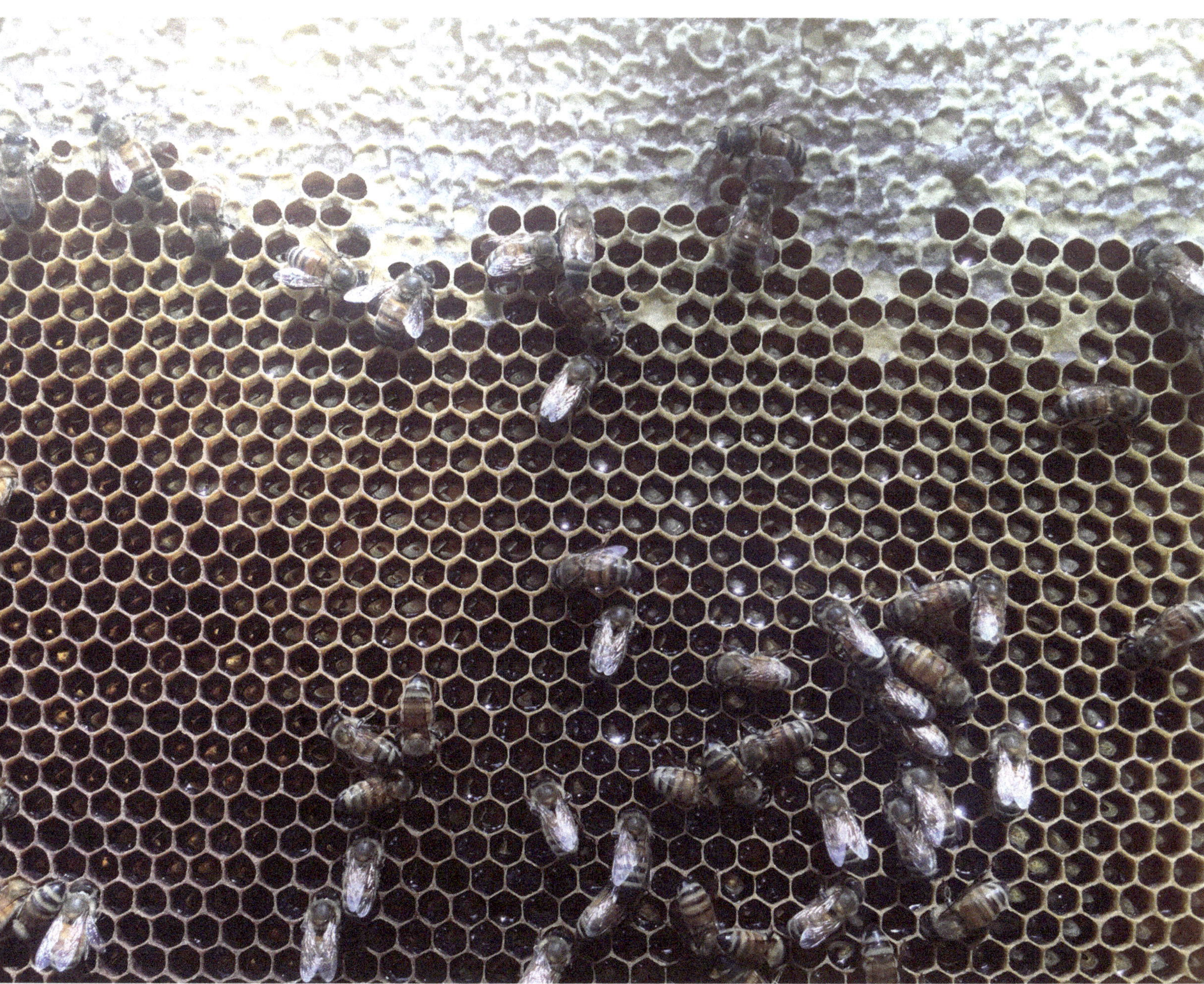

Feral bees or wild honeybees are those that live in a tree, in an old barn rooftop, or in someone's attic or old shed. Many years ago, wild honeybees were very common. Unfortunately, certain circumstances today such as attacks by different types of mites and environmental issues have adversely affected the population of wild honeybees. Mites weaken the immune system of bees. This causes them to be born without wings or with deformed ones, preventing them from flying so that they can do their job of collecting food for the colony. The result is that this dramatically weakens the colony.

*Page 8 top and bottom: Gravid queen bee; worker honeybee tending and feeding the queen.*

*Above: Bees capping honeycomb.*

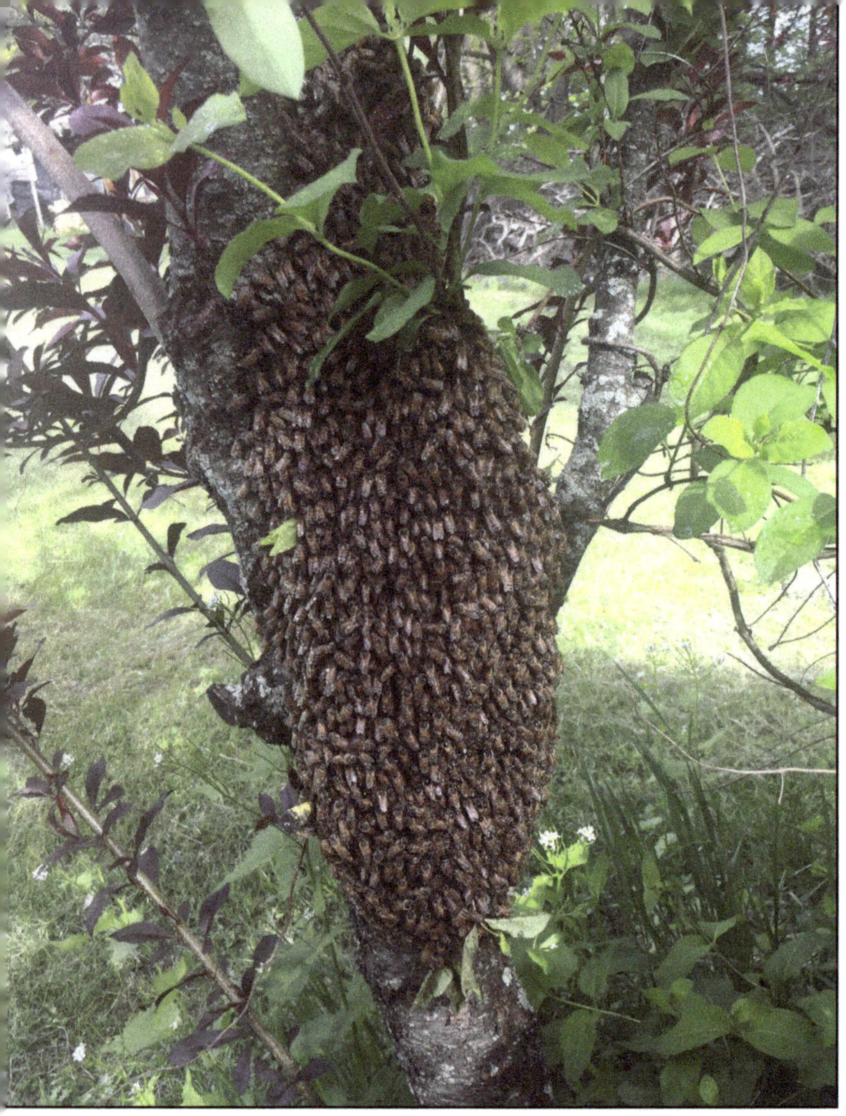

*Honeybee swarm.*

By finding the swarms when they split off from their former colony and introducing them to a man-made hive, a beekeeper can then collect and treat those feral bees. You're now preventing mite attacks on the bees. You're also providing a safe haven for the colony. Bees will often build in a rotted or decayed log. If that wood falls down, the colony is scattered and in disarray. Beekeepers give the honeybees a better chance by putting them in a hive. It gives them a safe home, and they receive treatment for the various parasites that attack them. Here's a situation that by taking an animal out of the wild, you're giving them a better opportunity to live and prosper.

Once you capture a swarm with a good number of bees and a queen, you shake the colony into the hive. When they become established, you can look in and see when the queen is depositing eggs in the cells. You can take a second box and attach it to the hive. The queen lives in the brood chamber. By attaching the second box that contains 10 frames with foundation, it becomes the second brood chamber, and the colony can grow. Younger bees draw out waxy comb that the queen will inhabit. Once she moves in and lays several thousand eggs, they develop into larvae and become nurse bees and foraging bees. Later in the season, you can add a honey super, which encourages the production of comb honey.

If you aren't ready to go searching for a swarm, there are other ways to start a hive. In the spring, you can form a hive either by obtaining a nucleus colony from a beekeeper you know or buying a package of bees. You purchase the package from an apiary, and it contains three pounds of bees and a queen. If you live in a northern area of the country, I don't recommend buying a package of bees because they might be from a warmer climate. They won't adapt to the cooler area in which you'd keep your hive.

I always recommend getting local honeybees from an apiary or a beekeeper that you get to know and with whom you're familiar. He can supply you with a nucleus colony, a hive split, or a swarm. Those bees will be more adaptable to settle in, be hardier, and winter much better than a package of bees from Northern California or Georgia.

About the first week of May is the best time in the Northeastern area to start a hive. The apple blossoms and dandelions provide the first good flow of nectar at that time of the year. The bees need this source of flowers in the early spring to build up and produce honeycomb. They gather the nectar, and the queen starts to lay and raise larva.

## *Harvesting a Swarm*

The development of a swarm usually occurs in May. It's part of their reproductive cycle.

The bees select an egg and feed it royal jelly produced by a gland in the nurse bee's head. In fact, they do this with two or three queen eggs because they need to produce "queen insurance cells."

The first queen to emerge and develop becomes the queen of the hive. When she's ready to hatch out, she begins making a "piping" noise. It's both a signal and a sound: "Bzz, bzz, bzz, bzz." I've heard it many times through the hive, and it's amazing.

As soon as the bees hear this, they rip down the other queen cells and destroy them. When the new queen starts making that noise, she's telling the old queen, "It's time to go and cast off your new colony."

This is when the swarming happens. The old queen bee is about to take off on her first flight in three years or so. Before she leaves, she sits at the entrance of the hive. Then, she'll make a short flight and land on a tree. Half the colony will surround her and go with her.

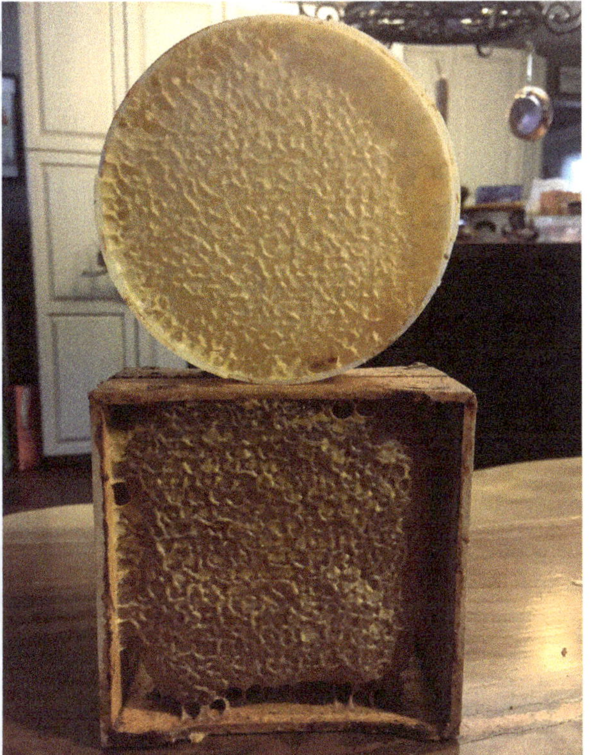

The other bees have been preparing since she began piping. They begin to drink honey, knowing they'll be homeless for several days until they find a new home. By the time they leave, they have a full belly of it.

This is why swarms are usually very docile. They're in between their old hive and starting a new one. You might see a swarm in or on a tree. You could put out your hand to them, and you won't need any protection. They're so full of honey that they can't sting. They're very lethargic, and they're not looking to defend anything.

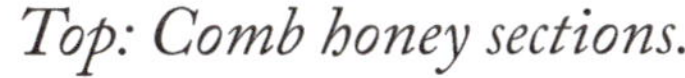

*Top: Comb honey sections.*

*Bottom: Ross Rounds are the new and modern way of producing comb honey. The wooden sections constructed of basswood is the way it was done back in the 1930s. I still do it this way.*

*Page 13: Beautifully capped honeycomb harvested in June.*

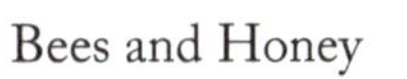

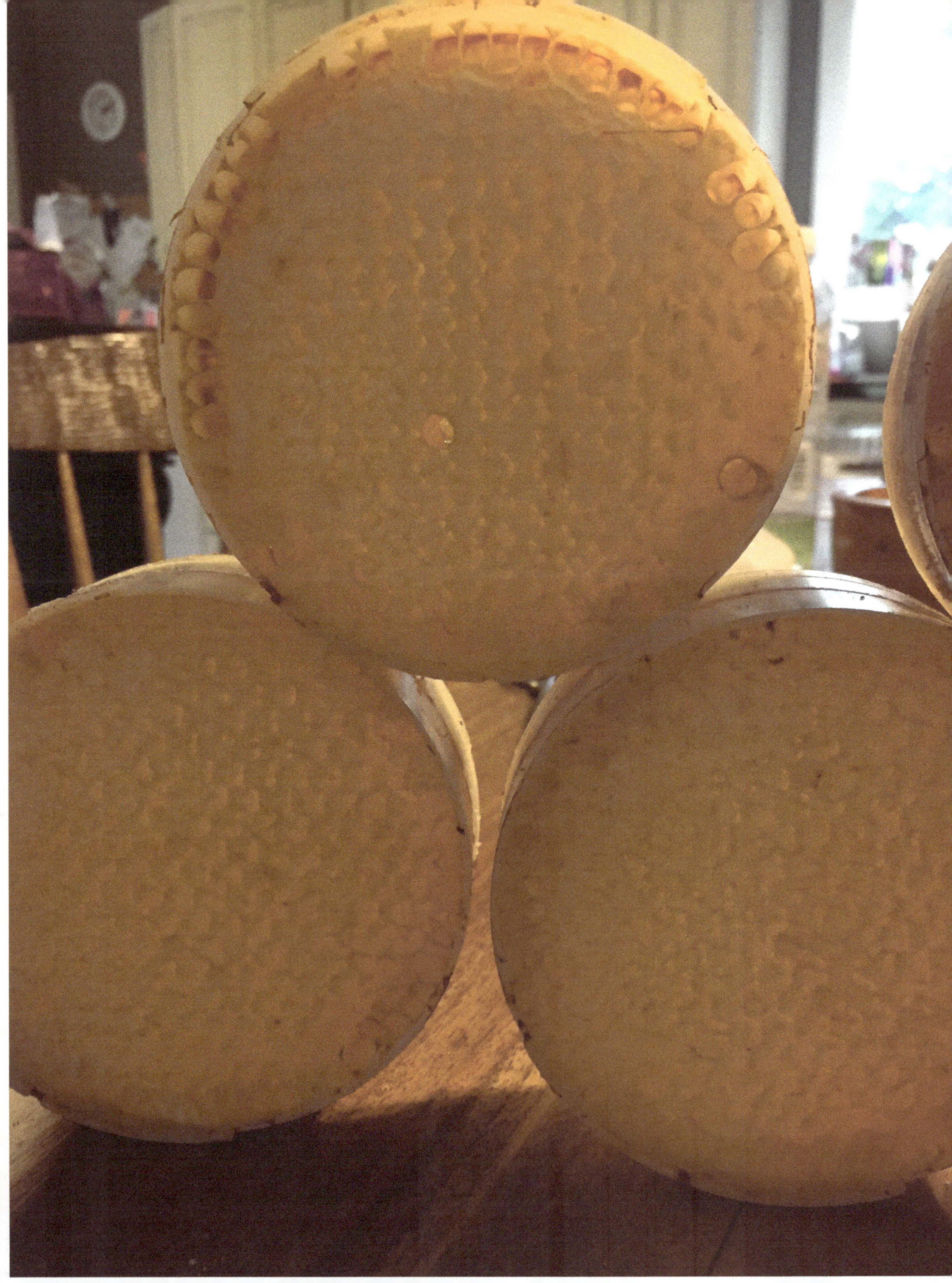

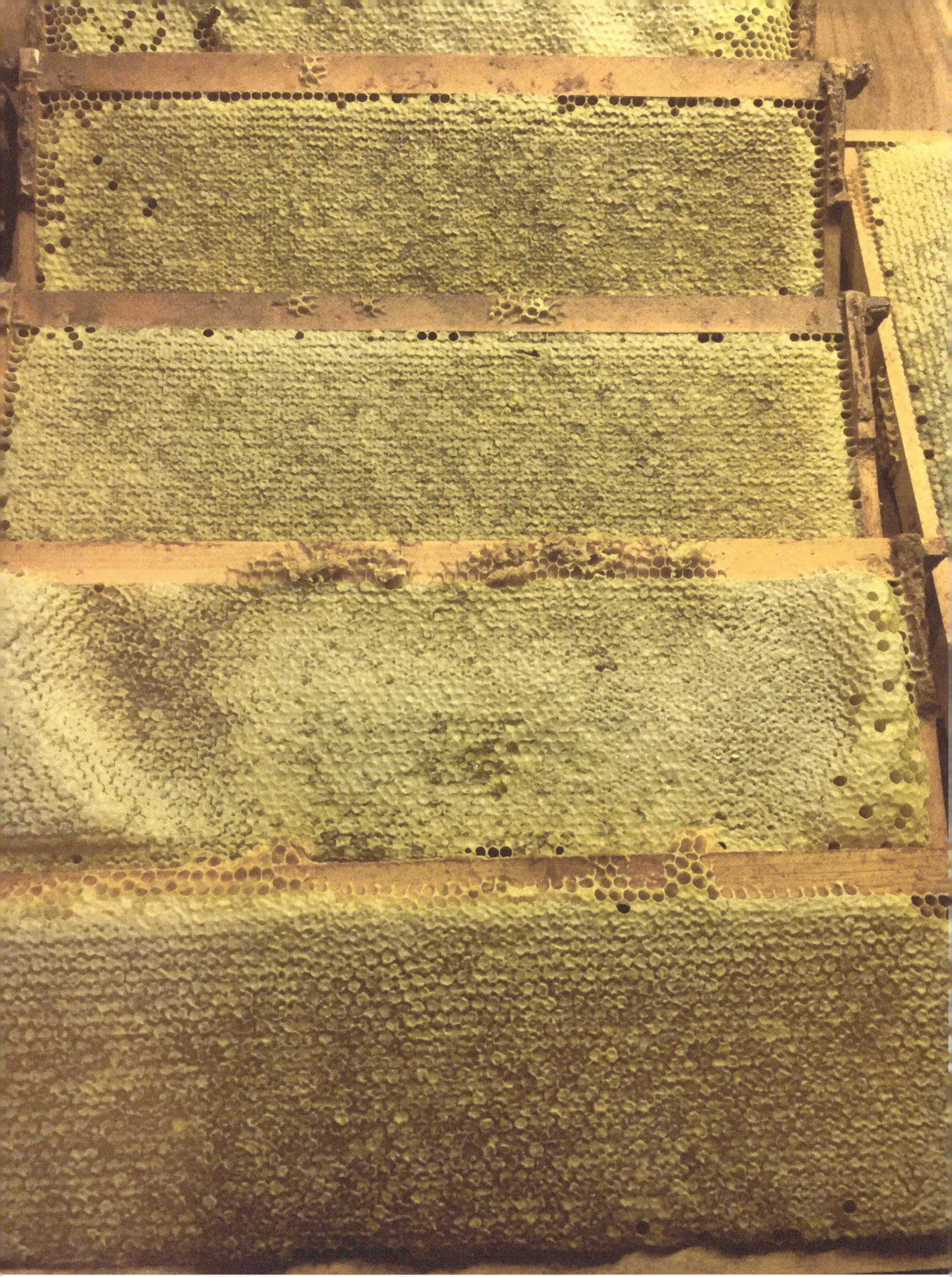

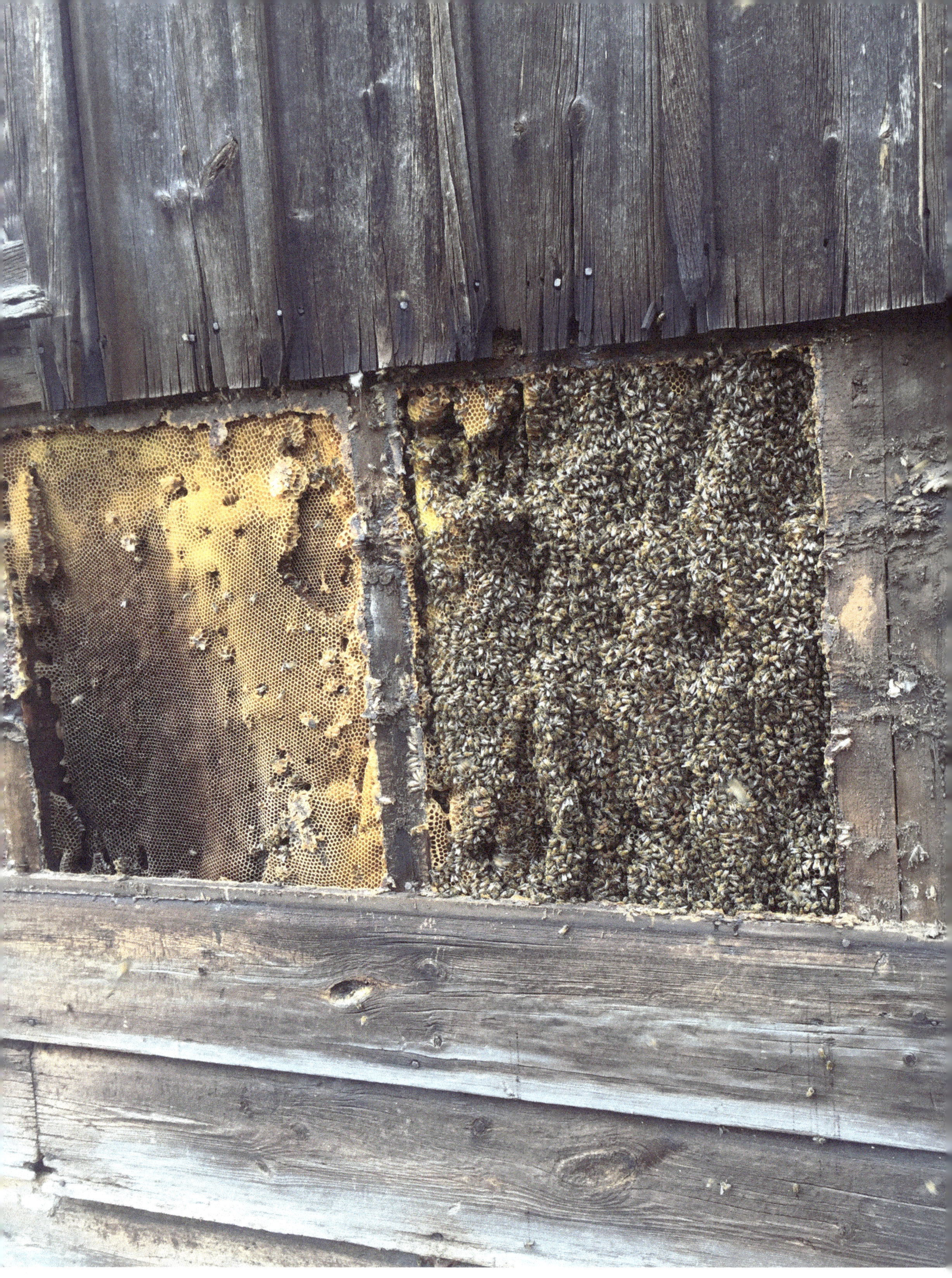

When I get a call to capture a swarm, it usually means that it's about 24 hours old. At this point, the scout bees have been searching for a new location but haven't found anything yet. If they're hanging on a tree, it means they've ingested all their honey. They're what I call "hot." They can be a little more aggressive than a fresh swarm and they're more apt to sting.

I usually carry a spray can of sugar water, and I spray them down. It makes them a little more flightless, and it also gives them something to eat. Next, I hold my swarm box underneath them. This consists of two or three frames of drawn comb, and it's very inviting to them. It's easy to entice homeless bees. I use a turkey quill to brush the bees into the swarm box. If I notice the queen, I grab her with a little queen catcher and put her in that box. As soon as I do that, the other bees in the box start flaring. This is when they all start fanning their wings and sending the air up to the other bees in the swarm. They're sending up the pheromone of the queen. When the other bees sense where the queen is, they all start heading for the box. They look like lava moving in slow motion down a hillside. It's cool to watch.

When you catch a swarm in spring, they have plenty of time to reproduce and build up their numbers and their strength. This way they'll be prepared to face the winter and survive the cold months.

The swarm box contains five frames as opposed to a standard hive with ten. Basically, it's half of a hive. I load the swarm box on the truck and bring them back to the apiary. I open a brand new 10-frame hive for them. I take five frames out and replace them with the frames from the swarm box. I take my time and work methodically to get all the bees into the new hive. I now have five frames occupied with bees and their queen. They have five blank frames in which to expand the colony.

I also get called to take a hive out of a barn on occasion. Now, I'm dealing with an established hive. I must actually go into the barn, cut the comb out, and then rubber band it into a frame. I gently and carefully measure the comb and cut it out with the brood still on there.

It's a tedious job. You're sweating, and you must be careful not to hurt any bees. Once you rubber band the comb into a frame, you put them into a hive. You leave the hive there for a week or two, while the bees build a brace comb all around the frames to lock the comb in place with wax. If I move them too early, those chunks of wax will move around in the frames and mess up the hive.

By leaving the hive there, they have time to put the brace comb all around the frames. They fix and repair everything! A week later, I can put the hive on the truck because everything is solid. Nothing is going to fall out of the frames now.

I take the hive away at night. By nightfall, all the foraging bees have returned to the hive. I put a piece of window screen in front of the hive to keep its entire colony inside. This way, I have all the bees, and there aren't any stragglers coming back to the hive to find out their home is gone.

*Left: These honeybees swarmed and settled into a barn and had made this their home. Unfortunately, the barn had to come down. I removed them and gave them a happy home in a hive.*

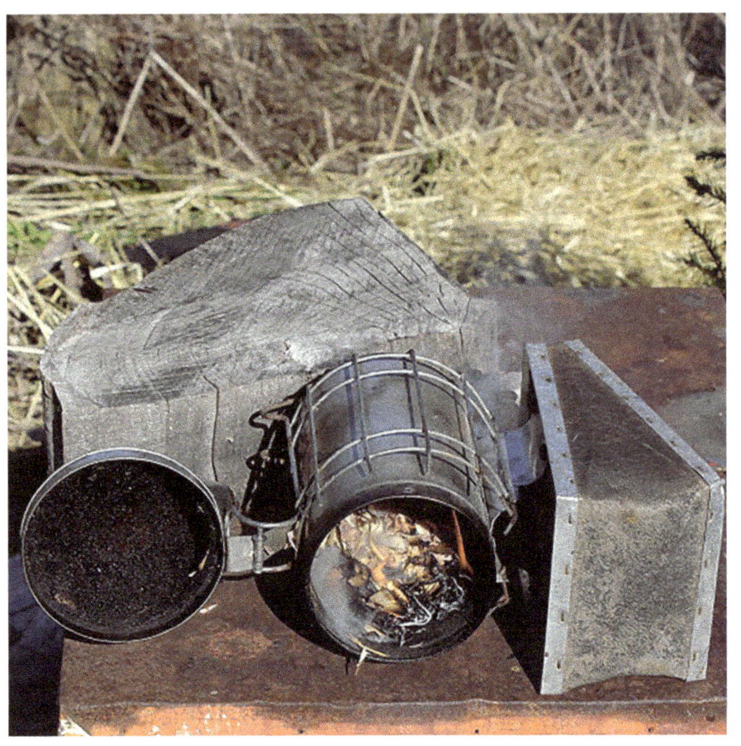

Let's start with the smoker. Any time I approach my hives, I use a smoker that I usually fill with cedar chips. You can easily find them in any Agway or a garden store. This simple device works by producing smoke and tricks the bees into thinking there's a forest fire. Unlike most critters that flee at the first threat of fire, a bee's initial inclination is to stick its head in the cells and start drinking up the honey it helped produce. They do this because they think they have to flee, but they need to fill up on the honey first. As they start to drink it up, they become very calm and easy to work with. Once a bee engorges itself with honey, it isn't likely to sting. It's too difficult to do when the bee is so full.

In the springtime, when the bees are busy collecting pollen and bringing a great deal of it back to the hive, I usually don't wear gloves for protection. In fact, when it comes to gloves, I generally don't wear them for the entire season. My motivation for this is to protect the bees. I feel that if I'm handling the frames of the hive without gloves, I'm less likely to pinch or crush a bee. When that happens, it triggers the other bees to flock to the scent of the crushed bee. This is when they start to sting whatever is around to protect the hive…even if it's the beekeeper. Think of it as a crowd assembling at some special event. For humans, emotions run high in that situation, and so do the honeybees' reactions. By being careful around my bees, I can avoid them wanting to attack me.

At all times, I usually wear a veil to protect my eyes just in case I have a foreign bee that decides it wants to sting me. It's always important to protect your face. I use what beekeepers call a "half suit." It's a long-sleeve jacket with a veil. This way you're protecting your face, chest, and body area. Gloves are up to you.

I always carry a hive tool with me. It's a great multi-purpose tool that I use to open a hive and remove the frames for inspection. Besides loosening up the hive bodies and frames, a hive tool is also great for scraping off excess comb from parts of the hive, and even for removing a bee sting from the body.

When you're doing an inspection on the honeycomb or the brood in your hive, sometimes you must move some of the bees away gently. One instrument to do this with is the bee brush. It works, but I find that it can aggravate the bees. My solution to keeping the bees calm is to use a turkey quill. I have a large turkey feather that I keep in my arsenal of tools. As I'm doing an inspection to look at the larva and making sure that the queen is laying properly, I use that feather to move the bees over so I can get a closer look. This usually happens in the early spring when the queen and brood production begins to pick up.

Now I want to go into more detail on the actual hive where the bees live and work. What I use is the Langstroth hive, which is an eight-frame or 10-frame hive. Patented in October 1852, it's the standard in beekeeping. Beekeepers use them all over the world. The advantage of this hive is that the bees build honeycomb into the frames, which you can easily move around. The design prevents bees from attaching honeycombs where they would either connect adjacent frames or connect frames to the walls of the hive.

The hive consists of several different pieces. The initial two parts are the bottom board and the deep super. The bottom board is the first piece. The hive body, or deep super, sits here. The deep super is the square box that holds ten frames. These frames contain a wax foundation that goes into the deep super.

The deep super is where the queen lives and raises her young. Once she occupies it, you can add a second deep super, which she will also utilize. This enables the queen to lay even more eggs and raise more young. When she has occupied all ten frames, you can go ahead and put on the smaller boxes, called honey supers. These are small boxes placed on top of the double brood chamber.

Between the double brood chambers is a thin piece of plastic or metal. It has very thin slots in it enabling the worker bees to pass through, but not the queen. You do not want the queen to go through and up into the honey supers to deposit eggs because having larva and eggs in your honey isn't fun when it comes time to extract the honey. You want to eliminate the queen from going up into those areas to drop eggs. You need to keep it for honey and nectar deposits only. You can add your honey supers when the colony becomes established. You'll be able to harvest honey in mid-summer right up until the fall.

If the hive is strong and the colony successfully weathered the winter, you'll be able to add two or three honey supers. Be aware that when the honey fills them, they could weigh anywhere between 50 and 55 pounds! We aren't talking a jarful of honey here — more like a barrel.

In the early spring, install bees into a new hive. They'll start to draw new comb on the wax foundation in the hives. Once they establish a wax foundation on all 10 frames, add the second box. The bees will collect nectar from flowers in the area. Then they bring it back to the hive and evaporate it into the cells, which produce the honey.

Bees also collect pollen and ferment it into cells. This produces bee bread, which is what they feed to the larvae bees. Comb honey production occurs in early spring; juvenile bees make it when they're 17 days old. The young bees draw out wax cells from their underlying platelets, pass them along to one another, and make the white honeycombs. As the season progresses, you can put comb on top of the hive to catch the nectar flow. When the bees cap the honey in mid-August, it's time to harvest the honey and run it through the extractor.

Other pieces of the hive are an inner cover and then the telescoping outer cover. You'll begin to realize what works best for you and your bees. The Internet has plenty of resources for both information and purchasing the items you need, and instructions on how to construct a hive. Beekeepers love to share their knowledge, so look for one in your area as a resource.

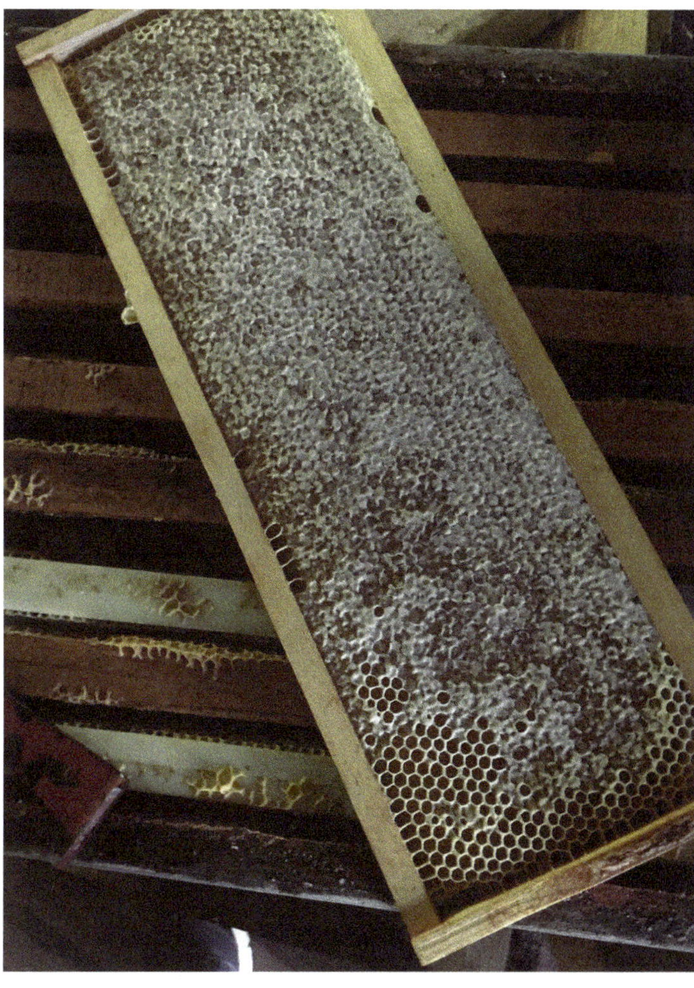

*Page 16: Smoker.*

*Right: Freshly harvested honeycomb.*

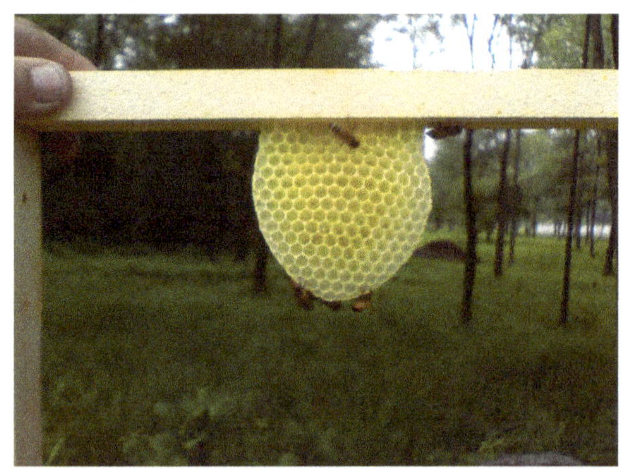

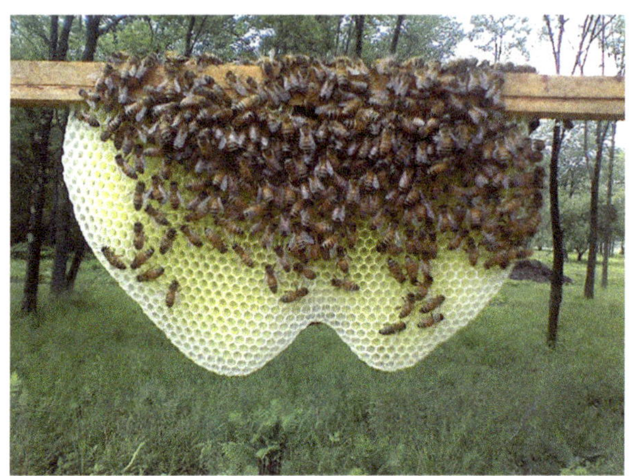

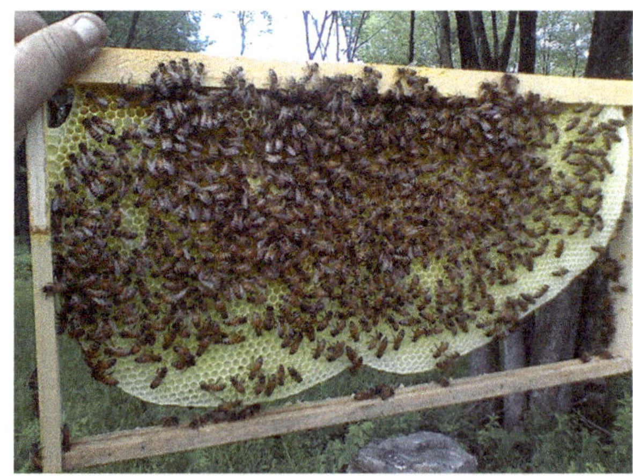

*Comb, first, second, and third week.*

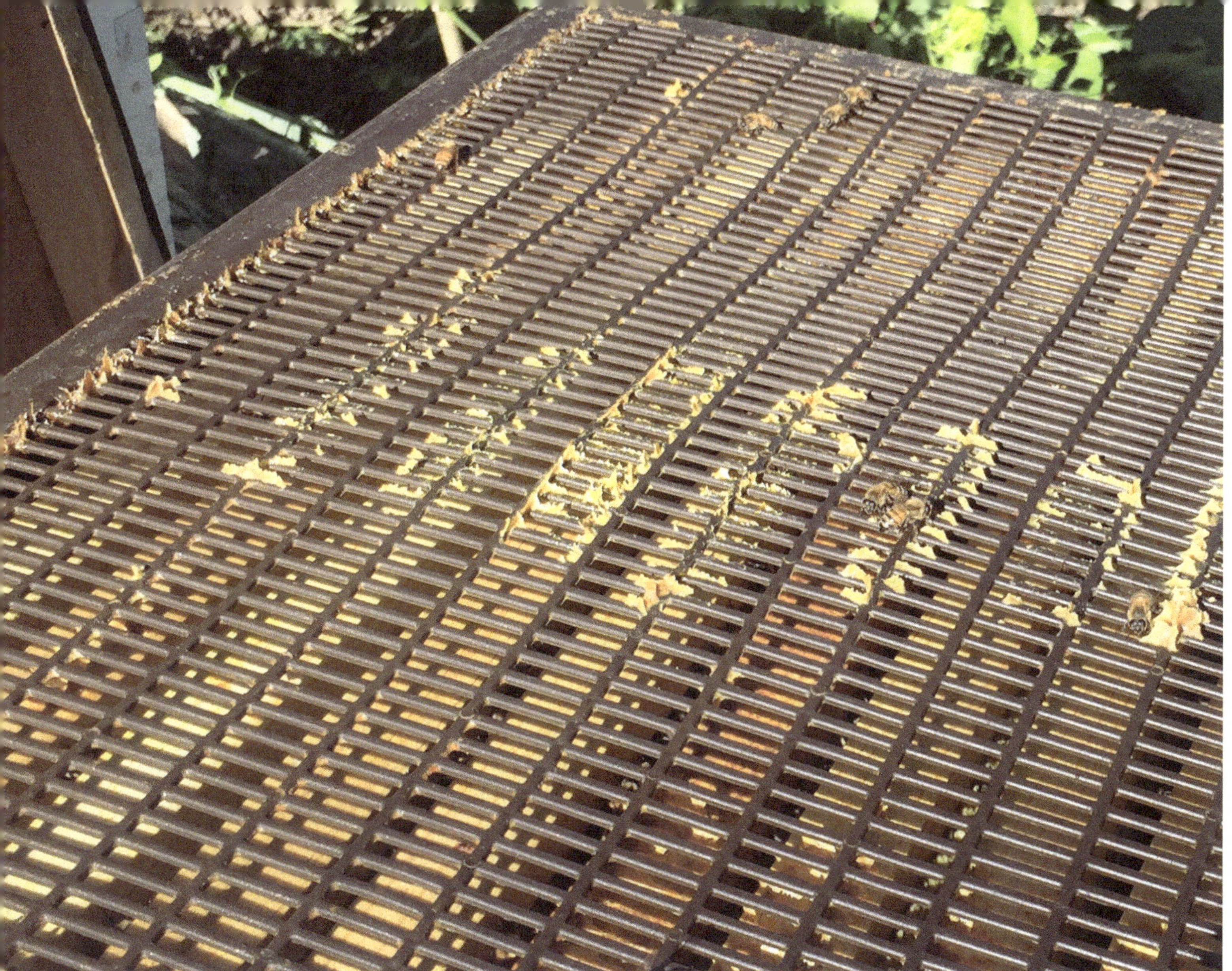

*Above: Queen excluder to prevent the queen from laying eggs in the honey super.*

*Page 20: Beautifully capped larva-free honey above the queen excluder.*

*Page 21: Full honey super ready to harvest.*

*Page 22: Early season black locust honeycomb.*

*Page 23: Hives in winter.*

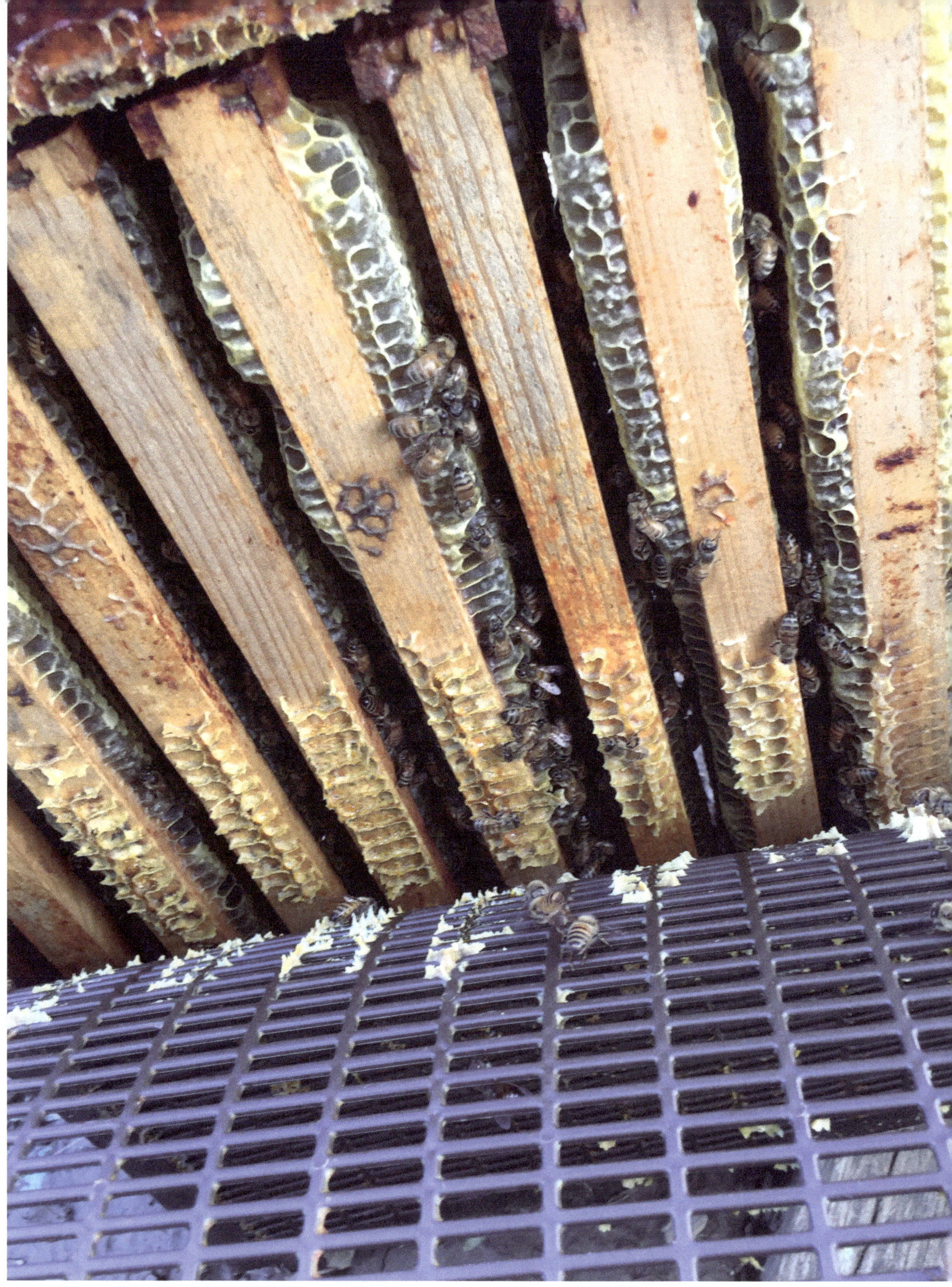

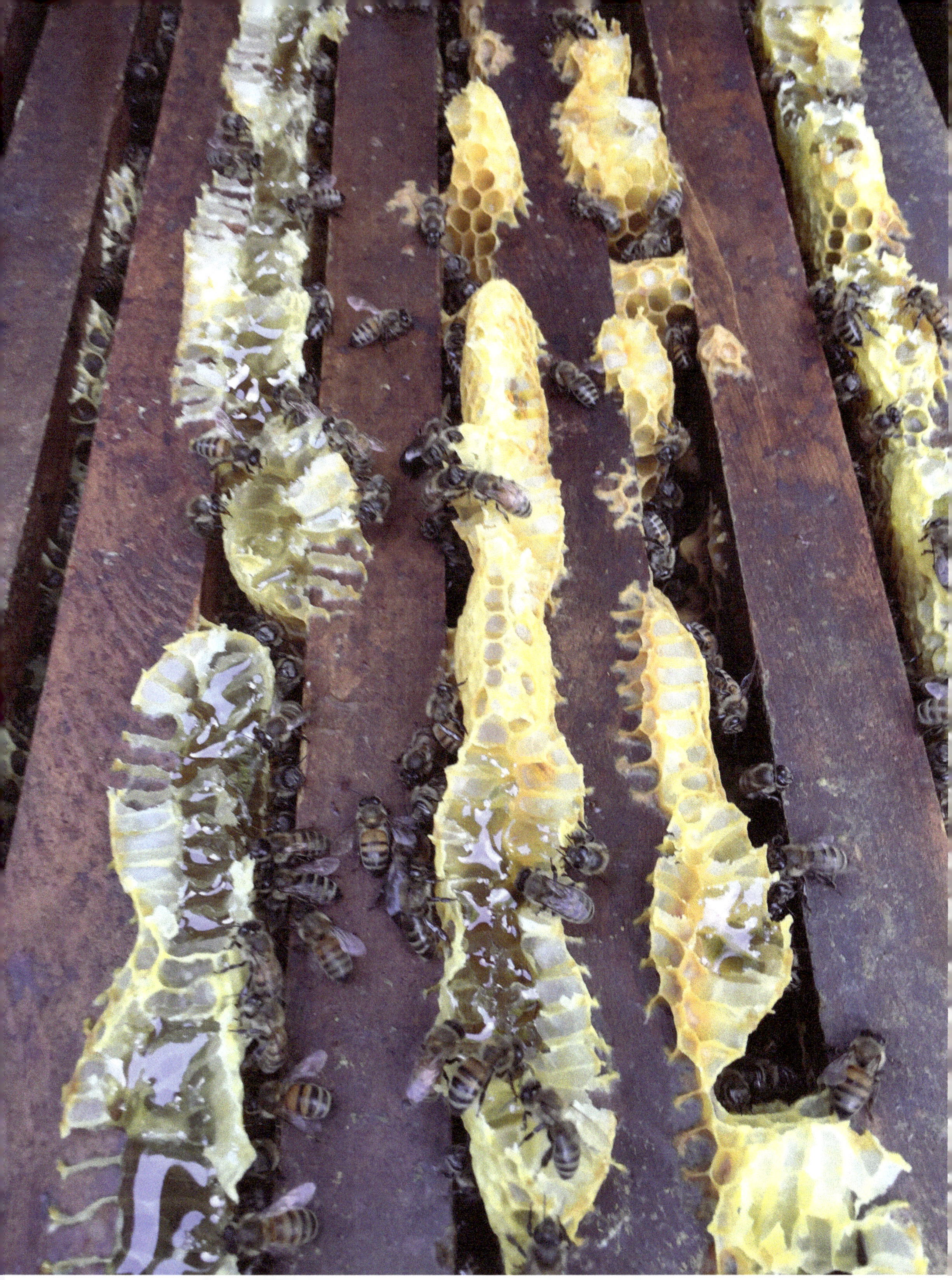

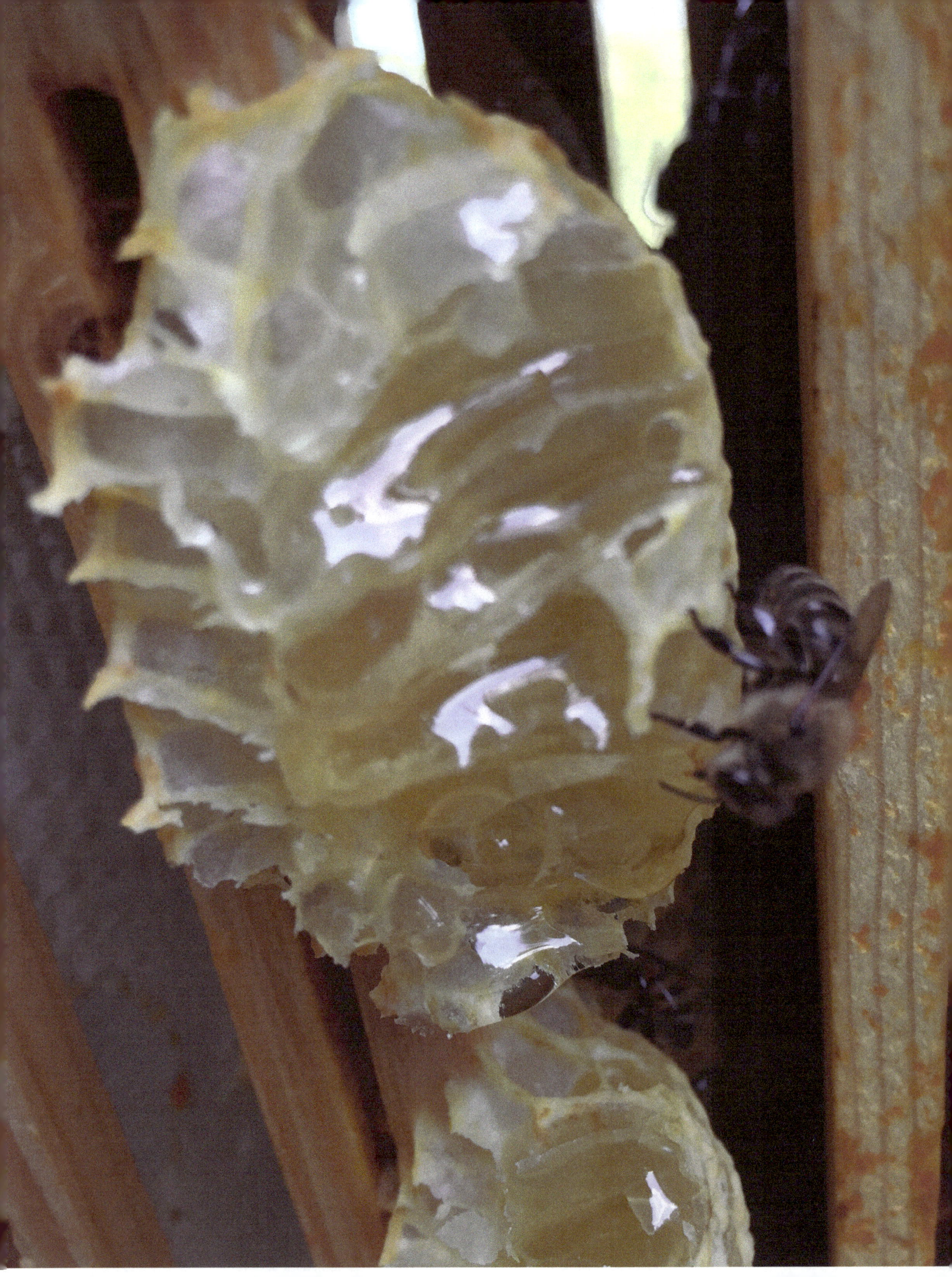

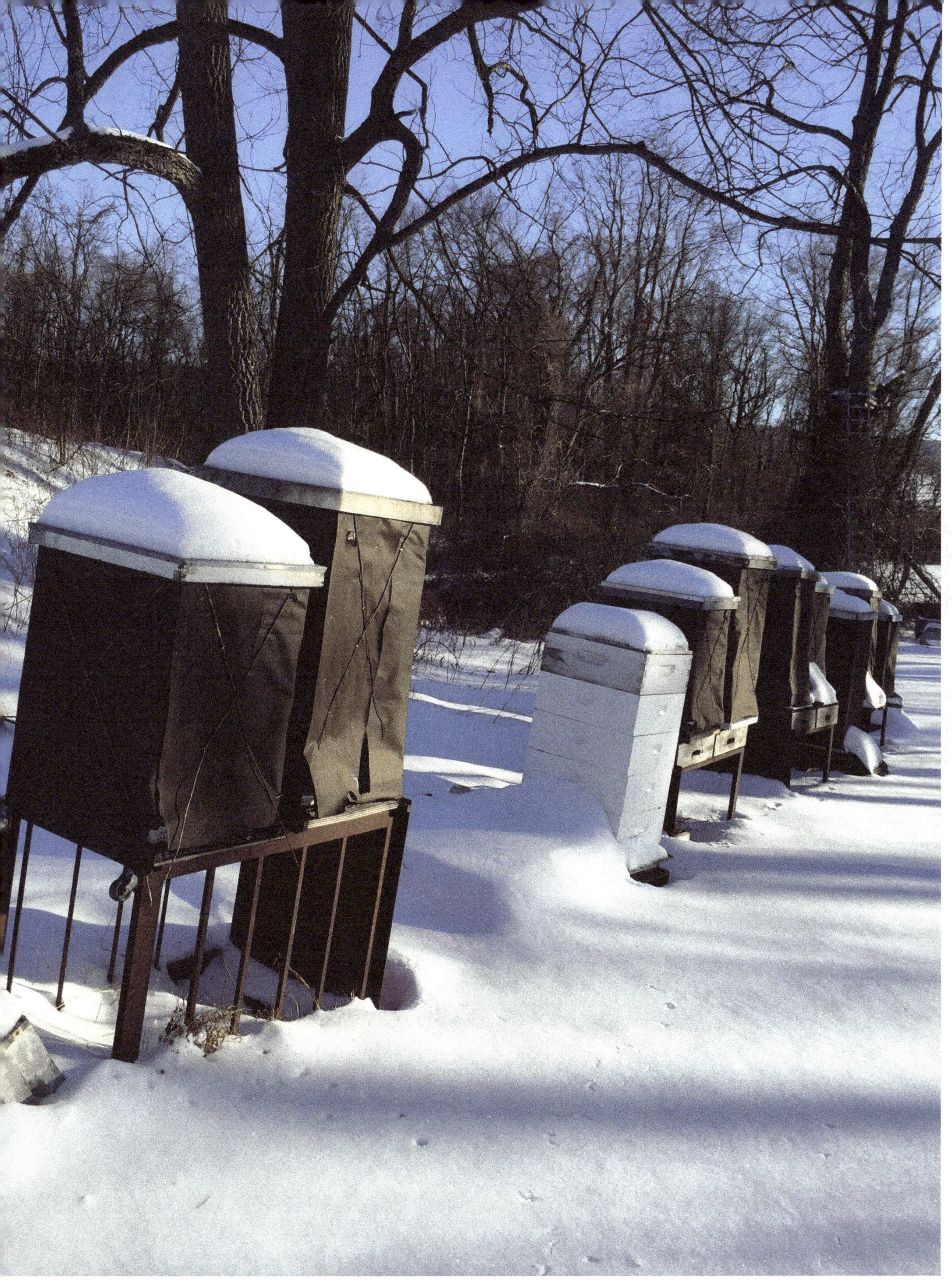

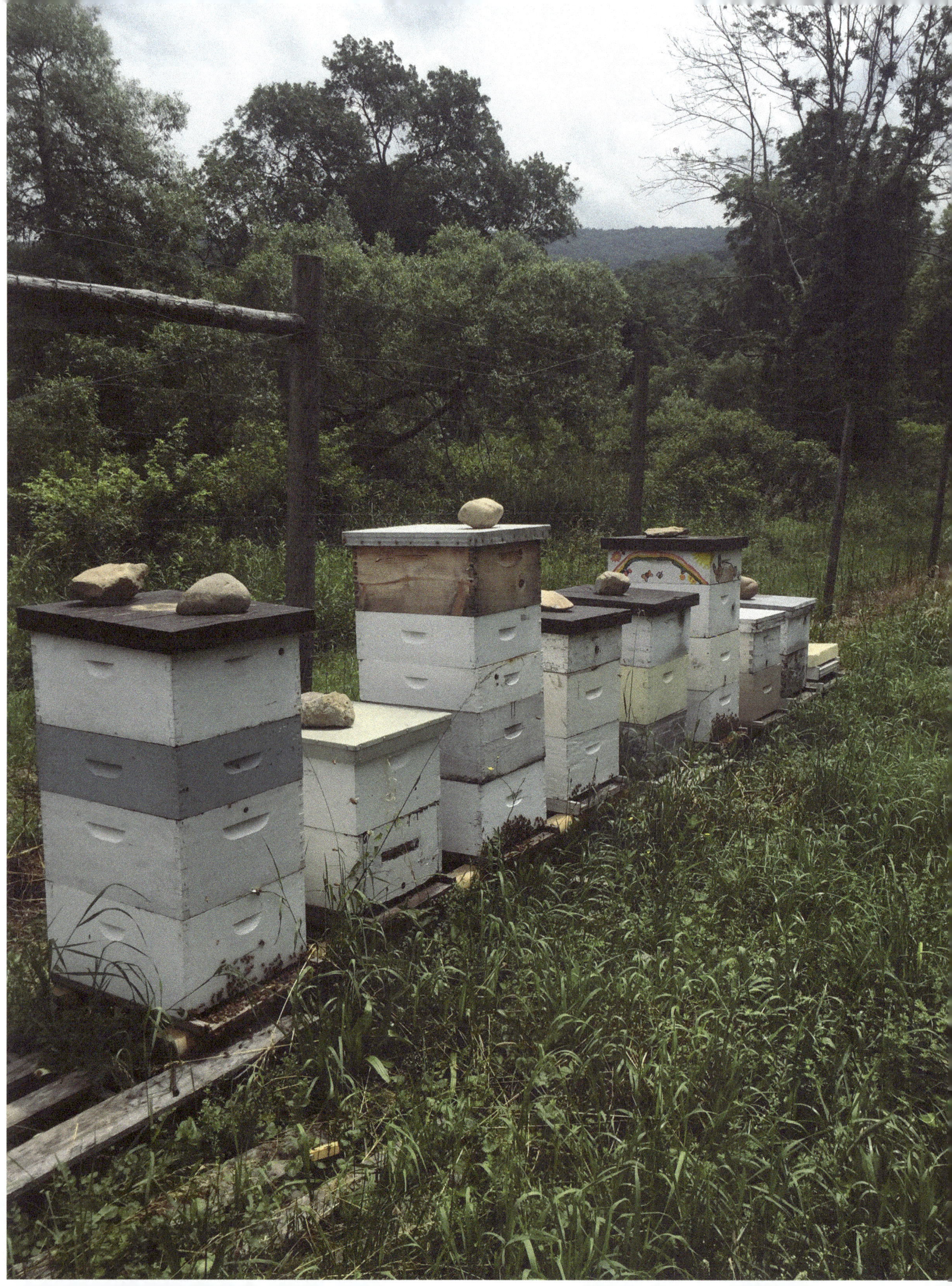

## *Placing Your Hives*

I told you that I first became interested in beekeeping when I was ten years old. I've been a beekeeper every year since and, as I hope you can tell by now, I thoroughly enjoy it. The bees brought me so much closer to nature, and they're incredibly fascinating to watch. Between observing bees and living in a rural setting, I've had a lot of practice in figuring out optimal locations for my hives. Besides bees, I've also gotten into producing many different varieties of stone fruit, such as peaches, plums, nectarines, and apricots. By increasing pollination with additional hives on my property and several farms that I've established nearby, I've noticed a big increase in fruit production. Besides honey production, your bees can make a huge difference in the ecosystem around where you set up your hives. Not only fruit trees but also plants like melons and cucumbers increase their yield dramatically when they're near bees.

Here's a good time to mention that not all honey tastes the same. It depends on the flowers the bees use to produce the honey. Honey from clover is going to taste different from honey produced by a hive on the edge of a blueberry farm. This is one of the reasons you see honey with different colors and textures. Where you locate your hives is going to have a direct bearing on how the honey tastes.

As a matter of practice, I like to situate my hives alongside a field that receives at least a half-day of sun. I also think that having a great deal of pasture and swampland in the area, when possible, is a good place to establish your hives. This way you have plenty of wildflowers growing in the surrounding areas of the fields, and wetlands where the bees can forage and produce a wildflower honey.

The biggest problem I have today, after raising bees for 35 years, is avoiding pesticides and Varroa mites. Back in the 1980s, bees were plentiful and strong. I had to prop my hives up with 2x4s because they were so heavy with honey. Mites and chemicals have greatly reduced the size of hives. I suggest treating hives with oxalic acid or formic acid in the spring or fall to stem the mite issue. As for insecticides, you need to know what's going on around you. For example, I live near a great deal of farmland. I have to be aware of what the different farmers use when deciding on locations for my hives.

## *Threats to Bees*

When it comes to beekeeping, many people neglect the Varroa mite. This mite is a pest that the bees obtain out in the fields and the wild. If bees bring any Varroa mites back into the colony, the mites will start reproducing quite rapidly. The mite cycle begins when you get your bees going in the spring and the queen starts laying.

Varroa mites go into the cells of the larva. They usually end up in with the drone brood, which is a bigger cell. These are the male bees, and the mites begin to multiply quickly by laying eggs in the cells. The mites cause havoc by weakening the bees. They feed on the blood of the larva and then the forage bees and the nurse bees that hatch will have deformed wings. Eventually, when enough bees are affected, the entire colony becomes weakened.

*Some of my hives.*

Many new beekeepers overlook this problem, thinking that the colony is becoming stronger as the season progresses. What happens is that the colony doesn't make it into winter because it has decreased in size so much. When you have a reduced cluster, there aren't enough bees to generate enough heat when the weather turns colder, and they will die. The mites can carry different types of viruses that can also adversely affect the bees.

The good news is that you can block the threat of the Varroa mite fairly easily. You must treat a hive twice every year to prevent the mites. There are several ways to do this. You can use an insecticide treatment. I tend to shy away from these, but you can research the different varieties and see if you want to try one.

What works best for me is that once the temperature reaches about 65 to 70 degrees late in the spring, I do a hive check for mites. At this point, the queen should be off to a good start, laying eggs and raising the young. When you first install your hive, you have a solid bottom board. This is where your hive super, or first brood chamber, sits. That's where all the frames are and where the queen will raise the young.

Some hive bottoms now come equipped with a screen bottom in which you can put a mite board that slides in underneath the super. You could rub that with Vaseline. The mites will fall off, get trapped in the Vaseline, and become smothered. Periodically, you can slide that out, and you can see and count the dead mites. When you see many mites, then you know it's time for a treatment. You can never get rid of the mites completely; there always seems to be a few in the colony.

By treating them in the spring and autumn, you'll greatly reduce the mite population and keep your colony much healthier to survive the winter by keeping a larger cluster in the hive. The way I usually treat for Varroa mites is formic acid or using an oxalic acid vaporizer. That's the best method I've discovered and I've had much success with keeping the mites down.

My treatment in the late spring is to use Mite-Away Quick Strips. They are formic acid, and you can buy them from many different bee suppliers. One of the suppliers I use frequently is Mann Lake Ltd. located in Wilkes-Barre, Pennsylvania. They also have a few other satellite distribution centers. They carry honeybees, and I've been buying my products there for several years now. They're very courteous, helpful, and ship quickly. One of their attributes is that all their shipping is free!

I also treat with another product called HopGuard. I alternate the treatments for the Varroa mites because they can build a resistance if you continuously use the same product. It pays to have several different methods to combat the parasite.

One thing I do with my bees throughout the season as they're prospering and the queen is laying eggs is to dust them with sugar. I do this about twice a month when I go into the hives to do an inspection. I use powdered sugar and sprinkle it over the colony. The dusting coats many of the bees. What they do is preen themselves, because they enjoy eating the sugar as a snack. By doing so, the bees will knock off any mites during the process. Once the mites are knocked off, the bees will discard them from the hive, or they'll fall through to the bottom of the hive and stick in the Vaseline.

A common problem you'll face is that neighboring beekeepers might not treat their hives for Varroa mites. I know from personal experience that when that occurs, my clean and mite-free bees will visit flowers visited by bees from another hive that is mite-infested. Then my bees bring them back to the hive and start the whole mite cycle over again. It's very critical that everybody in your area have an approach to keeping the Varroa mite numbers in their hives down. Most areas have some bee club or association where local beekeepers can get together to talk about issues and trade ideas.

Some other pests that get into the colonies are small hive beetles. They're easily detected. They can be a nuisance, but they're generally in the southern part of the country, and they usually appear in winter. I've never had a problem with the small hive beetles in any of my colonies.

Other pests you might not think about as a threat to the hive are mice. When the first frost of autumn occurs, I put on the mouse guards. These are half-inch by half-inch hardware cloths that measure two inches wide. I put it across the entire mouth of the hive. It allows the bees to go in and out, but it doesn't allow the mice to go inside and find a warm spot in the corner of your hive where they'll create chaos. They like to chew the honeycomb and make a mess. I take the mouse guards off in the spring when I do my early season inspection.

Another problem that occurs on the opposite end of the mammal family is bears. The real animals aren't as disarming as Yogi or Pooh. They'll destroy your hive to get to the honey. I like to put up a solar-powered electric fence to prevent any bear invasions. I select an area where there's lots of sun, and I run the electric solar-powered transmitter out to it. I then corral the hives with an electric fence. That usually does the job of preventing any bears from entering the apiary.

In spring, once the weather gets warm and the bees start flying, I go into the hive and remove some of the older comb from below the brood chamber. You should replace this older comb in the brood chamber every year and a half to two years. You replace the old comb with new foundation. For the most part, I don't take out all the comb. I checkerboard it, which means I replace every other one. You put in the new foundation so the bees can draw out fresh comb and the queen will have a nice, fresh place to lay eggs that will be cocoon-free in pure beeswax. They can then start their circle of life all over again.

## *Bee Terms*

**Re-queening:** If I notice that the queen is sporadic in laying eggs, it might be time to re-queen the hive. If you don't, then she won't generate enough brood, larva, and field bees to sustain the colony over the winter in the cluster. I'll usually raise a new queen myself. However, if you don't have the time or energy to raise the queen, you could simply go through a bee supplier and order a mated queen. When the queen arrives, simply pop the cork on her cell. The queen usually comes shipped with fondant, and the initial bees you introduce to the hive will chew the fondant when you place the queen cell between the frames. The bees will take several days to become acquainted with the new queen as they eat the fondant. They'll accept the new queen when three days have passed and they have completely chewed through the fondant. This is not a virgin queen since she has already been mated. She'll go into the hive and have a battle with the existing queen. They'll fight to the death, and the younger queen will take over.

If you abhor violence, you can skip this method of re-queening. Simply remove the old queen and add the new queen a few days after the old queen is gone. The colony will accept the new queen once the existing pheromones from the old queen dissipate.

**Splitting Hives:** Start between April and May when it begins to warm up outside. I've found that this is the best time to start a new colony. Begin with a nucleus colony (called a "nuc"). A nuc colony builds very quickly. Use a queen bee that you raise from an initial hive.

**Garden Hive:** This is a simple way to encourage pollination for different plants and vegetables you're growing. You start this hive from an established hive and locate it near the garden.

**Beeswax:** As combs become old and weathered looking, you can collect the beeswax. Take the combs and place them in a solar melter to render them down. You can produce candles from the wax that are beautiful gifts and have a wonderful scent.

**Comb Honey:** This is honey produced for consumption while it's still contained in the original hexagonal-shaped beeswax cells. These cells are what form the honeycomb. It's pure honey without any processing, filtering, or any other human manipulation.

Before the invention of the honey extractor, almost all honey produced was in the form of comb honey. Producing comb honey requires rigorous attention from the beekeeper. It's more suitable for areas with an intense growth of poppies, sunflowers, sage, mint, lavender, and thyme. They're heavy nectar-producing plants and conducive for honeycomb production. Wooded areas aren't as suitable for comb honey production, as bees tend to collect more propolis, making the harvesting of comb honey more difficult.

To facilitate the collecting of comb honey, you use sections. These are little boxes constructed of basswood that you place in the supers. You add thin sheets of surplus foundation, which is a wax that gets the bees started to produce comb honey. Four of them will occupy one frame. I encourage the honeybees to draw that comb honey in early stages so that it's very tender with fresh new wax. To harvest comb honey, I regulate the hive to make sure there are enough field bees to bring back extra nectar so I can put in my honey supers during the first week of August. Once the nectar is ripened and capped, it's ready for harvest.

**Pollen:** While some people might sneeze their head off at certain pollens, it has important beneficial health properties. It helps build your immune system. I collect pollen utilizing a pollen trap in the early part of the season when bees are collecting a lot of it. This is dried pollen, and the bees bring it back to the hive in their pollen baskets, which are located on the back of their legs. What the pollen trap does is knock a little of the pollen from their baskets and into a collector. I then have the choice of dehydrating it, freezing it, or eating it fresh. All three forms can be used on yogurt, cereal, or oatmeal. It makes a great dietary supplement.

For the bees' use, they take the pollen down lower into the chamber to produce the bee bread. Bees collect pollen from different flowers throughout spring and summer and pack it with their heads. They mix it with nectar, and this is what they feed the larvae bees. Pollen contains many minerals for younger bees in development.

When it comes to pollination, honeybees are extremely important pollinators. They pollinate over 200 crops, including flowers and most of our agriculture food supply. If you put a dollar value on that, bees help produce about $14 billion of crops and fruit trees.

**Propolis:** This sticky substance is something that bees collect from tree buds, usually willow, poplar, and chestnut trees. They use it as a varnish to seal up the holes and cracks in the hive. It's also the main ingredient they use to waterproof their hive.

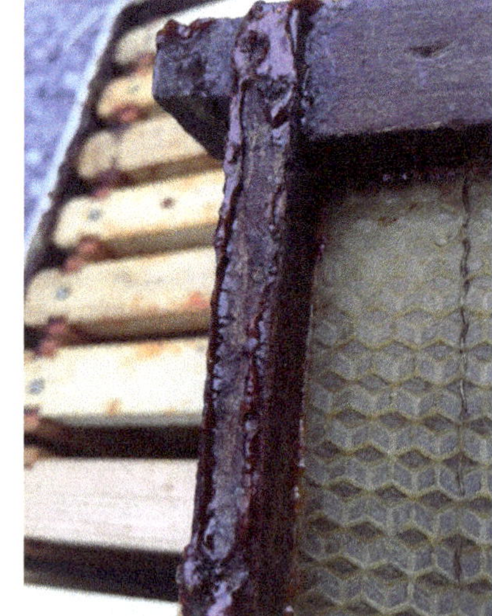

*Propolis.*

**Harvesting Honey:** Here, I'm specifically talking about removing the honey you run through an extractor. This centrifuge machine pulls the honey out of the comb. When you bring honey in for extraction, you must expose the cells. Remember that the bees bring in the nectar, fill up the cells, and fan the cells to evaporate the moisture of the nectar. Now you have honey. Once the nectar has become honey, they cap it with a thin sheet of wax. When capped, you know it's ready to harvest. If you take the honey too early, you risk the chance of it fermenting in the bottles, because there's too much moisture in the nectar.

When they cap the cells, give the bees a little smoke, brush the combs off, or use a bee escape. This tool is simply a thin sheet of wood that goes underneath the honey super. Bees pass through one way but cannot get in the other way. By the next morning, the honeycomb will be free of bees. Bring honey into your honey house. Remove the frames. Using a hot, sharp knife that you heat up in hot water, you can easily remove the cappings. I like using a capping fork. It goes underneath the capping and lifts it up gently, exposing the cells and the nectar. You can then put the frames into the extractor, which then separate the honey from the comb.

**Stingers:** The honeybee has a barbed stinger. Once it stings you, the bee flies off, and the stinger detaches from the bee's abdomen, which causes the bee's death. They risk their lives to protect what they have. If you follow the precautions I described in this book, they're usually very docile and easy to work with in the hive.

**Winter:** The biggest thing you must do in the fall to protect the hive for the upcoming cold season is to leave enough honey (60 pounds) to sustain your honeybees over the winter. To survive, the bees gather into a ball along the comb and become very lethargic. They vibrate their wings to stay warm and sustain themselves in a cold winter. They also constantly move from the inside of the cluster to the outside.

As a beekeeper, you can winterize a hive and keep the bees healthy by using a "top hat." It's a winter savior and consists of a single box without frames in it (Langstroth hive). In the fall, once I harvest the honey and conduct mite treatment, I prepare the top hat. I take an empty shallow box and put it on top of the hive with newspapers in the box. I prepare fondant, which is an insurance to help keep bees alive for the last few weeks of winter when they begin to exhaust their food supply. To make this, I mix five pounds of sugar with two cups of water and one tablespoon of apple cider vinegar. I then put it on wax paper and let it set up for a couple of days. With this concoction, if the bees run out of honey, they can sustain themselves on the fondant until the first blooms of spring appear. In my neck of the woods, skunk cabbage is usually the first to appear.

By placing the fondant on top of the newspapers and more paper on top of that, I then fill the rest of the box with cedar shavings. The cedar shavings wick the moisture from the colony and prevent moisture from dripping down on bees. I learned this the hard way after losing colonies from winterkill. If I put the top hat on, the bees move up to the top of the hive as they run out of honey and create condensation. Water would then drip down and saturate the bees, and they freeze to death. They can't keep themselves warm. By providing extra food and a way to absorb the moisture, I have big clusters of wintering bees that make a huge difference in the spring. Having a strong, healthy colony in spring allows me to do splits for myself or other beekeepers.

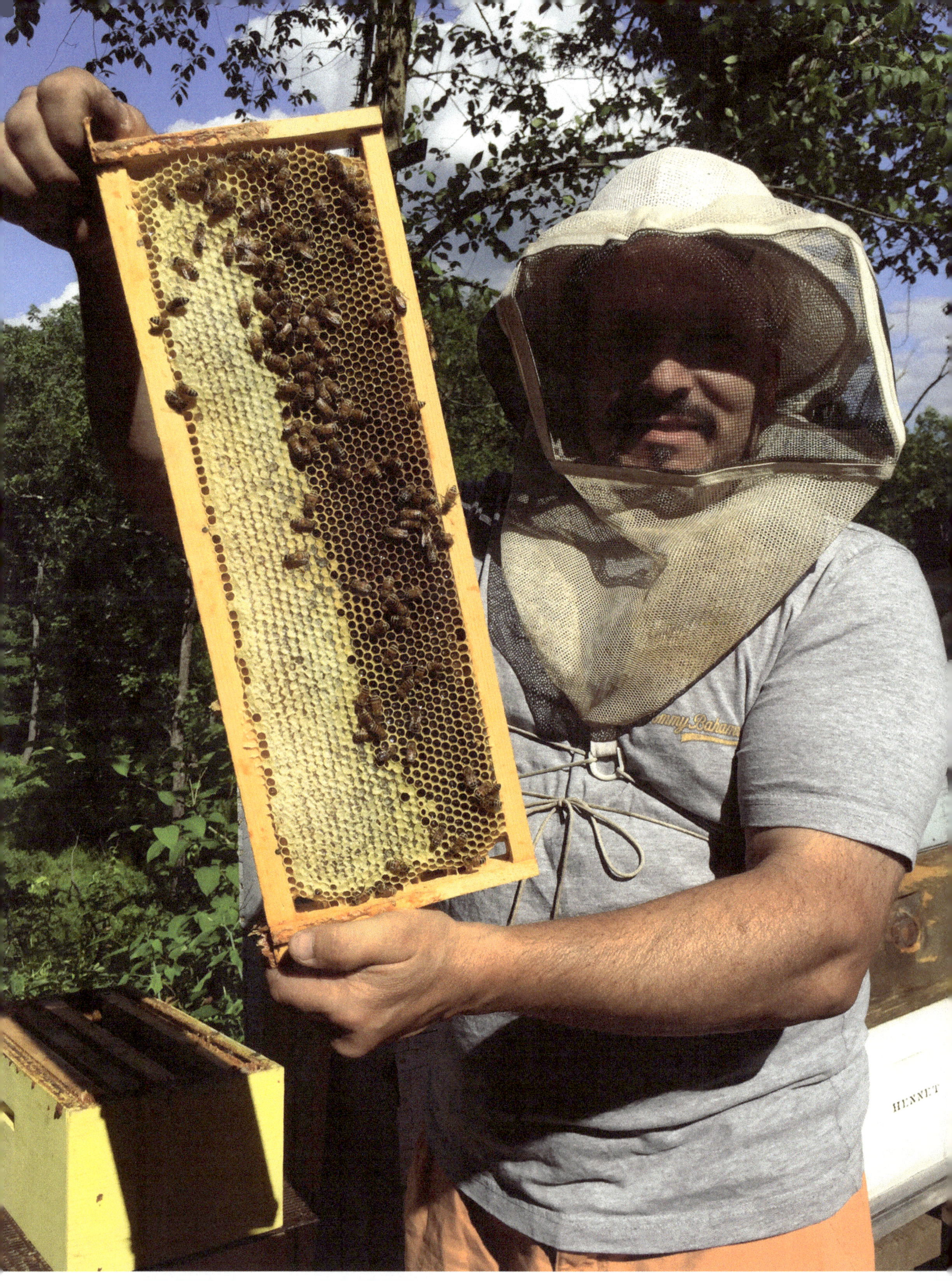

*Page 30: Honeycomb half capped with honey but not ready to harvest yet.*

*Below: Early spring hive inspection, clockwise from top left: 1. Checking frames for new comb development on foundation. 2. Adding pollen patties to provide food for developing brood to build up the colony as bees may be held back to forage due to spring snow and rain. This always helps them in the early spring. Once the weather warms up, they will collect their own pollen from blossoms. 3. Checking the brood development on the frame. 4. Holding up a drone honeybee. 5. Pointing out a drone honeybee; he's much larger than all the workers. 6. Pointing out the queen bee. (Courtesy JJ McKeever)*

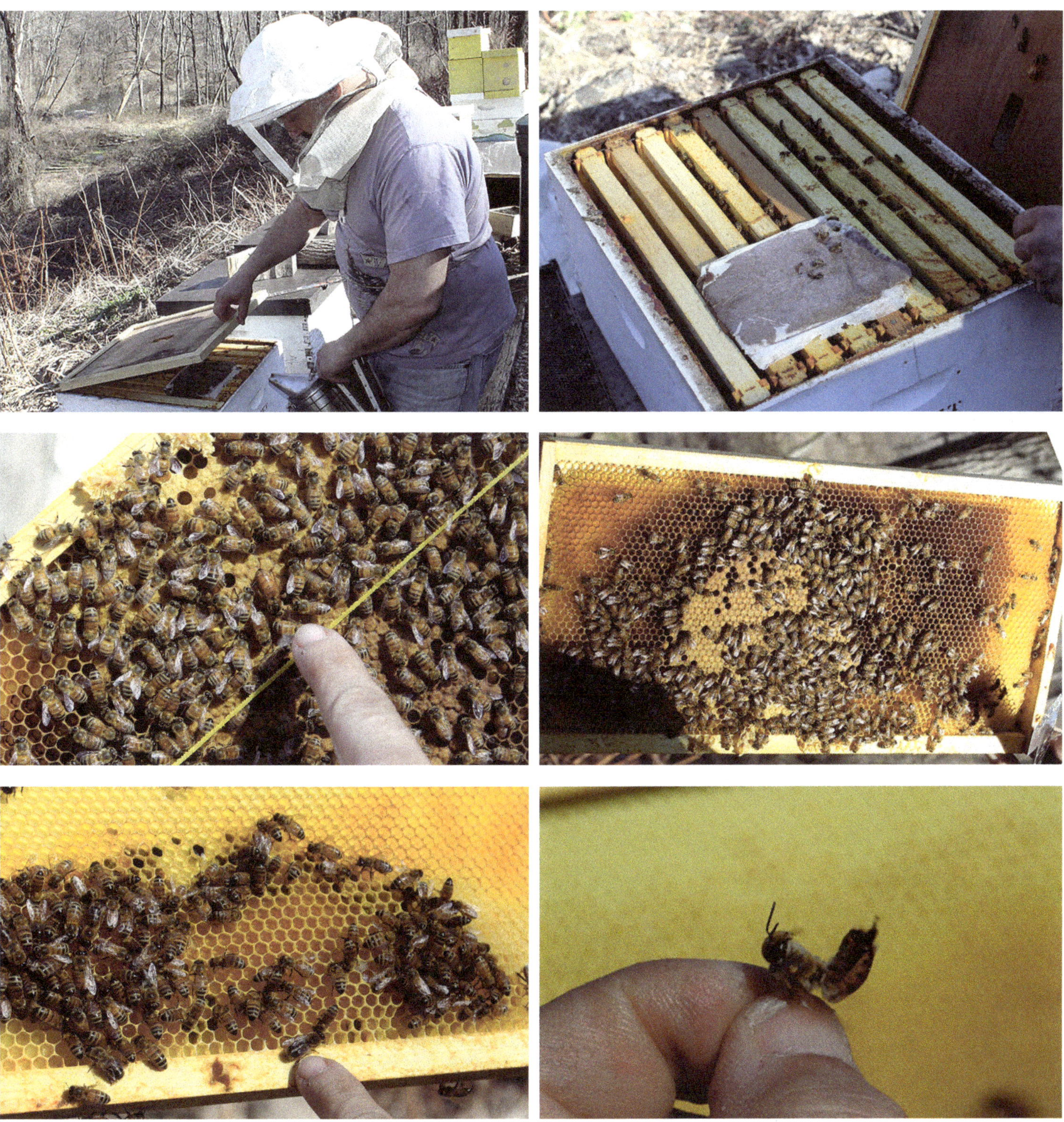

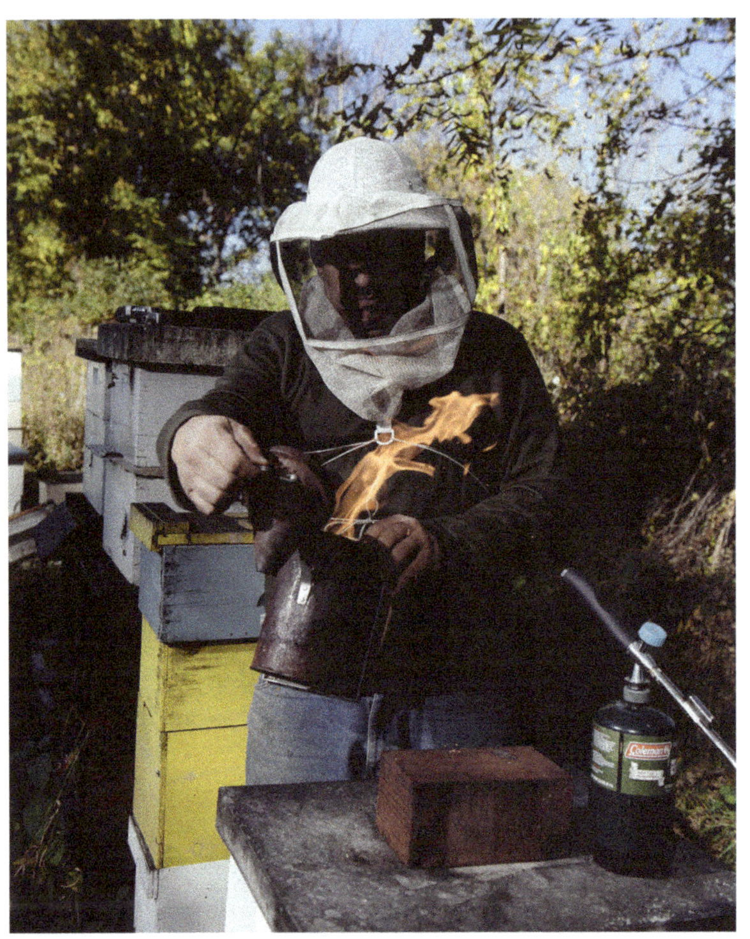


*Early spring hive inspection, with Bruno, clockwise, from top left: 1. Getting the smoker lit with cedar shavings. 2. Carrying over a frame of fondant to feed one of the weaker hives to strengthen them. 3. Looking down on ten frames in the super; I remove the brace comb on top of the frames to clean them for easier inspection and save that wax for the solar melter for candle making. 4. Frame inspection, checking if the queen is laying eggs around the band of capped honey. 5. Giving the hive a puff of smoke to calm them. (Courtesy Joe Carrotta)*

*Page 33: Spring swarm season, locating feral bees, and installing into their new hives as they settle in.*

*Page 34: Freshly harvested comb honey showing the varietal colors of nectar.*

*Page 35 and 36: Beeswax candle making and various candle shapes.*

*Page 37: Lucy making honey blossom cakes with her friend.*

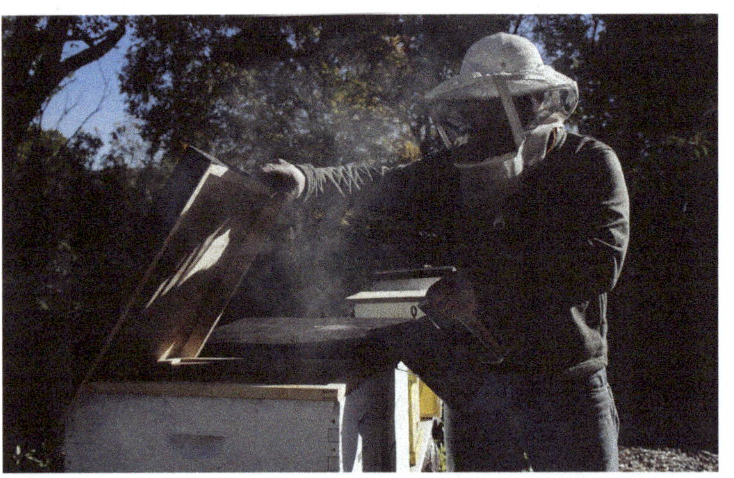

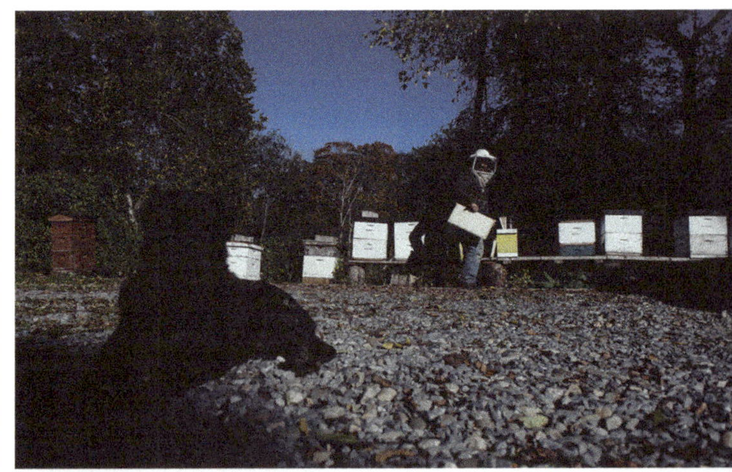

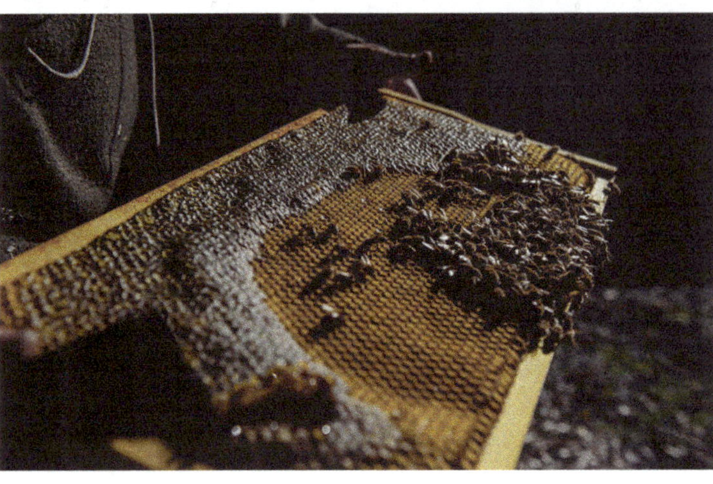

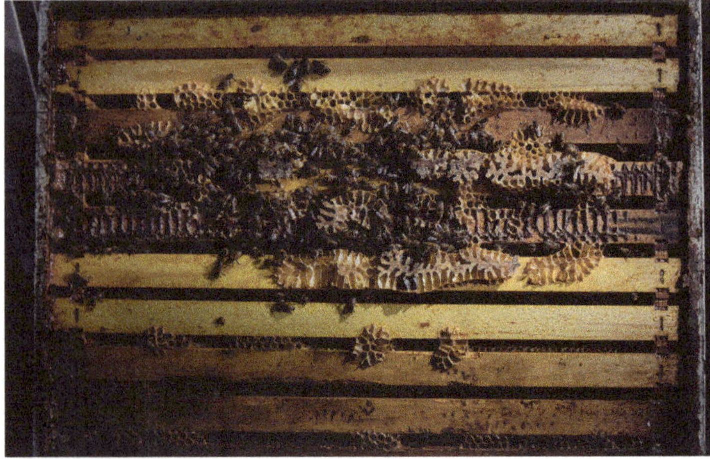

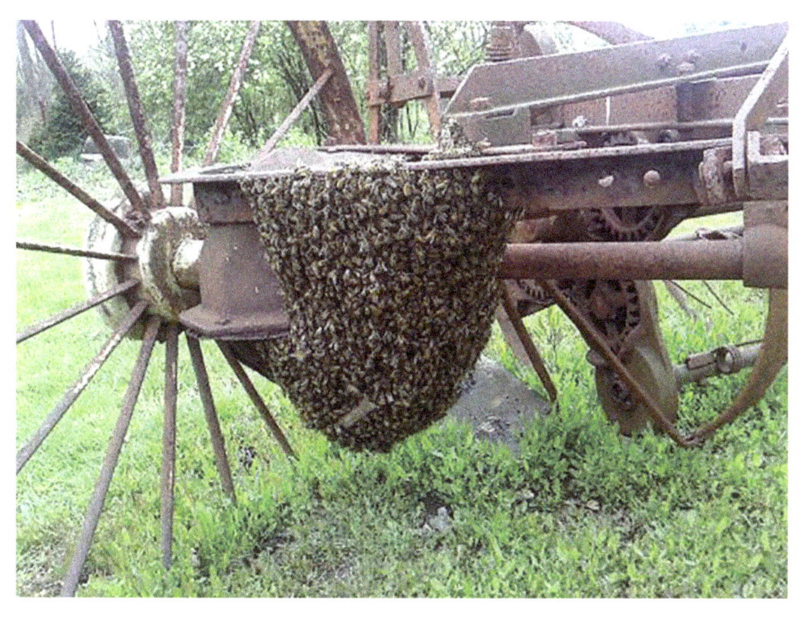

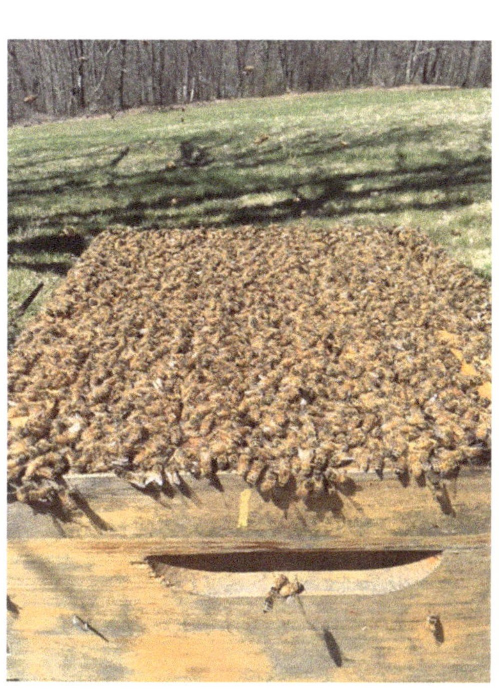

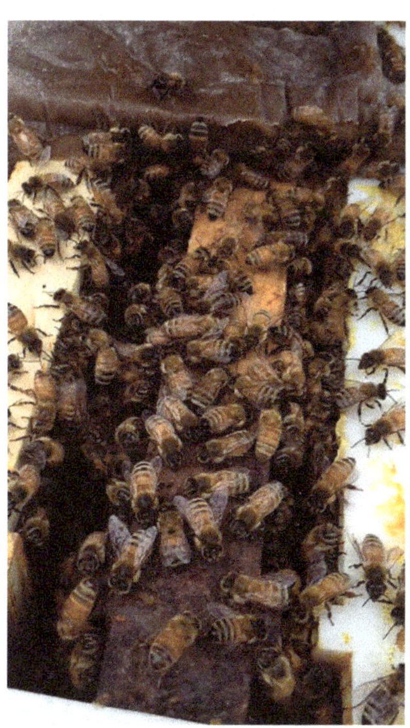

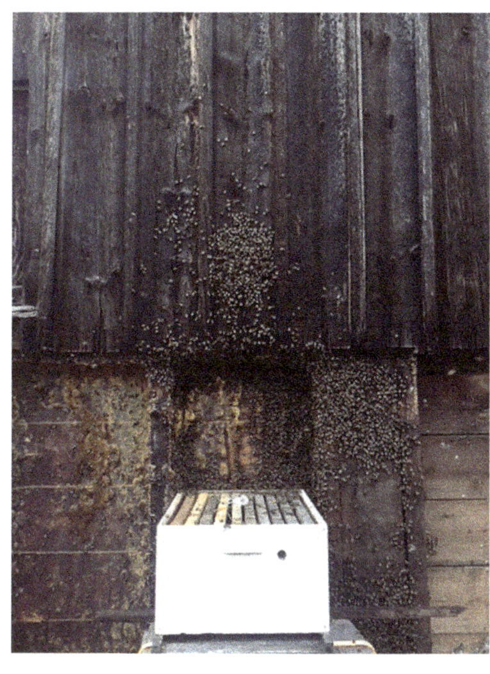

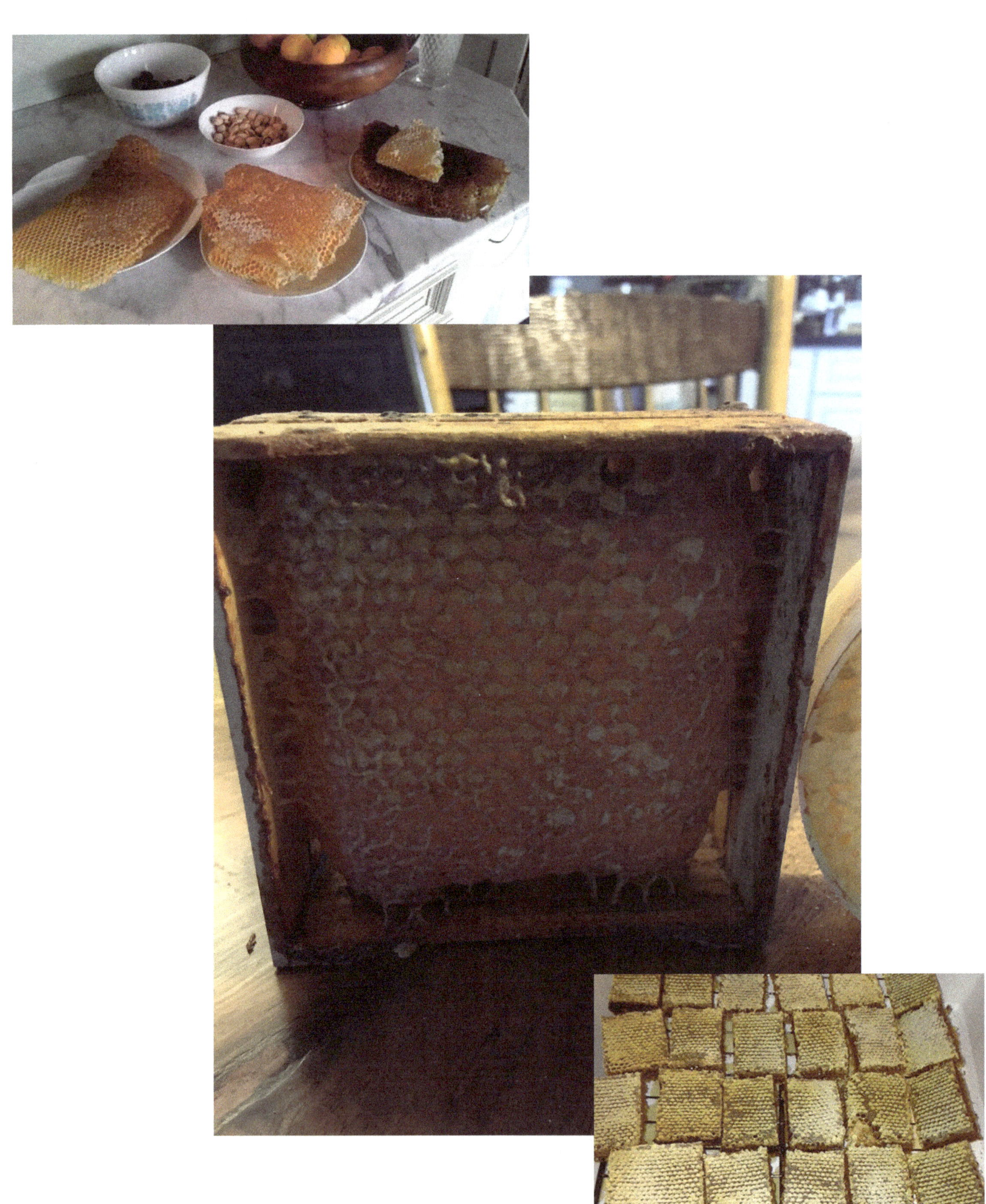

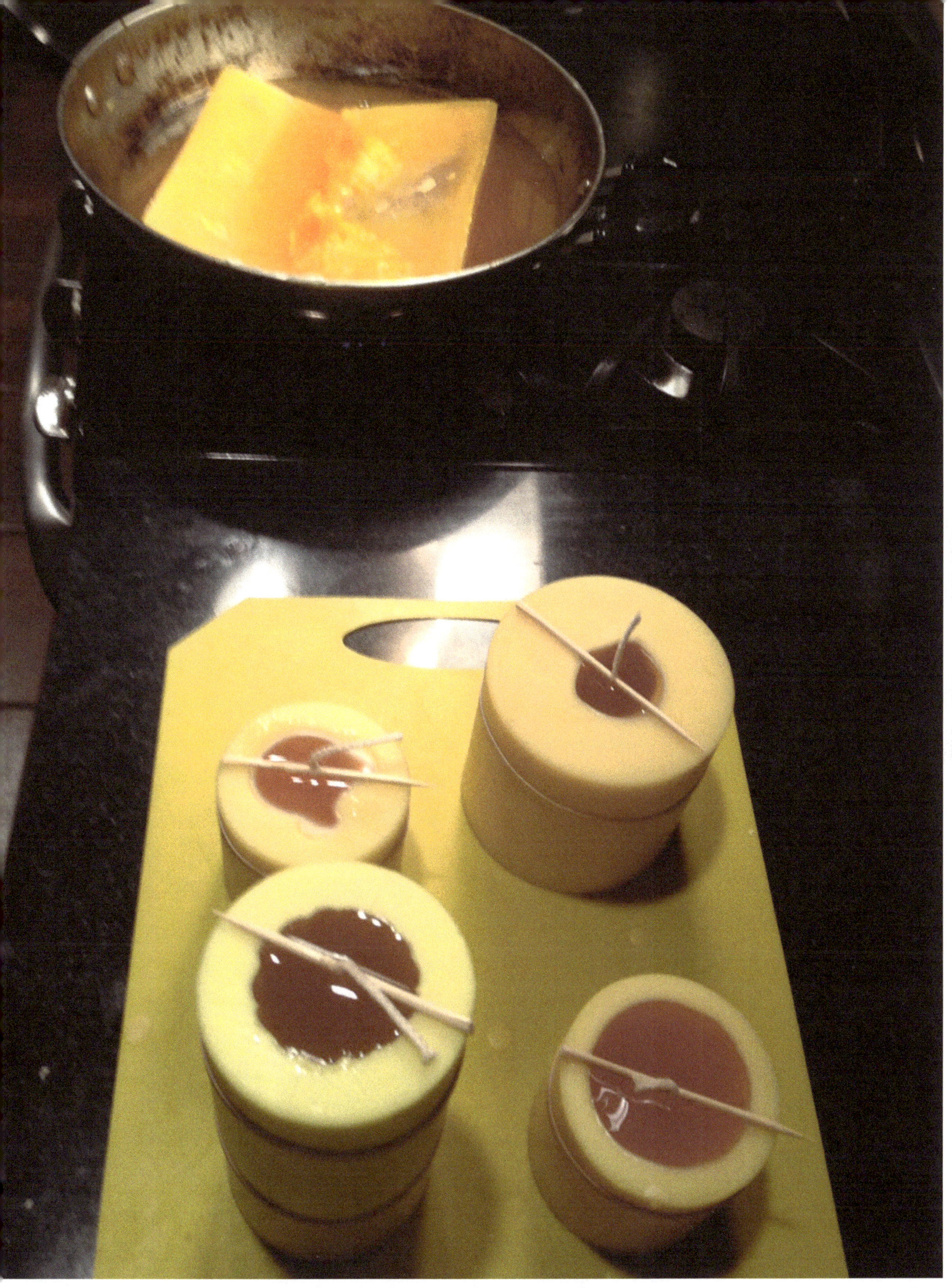

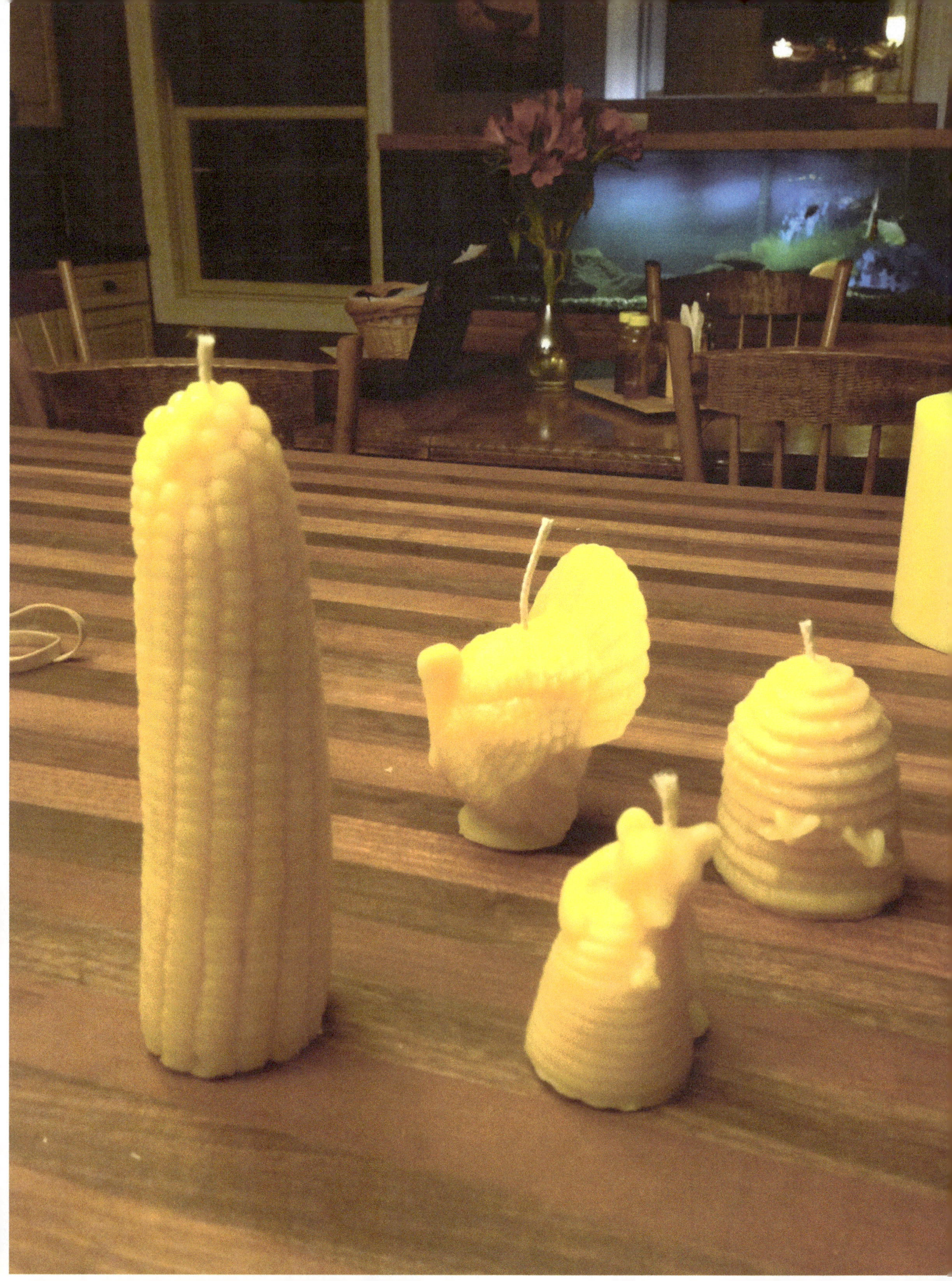

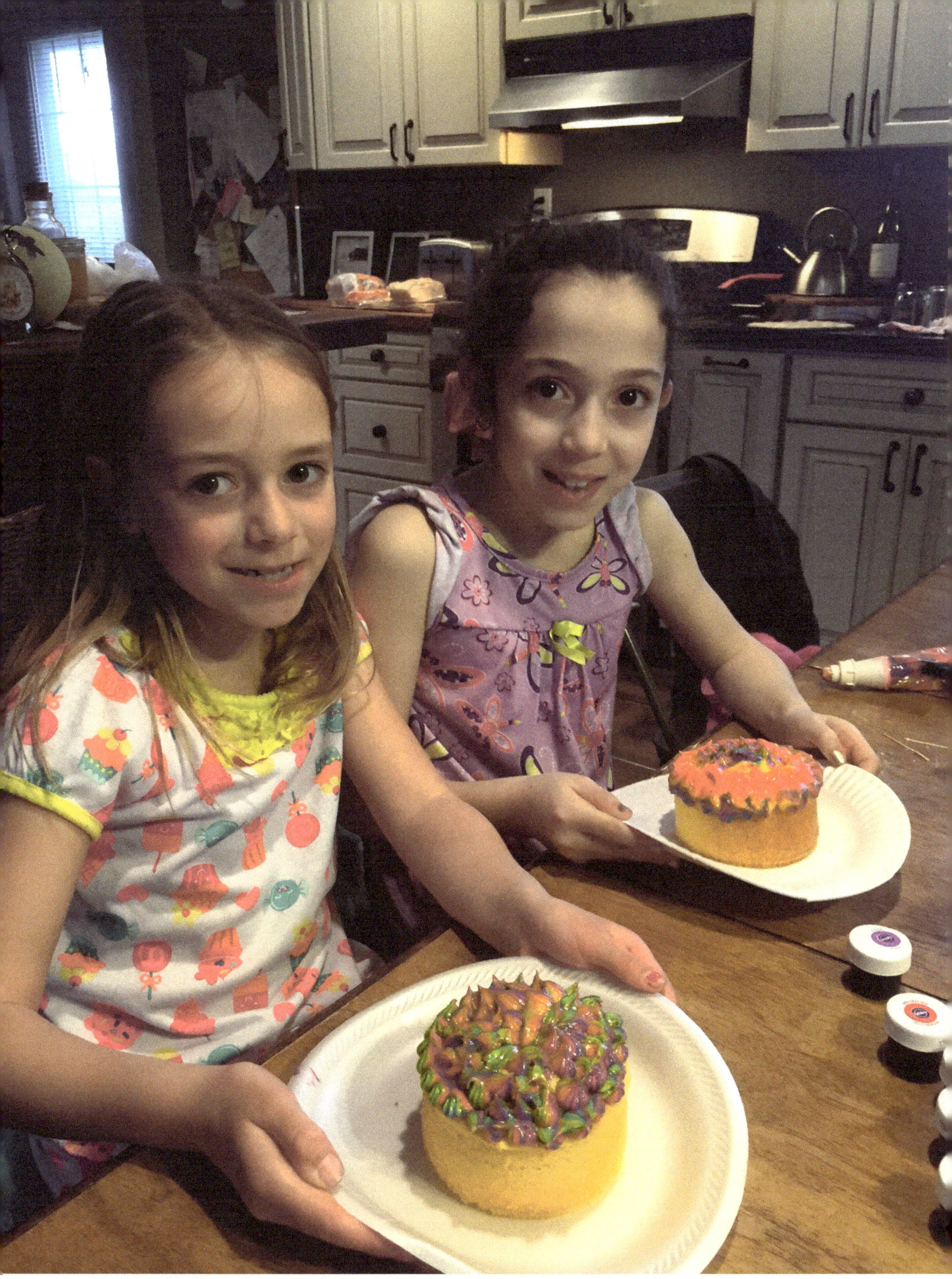

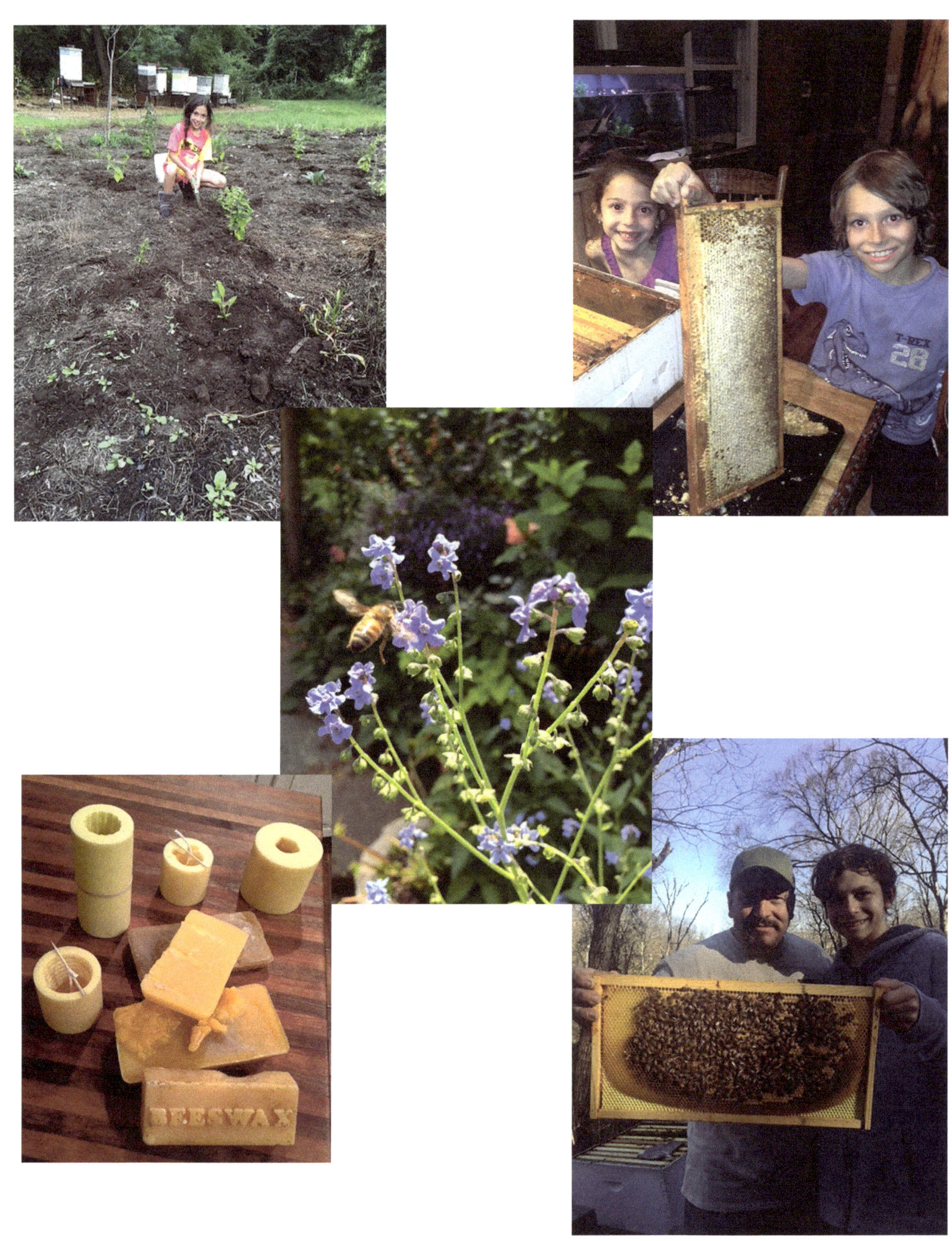
T-REX
28
BEESWAX

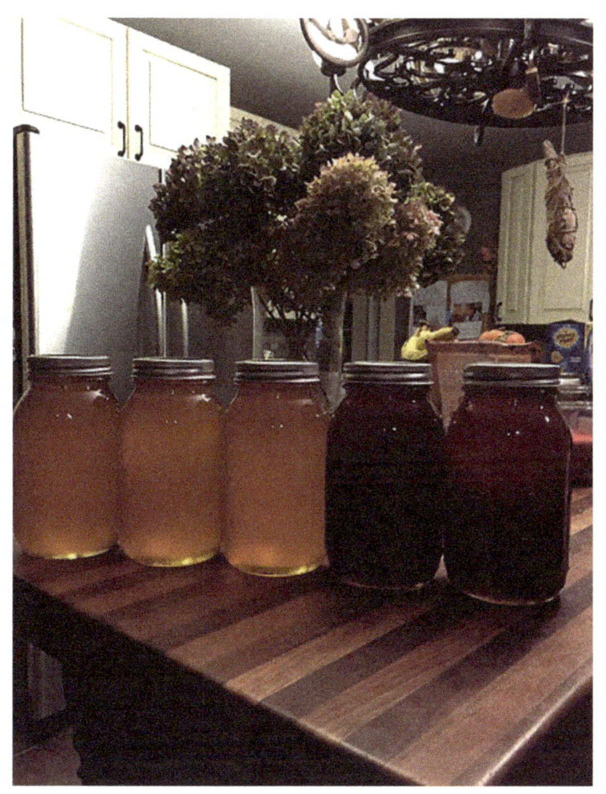

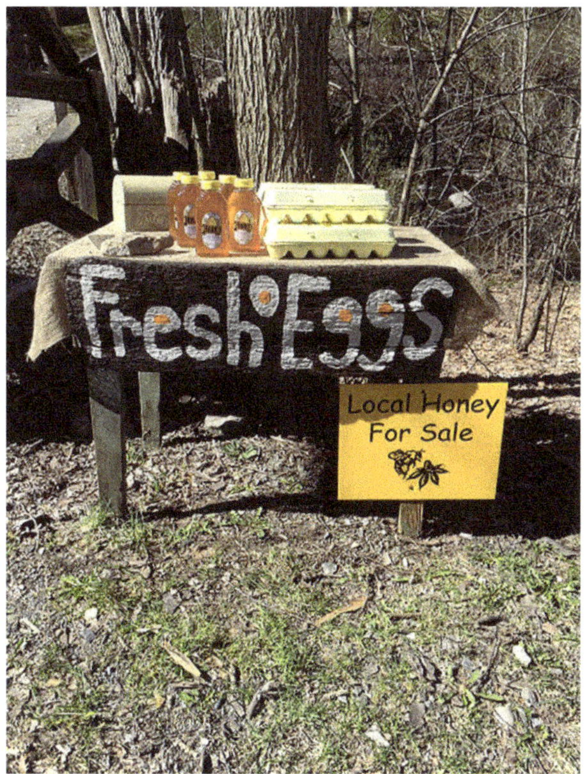


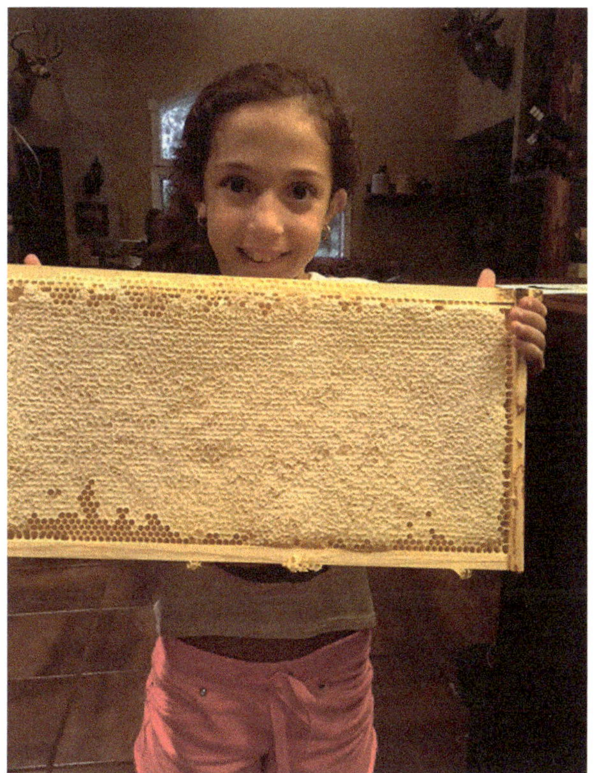

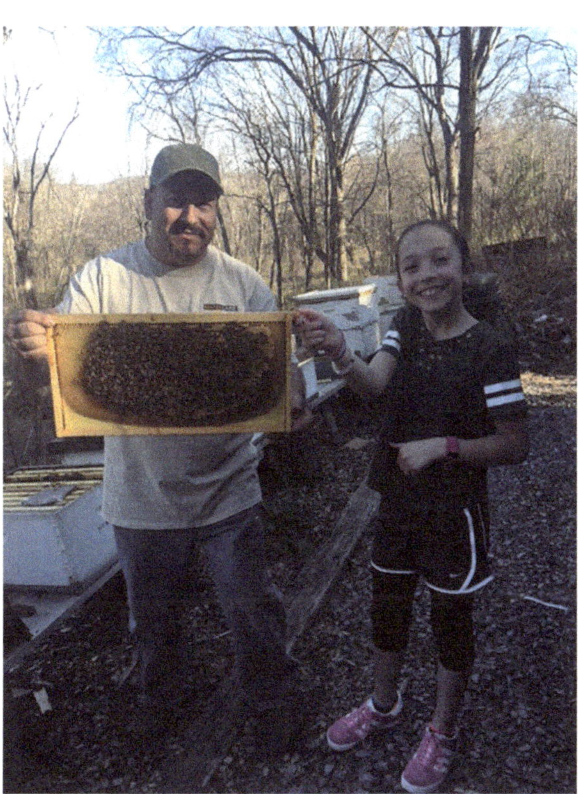

*Page 38: Lucy hard at work planting a bee garden. It pays off with a nice harvest of honey and golden beeswax.*

*Page 39: Fall harvest season and Lucy being brave during a hive inspection.*

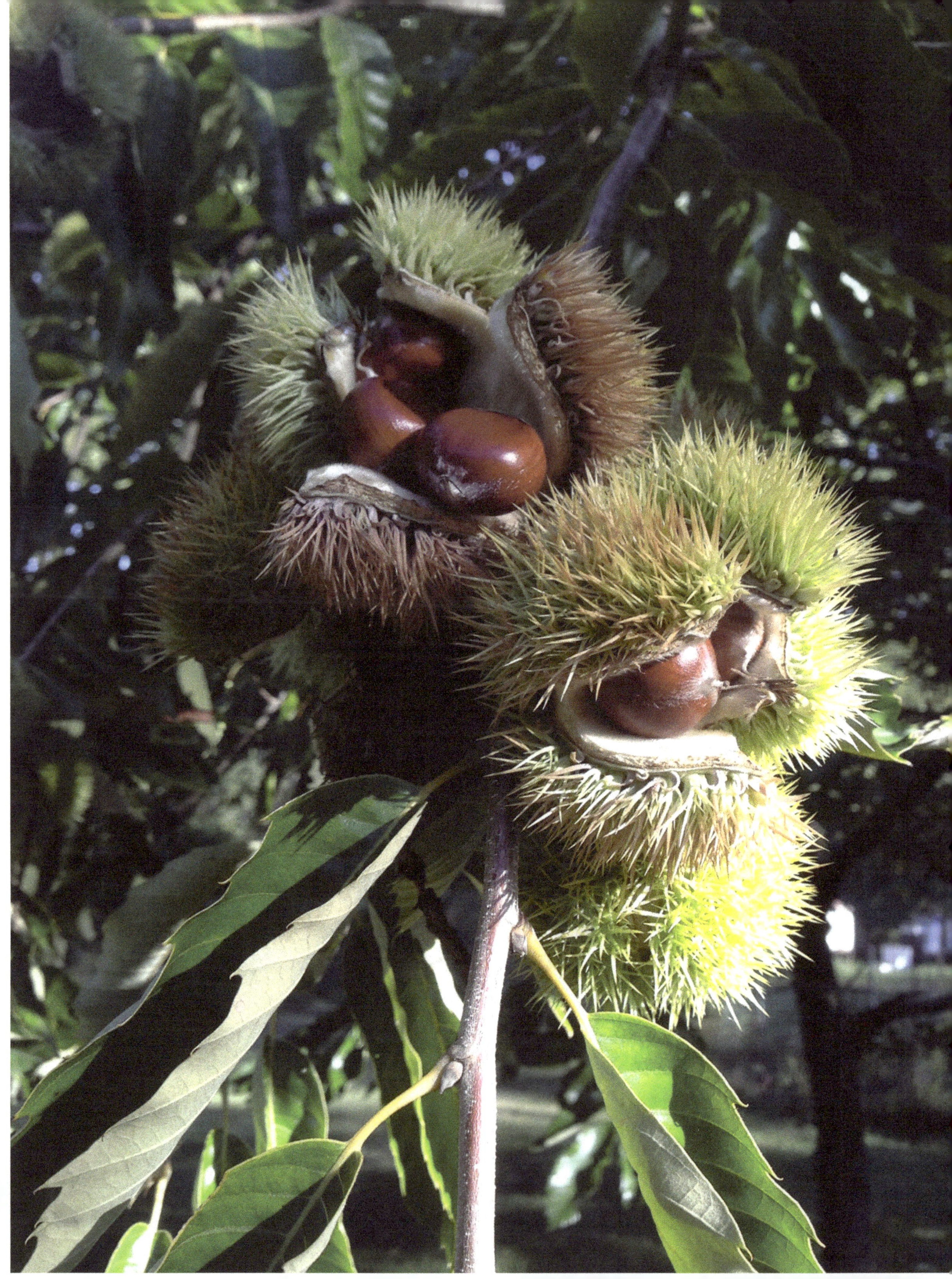

# Fruit Trees

*"Give me juicy autumnal fruit, ripe and red from the orchard."*

**— Walt Whitman**

In gardening and farming terms, a fruit tree produces fruit that people can consume. This includes certain nut-bearing trees such as chestnuts and walnuts. All trees with flowering blossoms produce fruit. By definition, fruit is the ripened ovaries of flowers containing one or more seeds. Fruit trees are a great addition to any landscape. I use fruit trees to add a lushness to the landscape. They produce beautiful blossoms in the spring, and you have nice fruit production through the summer and into the fall.

If you're getting started with honeybees, you'll find that the bees are a great help in the health and propagation of fruit trees. The bees I have in my apiary have greatly aided with the production of my fruit trees. The fruit trees I like to grow are peaches, plums, nectarines, apricots, and pears. I have a few unusual varieties as well. The pawpaw, which is also known as the Michigan banana, is an unusual fruit that I've grown for several years now. They produce a simply delicious banana custard-like fruit. They blossom in the spring. I notice my bees love to pollinate their blossoms, and that activity makes such a big difference in the fruit production.

A few properties I've worked on held a small collection of fruit trees. Their fruit yield was very low until I introduced honeybees near them. It seems as soon as I did that, the branches were bending and breaking. They became so fruitful that I had to cull some of the smaller fruit so that the branches wouldn't break.

I usually like to grow dwarf varieties of fruit trees. Since they're smaller than the standard, old-fashioned trees, you can tuck them into sunny little hot spots on your property. They're also easy to prune in the fall to keep their shape. You can purchase the dwarf variety of fruit trees through garden centers or via the Internet. One of my favorite companies is Stark Brothers. I've had very good success with their fruit trees. They ship well, and the trees establish very quickly and bear fruit at a young age.

Chestnut trees are another favorite of mine to grow. Some of the chestnut trees I have are bearing fruit at seven years old. They're wonderful. They add a great addition to the fall crop, along with the Asian pears and Bosc pears that we grow on the farm. The chestnuts provide nuts for us, as well as the wildlife. One thing I do, and have taught my children to do, is share. Chestnuts are delicious roasted, baked, boiled, and just a great addition to the fall crop.

When it comes to selecting a site for the fruit trees, you'll discover that they usually do best in full sunlight. I try to pick a well-drained area. I start by digging a hole twice the size of the root system. If you're buying through mail order and receive a bare tree root, it's best to double the size of the hole that you're digging. Place the tree in the hole with a combination of mixed top soil, hummus, or a good compost blend. Pack the soil firmly around the root system, creating a funnel-like shape, and then make a wall with the existing soil that's left. After that, put an ample amount of wood mulch over the area to retain moisture. This keeps the root system cool and allows the tree to get off to a good start. Water the area well.

I like to plant comfrey around the bases of my fruit tree. Comfrey is a plant that pulls nutrients from deep down in the soil and brings them to the surface. This helps fruit trees because most of them are shallow rooted. Comfrey also provides good organic matter. As the plant gets taller, the leaves can be cut and placed around the fruit trees.

For honeybees, the comfrey provides a beautiful blossom that is highly prized. The bees will soon pollinate them and gather the nectar from the blossom, and the whole cycle begins again. The plant will drop its seeds and create new comfrey plants around the fruit trees. This is another practice of permaculture.

Once the tree becomes established, generally after the first year, it may put out a few blossoms, and then the fruit will develop. Ideally, to get the tree off to a good start during the first year, the small fruit should be culled. By reducing the fruit the first year, the tree will generate a better root system for years to come. This will enable the tree to bear and produce an abundance of fruit.

When it comes to the fruit trees, I want to use the pear tree as an example of something I like to do. I take a piece of a producing pear tree and graft it onto an ornamental pear tree. Ornamental trees only produce a blossom that lasts for a week. There's a short window in the month of March where I can do this. I take a scion, which is last year's wood that grew from an existing fruiting pear tree. I prune that scion off in March and pare it down to a cleft, which is a small V. I prune off a branch from the ornamental pear and stick that little wedge of a V in an incision that I made on the ornamental tree. I apply some grafting wax on the junction and wrap it with grafting tape. What you now have is a branch on the ornamental pear tree that will produce edible pears. I've done this with several trees with great success. It works with peaches and apples also. They all tend to graft very easily.

I place other plants around fruit trees to prevent insects from getting on the tree and attacking the fruit. I like to plant garlic, chives, and some thyme. Oil from the thyme keeps away lots of pests. You can plant many edible flowers among the fruit trees or throughout the rest of your landscape.

Edible flowers have a short shelf life, but in addition to planting them around the fruit trees, you can grow them in a garden, in containers, and in window boxes. They're a lot of fun to grow. I like to grow borage. It's a blue flower with a cucumber-like taste and a blossom prized by the honeybees. You can also steep the leaves into a tea.

Calendula is another such flower. It comes in yellow or orange and is very sweet to the taste. It also can be steeped into tea, and it's good for the nervous system. You can mix it with beeswax and mineral oil and use it as a salve.

Arugula has a delicate white flower with a peppery flavor; I like to toss it in a salad with garlic. Nasturtiums taste very much like radishes, and are delicious in a tossed salad as well. Some others that are edible are geraniums, hibiscus, and violets. All are good to eat.

*Page 40: Chestnut tree.*

*Page 43: Some apples in the dwarf variety produce quickly, are easy to reach, and can fit in small spaces.*

*Page 44: Nice pawpaws developing.*

*Page 45: Lucy with dwarf ginger gold apple tree.*

*Page 46: Asian pears are maintenance free, easy to grow, and delicious.*

*Page 47: This Elberta peach tree has been heavily pollinated by honeybees after the introduction of a hive to the orchard.*

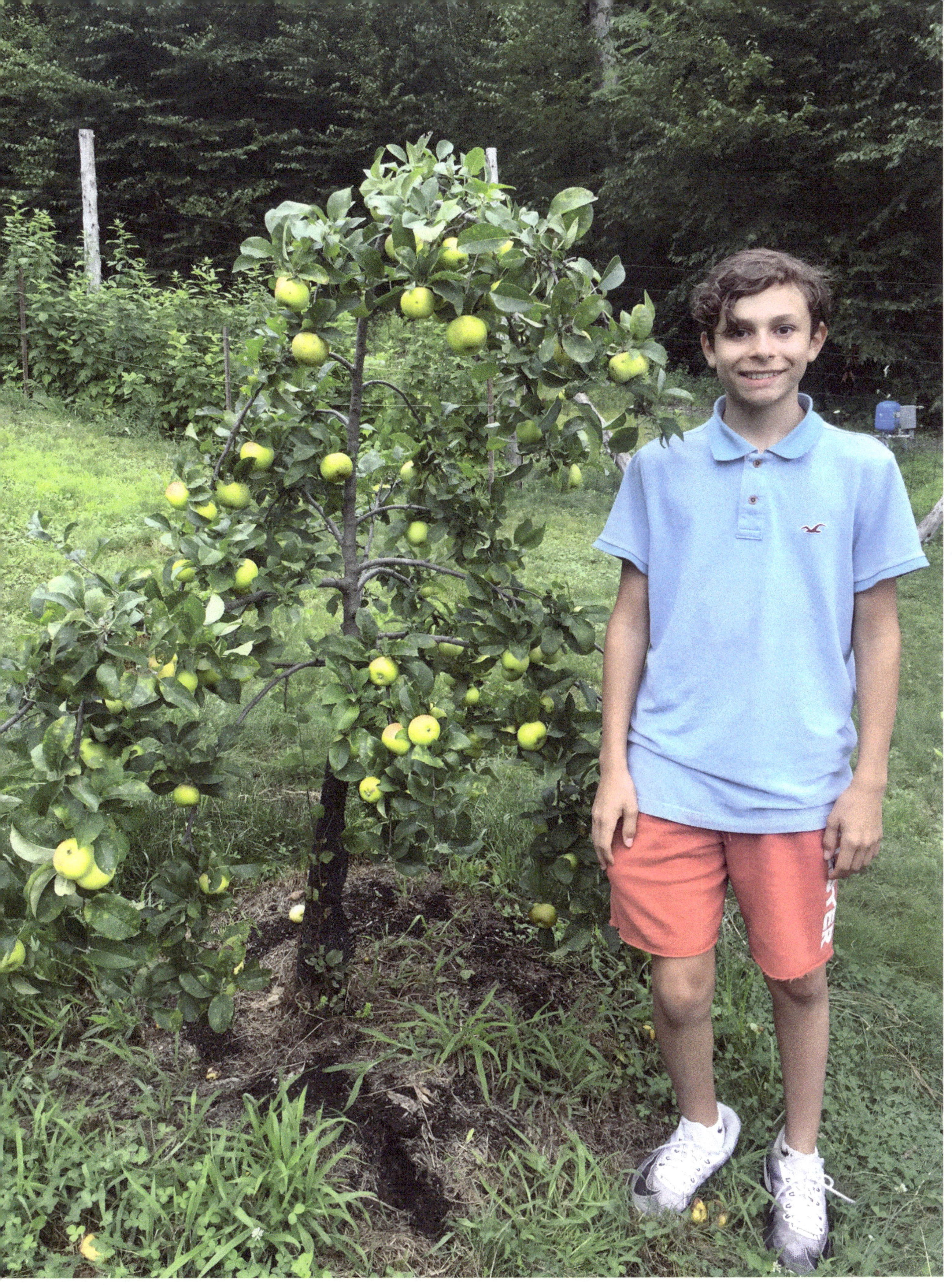

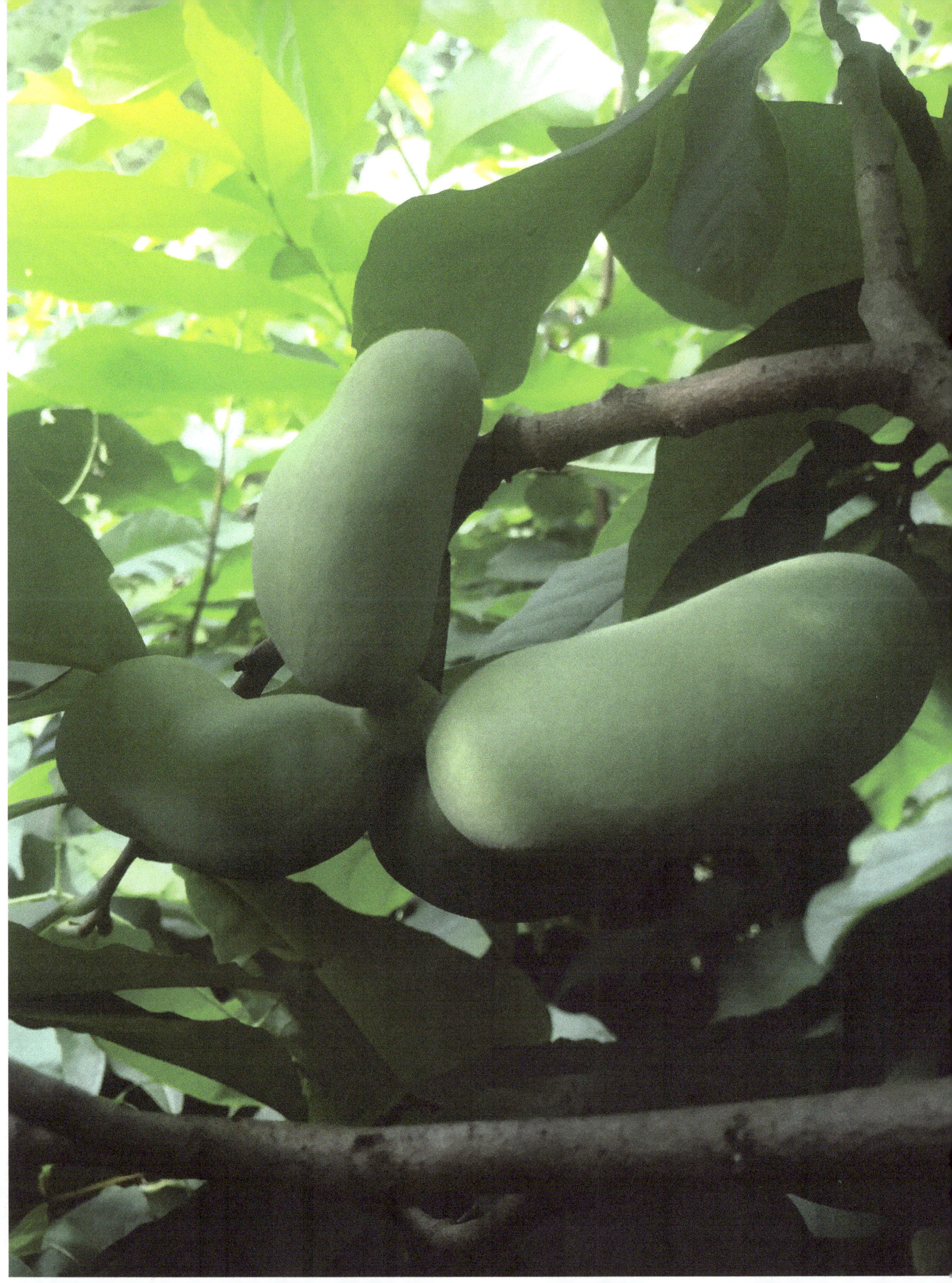

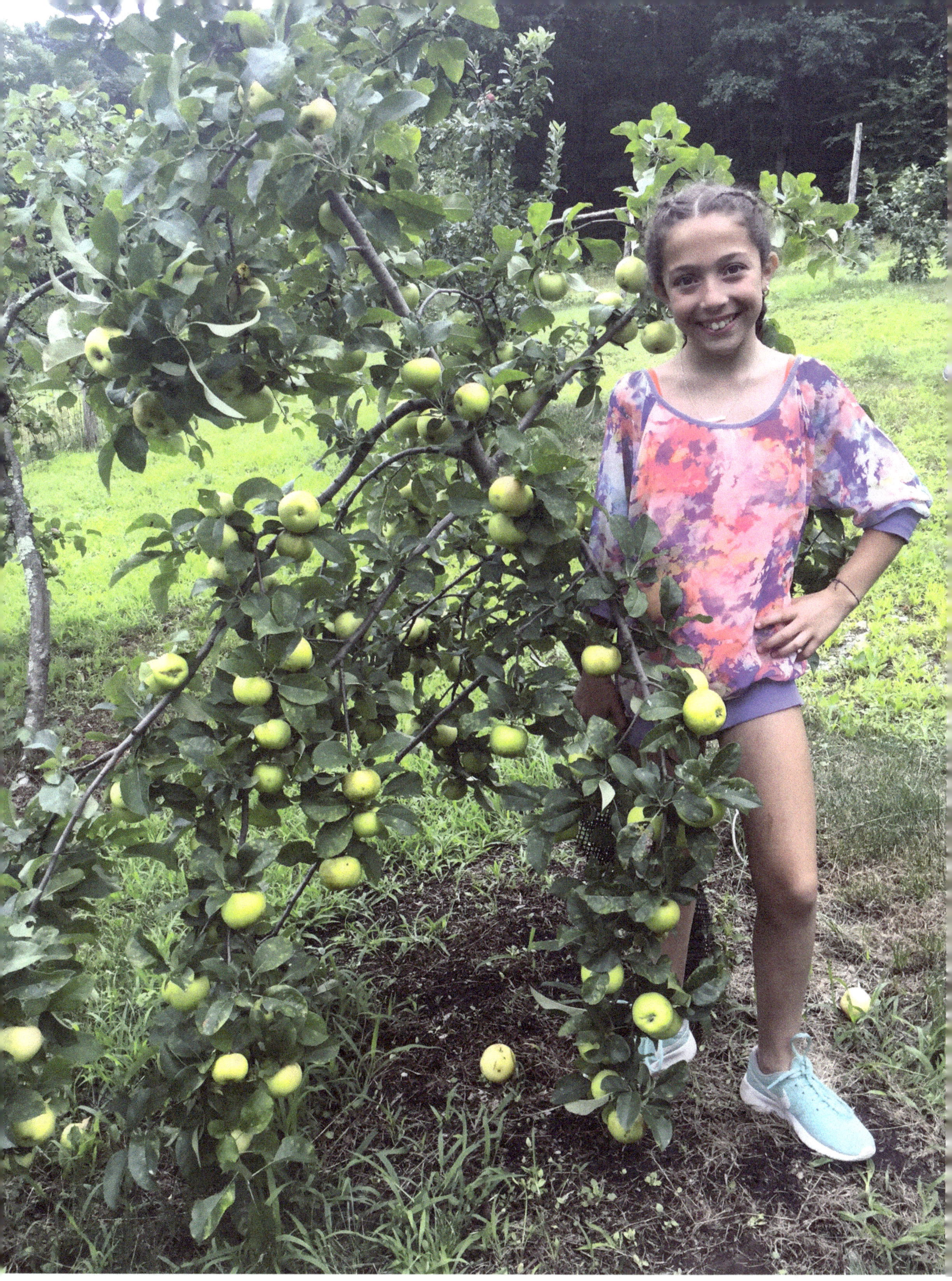

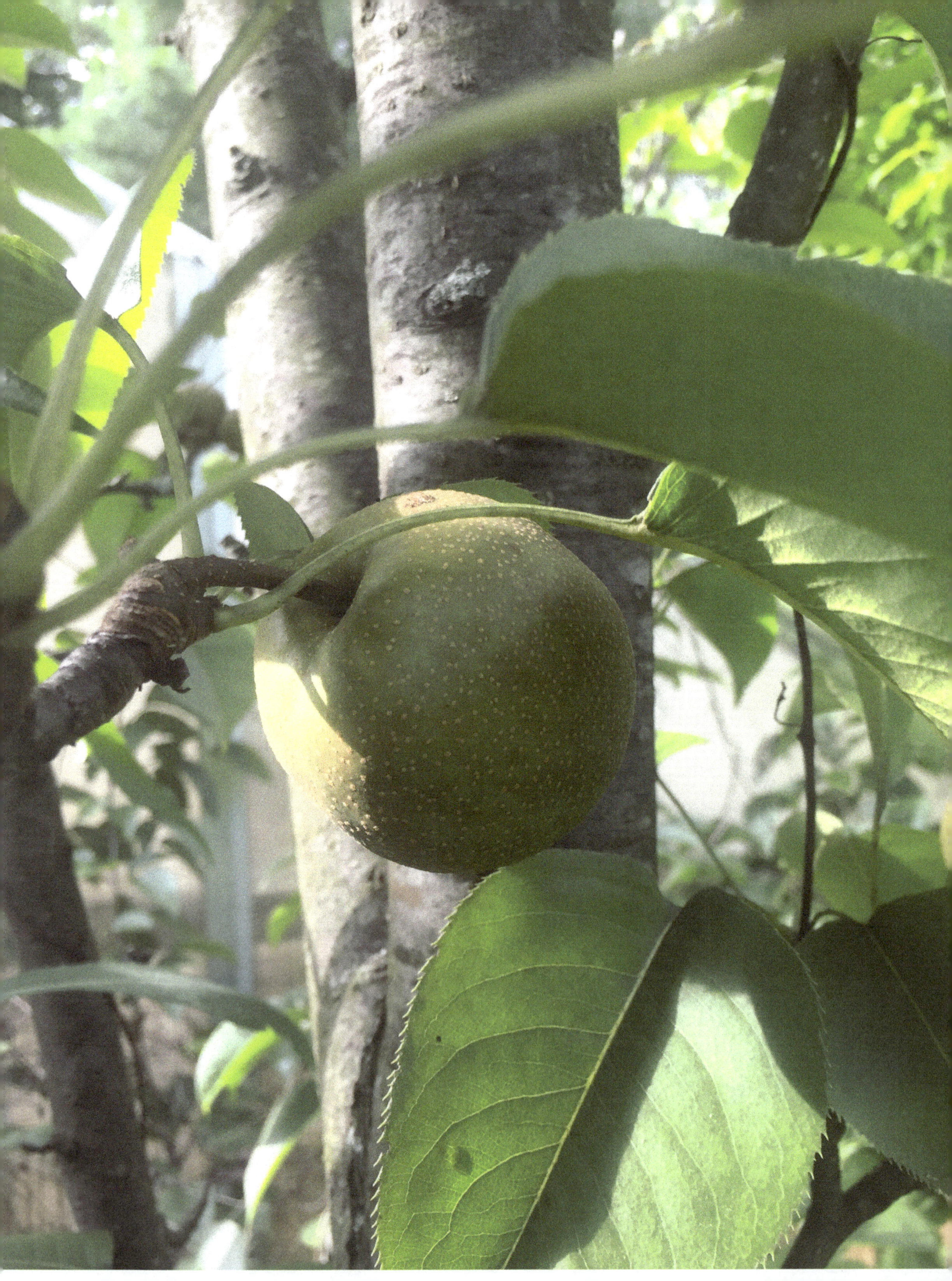

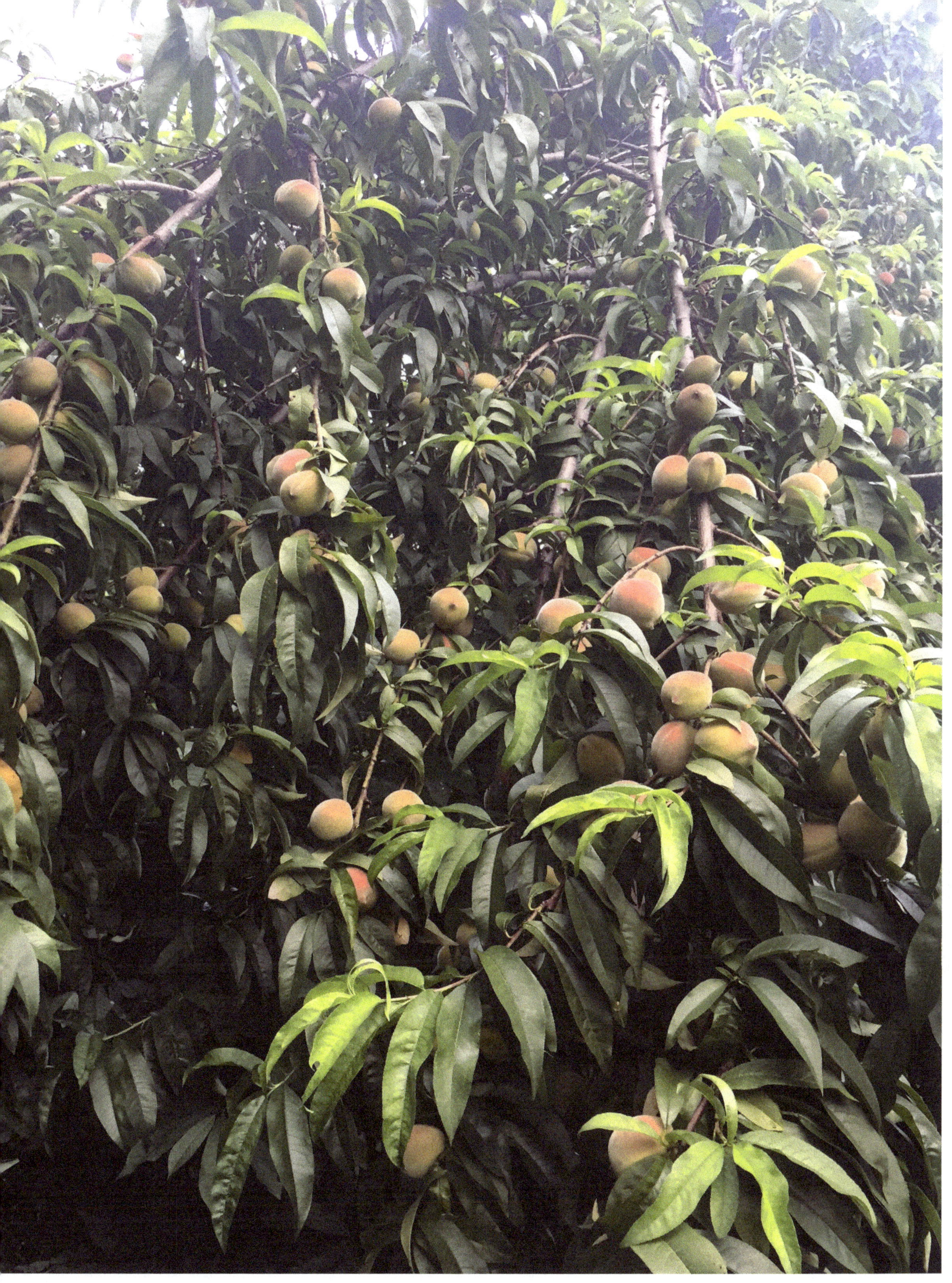

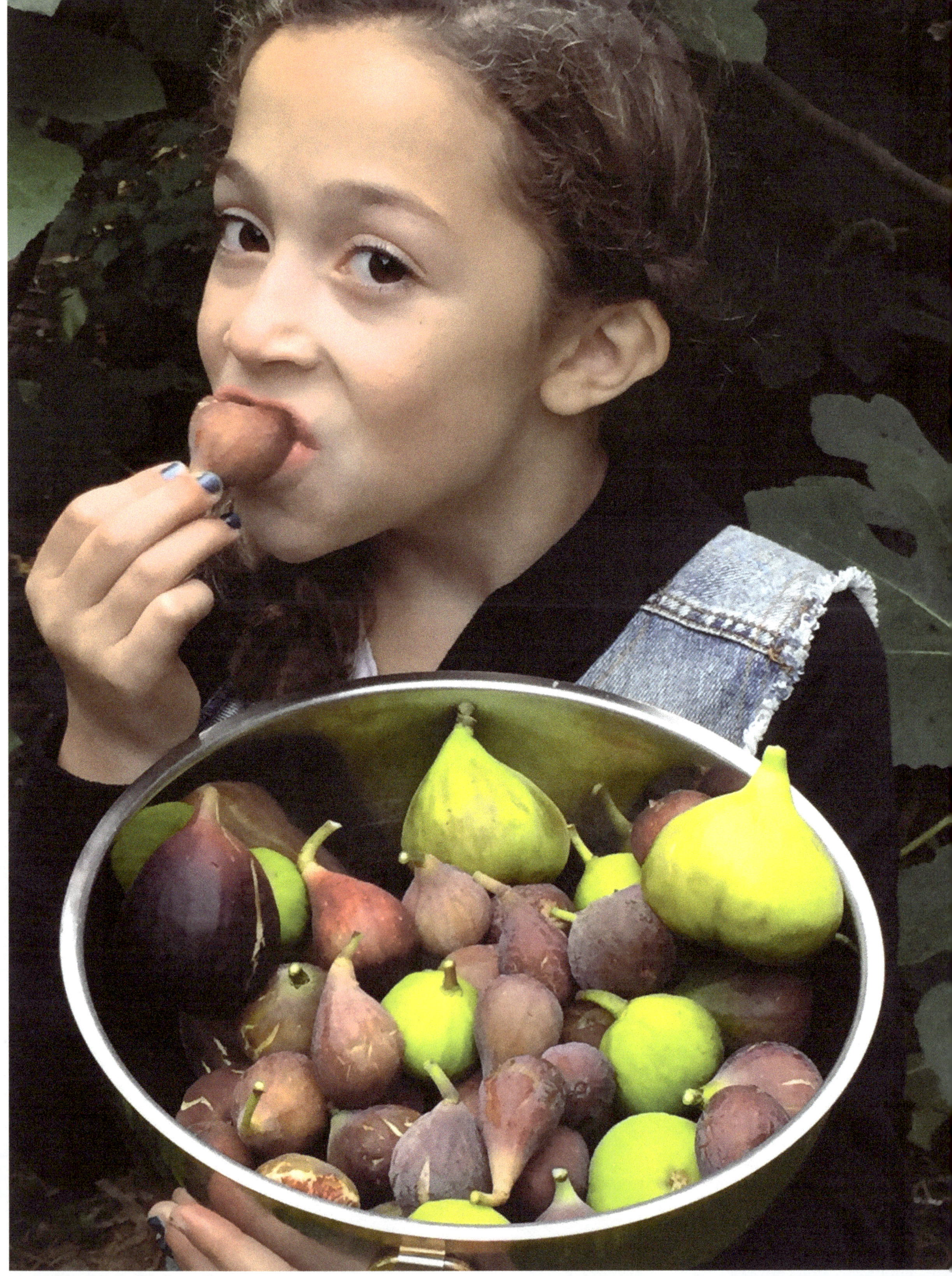

# Fig Trees

*"To eat figs off the tree in the very early morning, when they have been barely touched by the sun, is one of the exquisite pleasures of the Mediterranean."*

**— Elizabeth David**

It isn't just in the Mediterranean that this is true. I grow them not far from New York City and they're delightful. Figs are one of the most rewarding fruits you can grow. I raise several varieties of them. I started raising fig trees because I enjoy the fruit so much. I give them to my family once they ripen, as figs are a very perishable fruit. If you can't consume them right away, you can dry them, or make them into a jam. One of my favorite recipes with figs is to use them in chutney. You can see how to make that in the recipe section of this book.

The fig tree is an Asian species of flowering plants in the mulberry family, known as the common fig (or just the fig). Its fruit, also called the fig, is a key commercial crop when grown in orchards. The fig tree is an ancient fruit tree cultivated for centuries and continues to be popular today. While the Mediterranean area is its native habitat, the fig tree can grow throughout the world as an ornamental shrub and for its fruit.

The fig is one of the first plants early humans cultivated. Scientists have discovered fossilized figs in ancient villages dating back to 9400 BC. Growing figs might be the first indication of agriculture. Their production seems to predate the cultivation of wheat, beans, or barley. In fact, growing figs may have occurred a good thousand years before any other type of crop.

Figs were definitely common in ancient Greece, as philosophers such as Aristotle and Theophrastus commented on their cultivation and reproduction. Roman texts list several types of figs grown back then and their uses. Spanish missionaries brought the first figs trees to California. With a climate similar to the Mediterranean area, figs thrived there and continue to be popular.

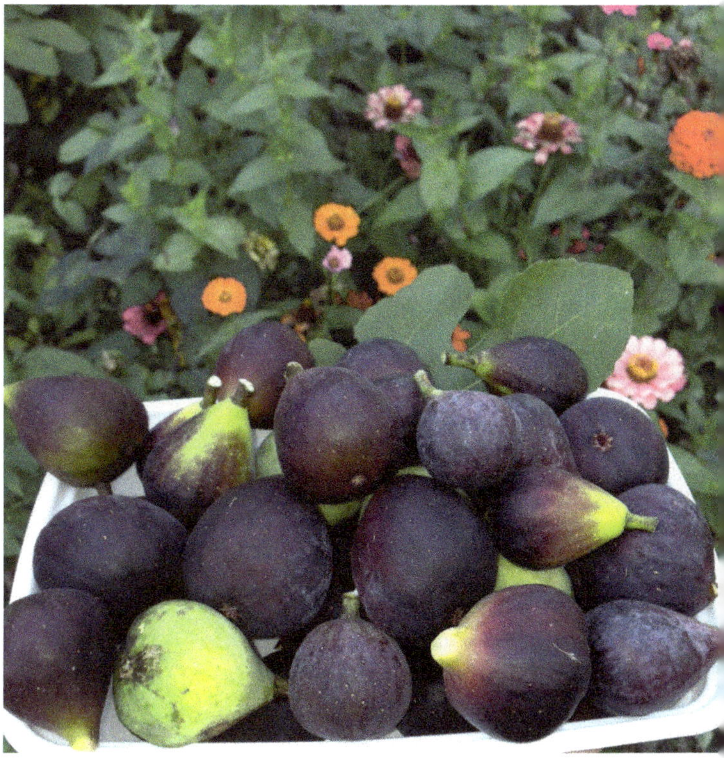

*Left: Lucy enjoying an array of figs.*

*Right: Brown turkish figs.*

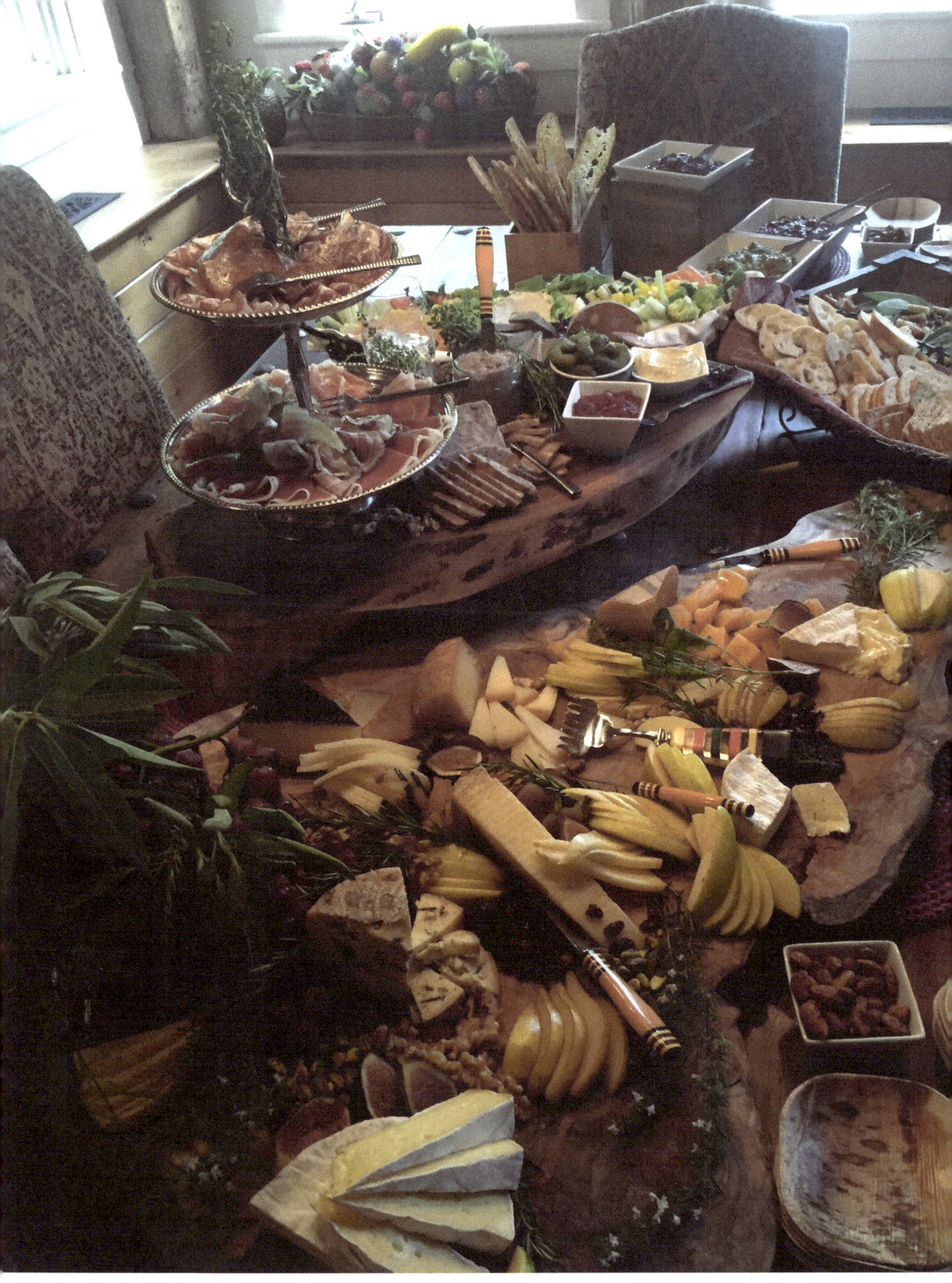

About 80 percent of the United States' fig production occurs in California. As a whole, America ranks low on the scale of fig-producing countries. Turkey is number one with the responsibility of growing 28 percent of the world's figs. That percentage equals about 275 thousand metric tons. That's a lot of figs! The other significant producers of figs center in North Africa with Morocco, Algeria, and Egypt leading the way.

Figs can be eaten fresh or dried. They're often used in jam-making and commercial products using dried or other processed forms of figs. Once a fig is picked, it doesn't keep very well and is hard to transport. Fresh figs tend to be in season from August through early October. The fresh figs used for cooking or baking should be soft and plump. They shouldn't have any bruises or splits. If a fig smells sour to you, then it has become over-ripe. If not quite ripe, you can keep figs at room temperature for a day or two to ripen before you serve them. Figs have their best flavor when served at room temperature.

I usually grow figs in containers. I've had great success doing this since I can move them around and store them in a cool, dark place in the winter during their dormancy. Figs grow best in the full sunlight, and that's where I put them when I take them out of their winter quarters in the springtime. This is also the time that I treat them by putting some composted manure into their pots, along with limestone. Their growing season gets off to a great start this way.

The spring is when the fig trees start to bud. The tiny embryo figs that have been dormant for the winter start to emerge. These are the breba figs. They are the first figs to emerge in the spring, and eventually ripen in early summer. These figs grow rather sporadically, but they are the largest figs.

In general, my fig trees produce two to three crops a year. They come in many different shapes, colors, and sizes. I happen to have just about all of them. I've been growing them for over 25 years, and have a collection of over 65 trees.

To many people in America, especially here in the Northeast, figs sound like a distant and exotic fruit. They aren't as hard to grow as you might think. In fact, they're fairly easy.

The first thing to ensure success with growing figs is to place them in the sun. It's imperative that they have at least six hours of full sun. After all, they are a Mediterranean plant, and they love the heat. I place a large coaster underneath the pots to catch any of the moisture that runs out of the pot. Fig trees have a very dynamic root system, and it can lap up any excess water throughout the hot, sunny day when I'm not there to water them. In general, I do set a schedule of watering them every morning to keep them lush, green, and happy.

Once a fig tree sets its buds and little figs start to form, then they will tolerate some drying out. To give you a size reference, this is when they're a little bit bigger than a Tic Tac breath mint. They slowly begin to develop when they're that size. As a fig's angle on the tree begins to change and they drop towards the ground, that's when it's ripe. At this point, you can feel the softness of the flesh, and that's a good indication they're ready for you to pick them.

Figs trees are also very conducive to propagate and increase your number of trees. Once a fig tree is established, you can select a couple canes from it for cutting. This happens to me when a friend or family member samples one of the fruits and comments how delicious it is. I often offer to give them one of my cuttings so they can start growing their own fig tree. In this way, you can share the bounty of the crop with a good friend or neighbor.

*Fresh figs served with cheese.*

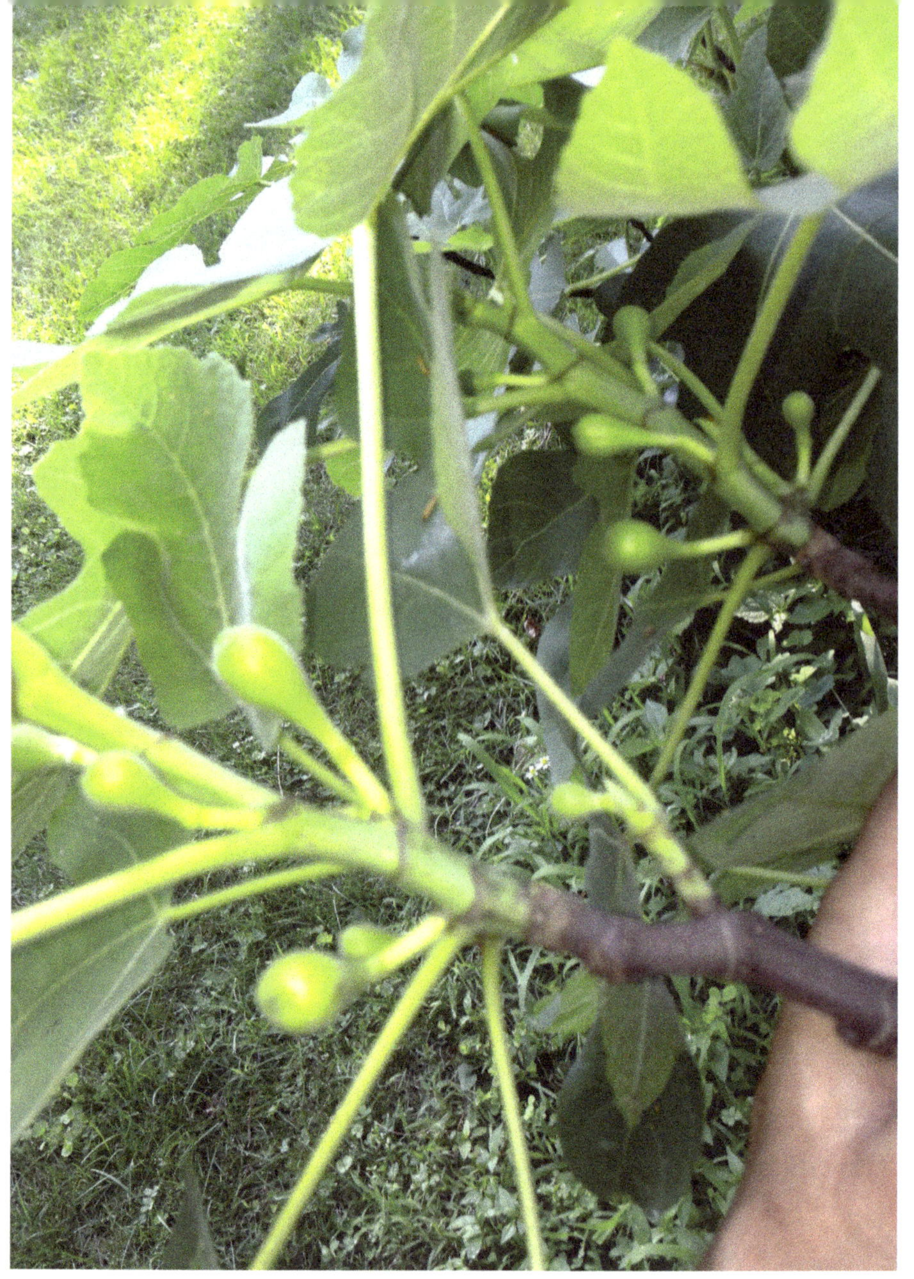

*Figs just starting.*

I have a few different methods to propagate my figs. I select a branch that's 10 to 12 inches long and is nice and straight. I prune it off the tree, remove most of the leaves, and scratch the bottom of the cane. Then I add a little bit of rooting hormone. The one that I like the best is Rootone. I dip it into the Rootone and then place it in some wet sand. This doesn't have to be a large pot; it can simply be a small container. I like to use a water bottle with the top cut off, because I can see the new roots emerging through the sand.

I place it in indirect sunlight at first. After about four weeks, you'll notice a few newer leaves start to emerge on the branch. When I see those white roots popping through and new leaves emerging, I transplant the fig tree cutting into a small pot with some soil. I water it and then move it into a sunny spot. I transfer it into a bigger pot when I notice it's starting to mature and putting out new shoots.

Another way I propagate fig trees to increase my collection or give to others is by a method called layering. Layering is when you take an existing mature plant and select one of the lower branches. You can then bend the branch into a container with fine potting soil mixed with sand. You do this so that the branch makes a depression when you lay it into the soil. I then put a brick or weight on the branch, holding it down into the soil. It takes a few weeks for the branch to begin rooting. Keeping the soil moist will encourage the root system to develop quickly on the branch that you want to get started.

This method ensures you 100 percent propagation. The branch that you bend into the container is still alive. The cambium, which is the bark of the small branch you're trying to root, is in contact with the damp soil. This encourages the growth of mature roots.

As soon as the branch is rooted and you remove the brick, gently tug on the branch. When you notice that its new roots are anchoring the branch, cut the branch below the root line. After you do this, stand the branch (your new tree) upright and pack fresh soil around it. Just like that, you have a newly propagated fig tree you could use for resale, to give away, or to increase your collection. The cutting from an existing plant is called a clone.

When you've potted and placed the plant upright, you can stake it with a piece of bamboo cane to train it to grow nice and straight. After its first year, when the plant goes into dormancy, you can snip the top bud off to encourage more branches to grow from your newly propagated fig tree. By doing this, you can train it to become more of a bush that is easier to grow in a container. This is all you have to do, and before you know it, the fig tree is ready to begin producing fruit. After the first year of producing fruit, when the plant is into its second year, you can propagate that one as well.

I like to keep my fig trees in the full sun. Once the trees grow through their season, you'll find their fruiting months are September and October. This is when you'll be picking your last crop of figs. After you've picked all your figs, it's time to let the trees go dormant.

Fig trees are deciduous, which means they lose their leaves. The first step of dormancy is when you notice that the larger leaves on a fig tree are starting to turn yellow and fall off. You must wait for all the leaves to fall off the tree before you prepare them for dormancy. If your tree is growing in the ground, you must wrap it to protect it from a harsh winter. If in a container, you need to tie it up and bring it indoors for protection.

I store my fig trees over the winter by letting them go through their dormancy and drop all their leaves. Only then do I tie them up with a piece of garden twine to make them more manageable. Their branches are very flexible at this time since they don't have any foliage on them and they're not frozen. I gather all the branches, tie them up, and put all the containers on a small dolly to bring them into my basement. I have a spot there that's very cool and dark. They stay there over the winter and complete their natural dormancy while being protected from the harsh elements of the season.

After I place them in the basement, I water them once a month, just keeping the soil moist and not allowing them to dry out. They store very well. In the spring, I bring them out of the basement as soon as there's no more danger of frost. I then fertilize the trees, water them very well, and place them in the sun, where they remain during the summer.

I have a large collection of fig trees and bushes. To facilitate their care, I decided to put my figs on a drip irrigation system. I know this might not sound simple, but it does save you a lot of time if you have a collection of six or more figs of different varieties. The method I devised is very simple. You can purchase what you need from any garden center or hardware store that carries irrigation supplies.

To build my system, I start out with a one-inch fitting that connects to my hose, which is similar to a regular garden hose. The fitting is connected to a three-quarter-inch black poly pipe, which is irrigation line, hooked up to a timer. The timer controls the water flow to the fig trees, which connect to the black poly pipe with water drippers. The drippers are little pieces of hose that come out of the main three-quarter-inch line. I set them up so that each one is dangling in one of the fig trees.

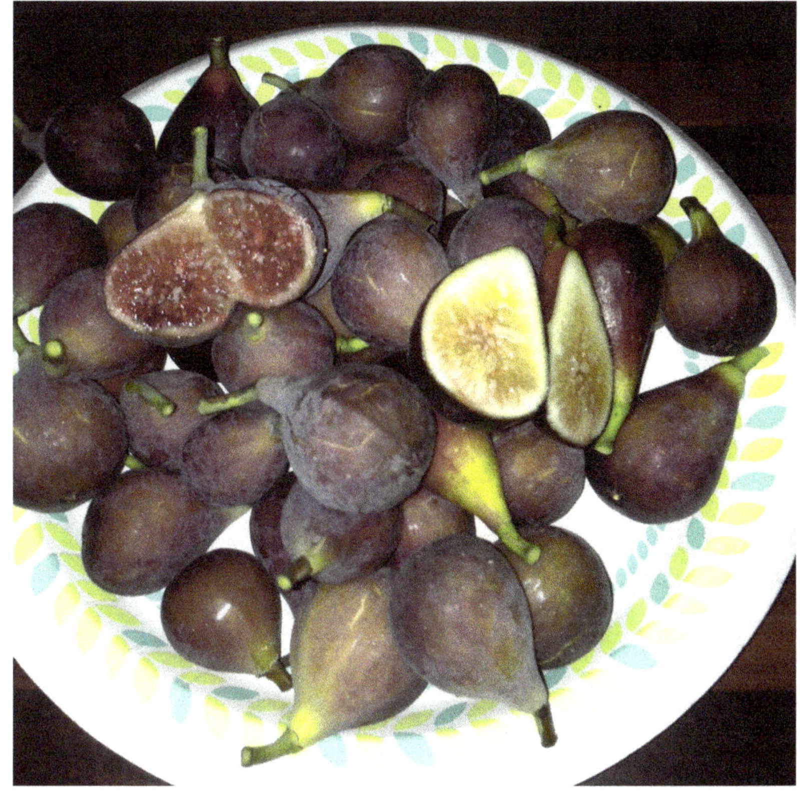

*Negronne figs on the left, and black Spanish figs on the right.*

I set the timer to water them an hour in the morning and an hour in the afternoon. It saves me a lot of time running around throughout the hot summer days when they need water the most. Now they're automatically provided with water in the morning, and then again in the afternoon. The fig trees stay very happy and healthy this way. It also gives me a chance to go away on the weekend without worrying about watering my figs.

Most of the fig trees I grow are in containers. In my climate, slightly north of New York City, the winters aren't favorable to keeping them alive. As fig trees are Mediterranean plants, I have to protect them. My trees produce an abundance of beautiful fruit twice a year. A dormant embryo fig first appears in late November. When the tree comes out of dormancy in spring, it produces its biggest figs from those embryos. This is the breba crop fig and they will be ripening around August. Once those ripen, the tree will bear many smaller figs that will result in ripe fruit at the end of September going into October.

The first thing I do in the spring when I take the fig trees out of dormancy is to fertilize them. I make a mixture of one part superphosphate, one part bone meal, one part lime, and one part of a fertilizer named "5-10-5." I mix it up in a bucket, and I give them each two cups. They're all potted up in 10- to 15-gallon containers, and they do very well in them. As I mentioned before, I set them out in full sun as this is important for growing fig trees.

In the autumn, I make my cuttings and do a lot of pruning. I take off many of the tips, which are scions. This is last year's growth and the prime choice canes for cutting. I place those cuttings in Ziploc bags and label them. I keep them in cold storage for a while, and then pot them up in a loamy mix with a little bit of rooting hormone on the bottom of the cane. I put them down in the root cellar, water them, and let them stay in dormancy until spring.

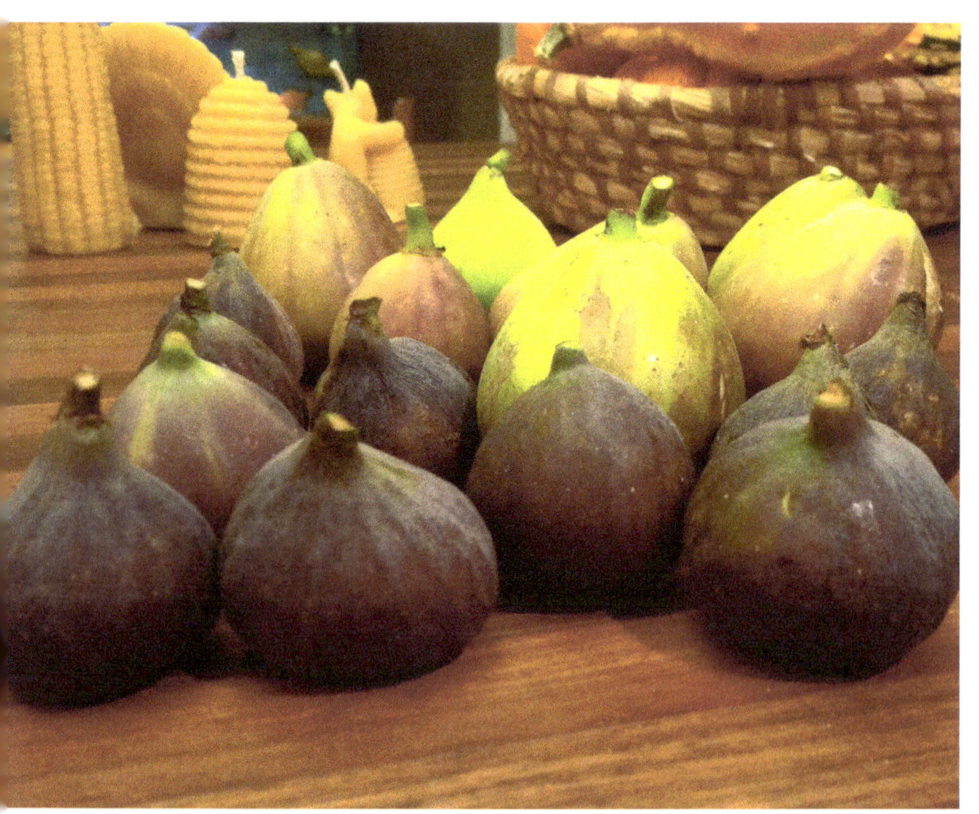

*Fresh picked figs.*

Once we are into spring, I take the canes out, along with the mother plants, and I give them some more humidity. I place them in a little bit of shelter and shade. If I have some room underneath the bench in the greenhouse, I'll store them there. When the buds start breaking, I give them a small amount of the fertilizer mixture that I mentioned earlier. That encourages them to gain a healthy root system leading to a hearty, fruit-producing tree.

For figs that ripen late in the season, I place them in a dehydrator. I dry them and store them for the fall and winter months to snack on. They're definitely one of my all-time favorite fruits to grow.

When the trees get a little bit bigger, I take them out of their pots, and I will slowly examine the root system. I then selectively prune the roots back. This process encourages fresh and new roots to develop. Where I took out the older roots, I repack with fresh soil.

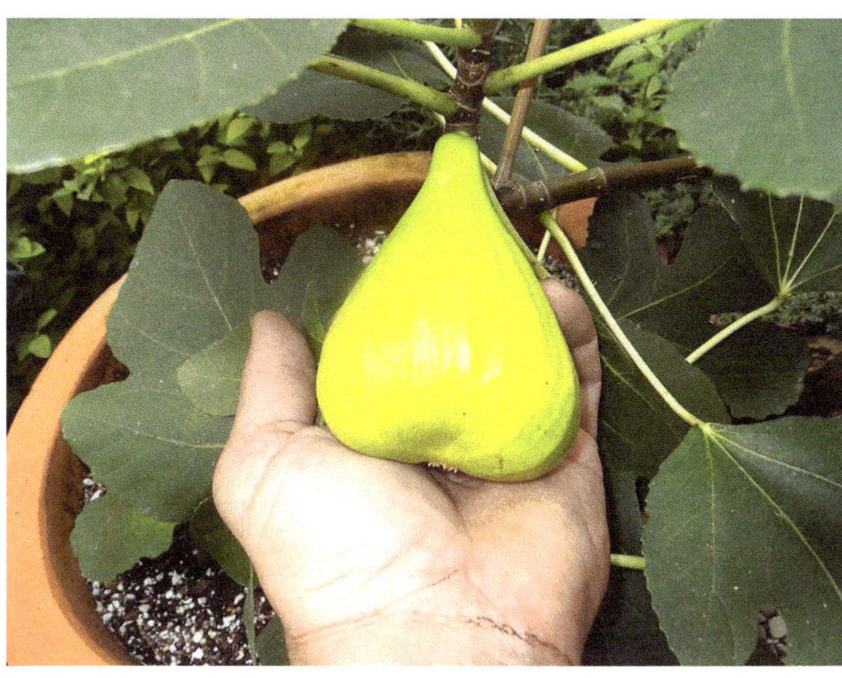

I know all of this might seem like a lot of work, but the fig tree is one of the most rewarding deciduous plants to grow. It does have to go into dormancy, and you need to help prepare it as we talked about. You can't just bring it in the house and let it stay and foliar and leaf. It needs to go to sleep and come back in the spring. If you get into a routine as I described, your trees will produce beautiful figs for you year after year.

Figs are a great source of fiber and very high in potassium and manganese. They're very delicious. You can use them in a variety of dishes from throwing them into a salad to serving with honey and goat cheese. Its flavor can enhance many dishes. If your palate isn't familiar with this incredible fruit, try some. You'll be captivated by its flavor and uses and might decide to grow your own figs as I've described.

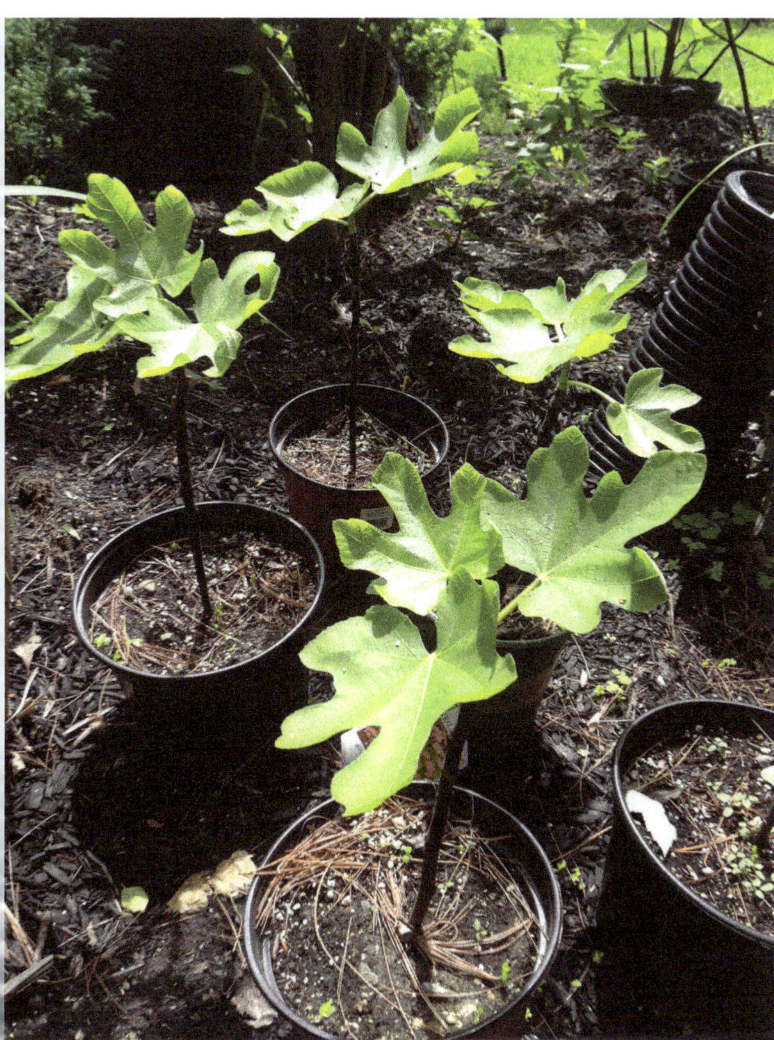

*Top: Pete's honey breba fig.*

*Bottom: Newly rooted fig tree propagations.*

*Page 56: Turkish figs ripening.*

*Page 57: Lucy with two giant Turkish breba figs.*

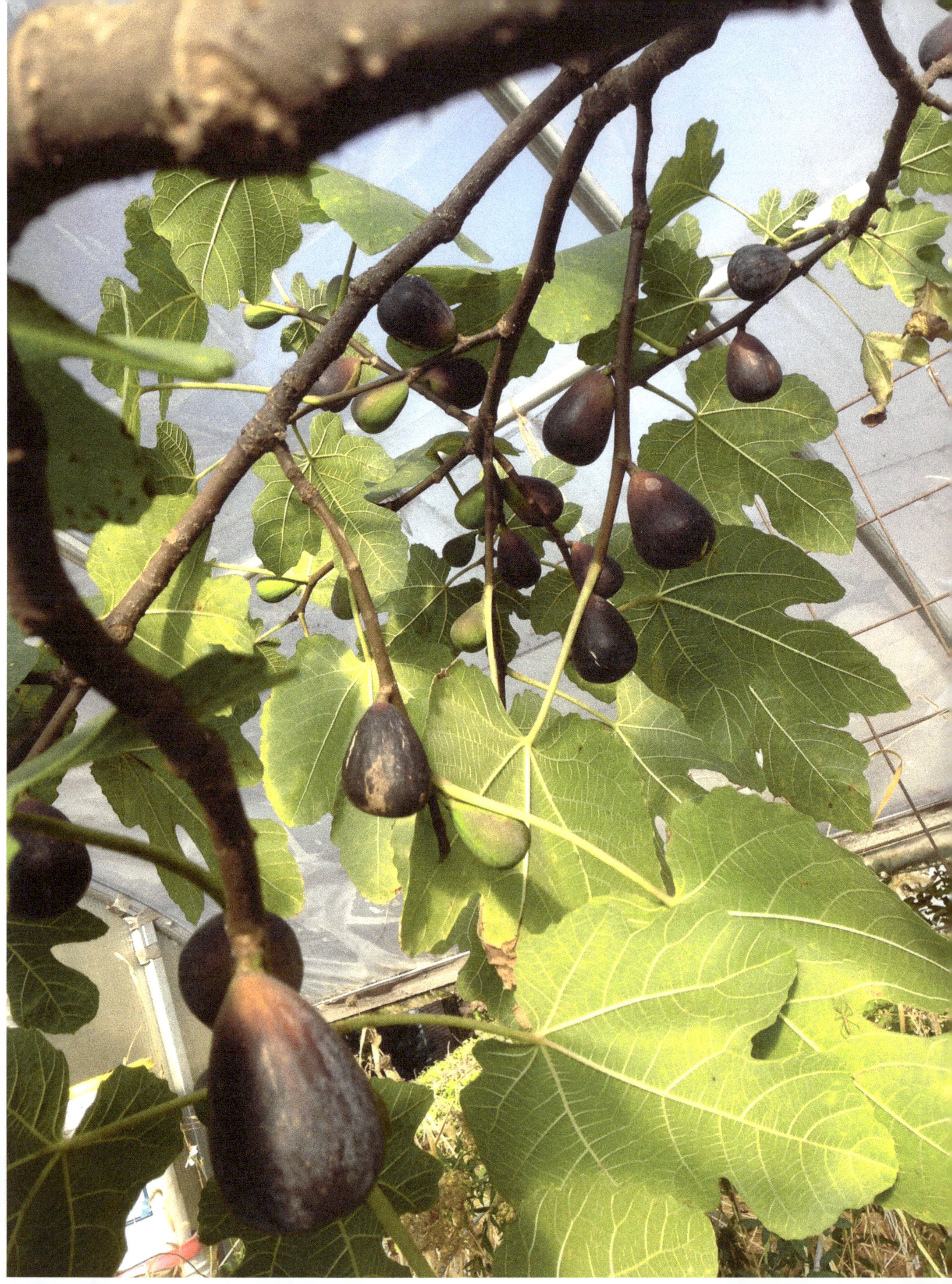

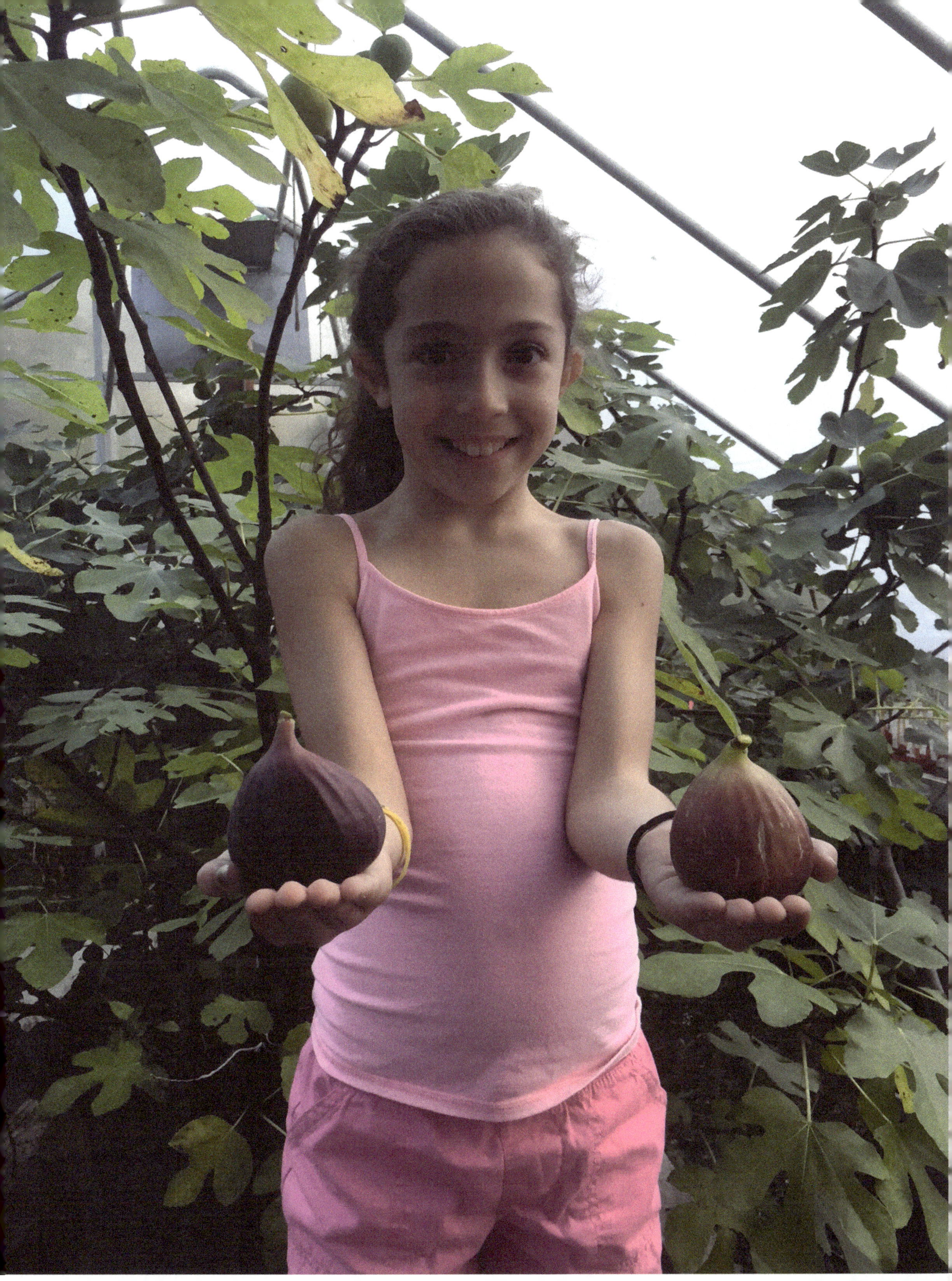

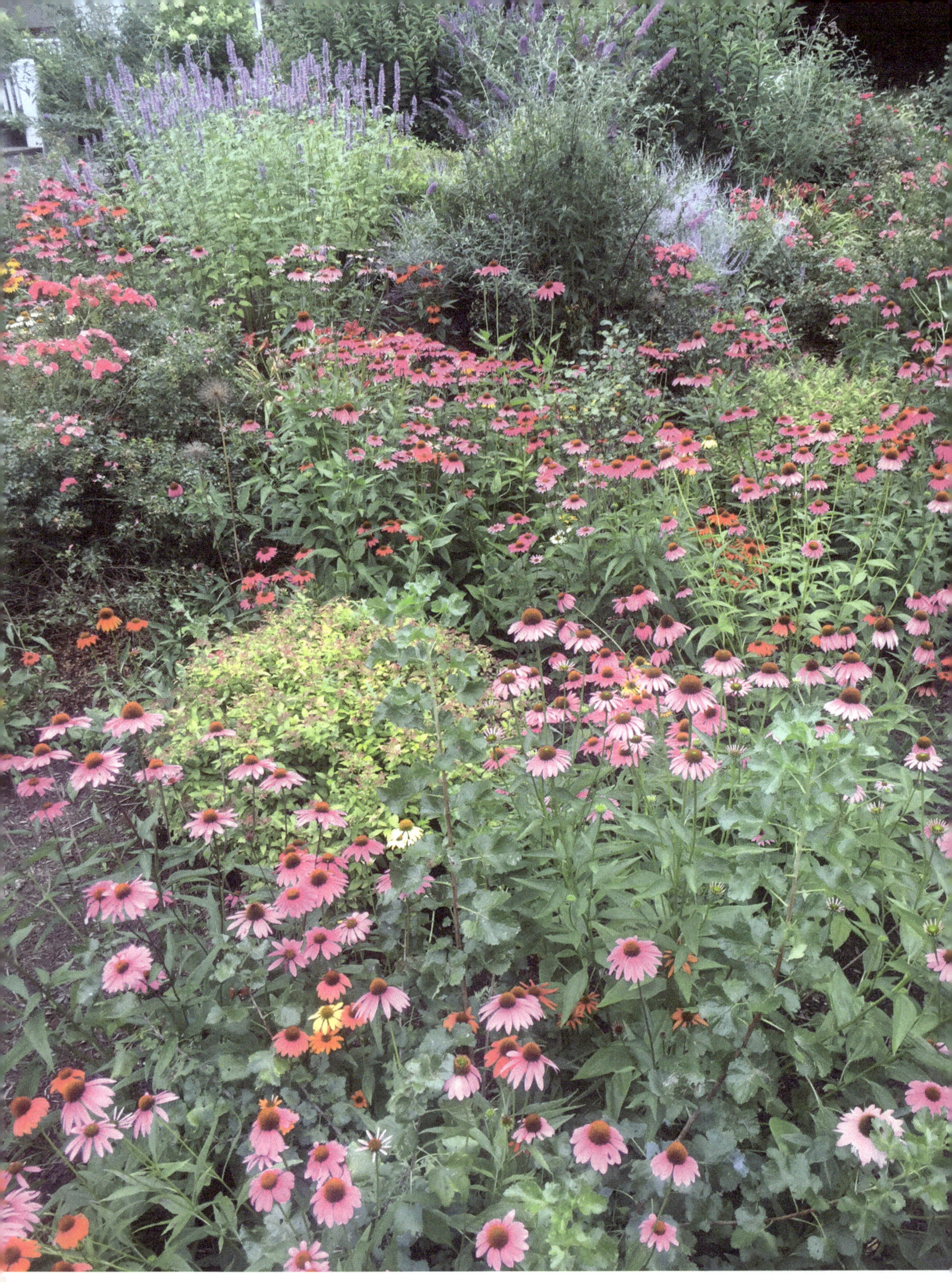

# Gardening

*"Gardening is cheaper than therapy, and you get tomatoes."*

**— Author Unknown**

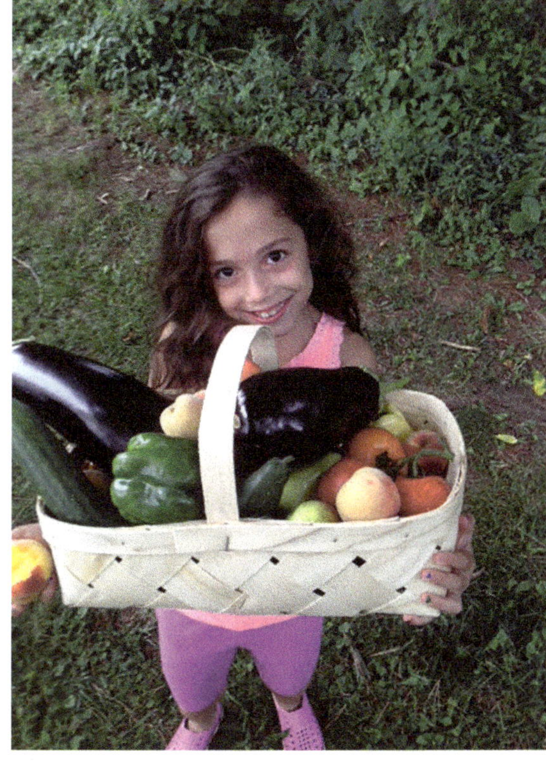

Gardening is the practice of growing plants. The reasons can be as varied as doing it for decoration, to grow vegetables and herbs, or a combination of reasons. Egyptian tombs show pictures of gardens from that ancient time. The Hanging Gardens of Babylon was one of the Seven Wonders of the Ancient World. The nature of gardening changed as the times changed. Sometimes gardens were strictly ornamental while others produced vegetables for survival. People also grew plants for medicinal purposes.

You can have your garden today for any or all of these reasons. You have a choice of ornamental plants grown for their flowers, foliage, or overall appearance. There are plants for consumption such as root vegetables, leaf vegetables, fruits, and herbs. Then you have very select plants that you can grow for dyes, for medicinal use, or even cosmetics.

When I grow vegetables, I like to pick out a site in the sun. If it's a new location and sod covers the area, it's a good idea to overturn the sod with a rototiller to cultivate the soil. When you do this, you're adding the sod back into the earth. This helps replenish nitrogen and nutrients.

I like to create a new garden in the springtime. As the weather warms up, I turn the sod into the soil, and I also add rotted leaves, compost, and manure in with the sod. This creates a raised bed. Once I establish the beds, I select the areas in which I'd like to grow specific vegetables.

If I'm growing root crops such as turnips, parsnips, beets, radishes, and carrots, I know that they require a deeper, sandier, and loamier soil. I like to keep those beds raised about 8 to 12 inches. I then seed my root crops directly into the beds in the spring. Some crops must be planted only when the soil reaches a temperature of at least 60 degrees. If you plant them when the ground is cooler, they'll go into shock. These plants are known as nightshades. Some examples are tomatoes, eggplants, and peppers. They do well in the warmer weather.

*Page 58: Bee and butterfly garden teeming with echinacea, Russian sage, agastache, buddleia, spirea, and hydrangea.*

*Above: Lucy with a basket of fresh bounty from the garden and orchard.*

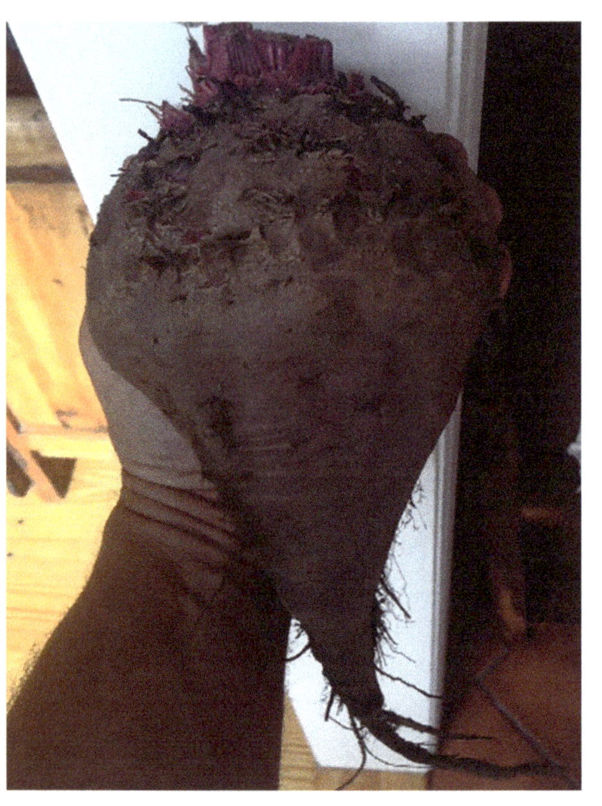

When the weather warms up and I can put the plants outside, I make a garden compost tea. This consists of at least 10 gallons of water. I add in four cups of chicken manure and six cups of compost. This forms a high-nitrogen solution that gets the plants off to a good start. My dad taught me how to make this, and he called it "Kickaba Juice." I apply it to the plants in the early stages, and it's excellent at getting their root system established. It does wonders if you're looking to grow large fruits and vegetables.

I've also grown a great deal of squash with this compost tea. Some of the butternut squash that I fed this tea weighed in at over 15 pounds! I've done a few other things to create bigger vegetables. I've grown tomatoes and sweet potatoes that looked like they were on steroids. You can achieve these maxed-out vegetables very naturally.

Culling has a lot to do with the success of my large produce. For example, if I'm growing a giant, prize-winning tomato, I grow the tomato plant with no competition. That means no weeds or other tomatoes. I give the plant plenty of room, with at least four feet on each side. It will also be in the full sun. This works on different varieties of tomatoes. I like to grow Big Zac, Mortgage Lifter, Beefsteak, and one of my all-time favorites, Belgium Giants. I feed the tomatoes composted tea throughout the growing season, and as the plant grows, I remove its suckers. These are the little shoots that grow between the leaves. I call it the armpit of the plant. The flowers are set alongside the main stem of the plant, and not the suckers. By removing all the suckers, a lot of the energy goes to the main stem of the plant.

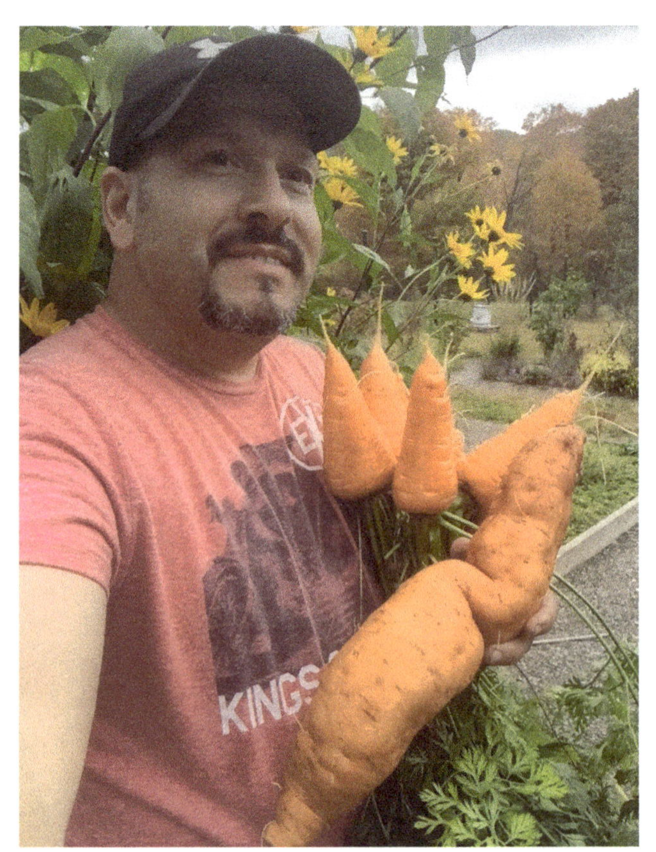

Once I notice that the tomato is starting to go into flower, I let it set the fruit. When the fruit is the size of a grape, I select some of it and remove the rest, only keeping four tomatoes on the vine. When the tomatoes reach golf ball size, I reduce it to two. I remove all other flowers and tomatoes. I keep two for insurance, in case one becomes damaged or eaten by a predator. It's unlikely, but things happen, so I always raise two on the vine. Now, all the plant's energy will go into those two pieces of fruit. I continue to remove all the suckers, which will compete with and take away nutrients from the actual tomato. By the end of the growing season in August when that tomato starts to turn ripe, it will be very large.

Tomatoes are one of my favorite plants to grow large. It's always fun to have the children enter them in the county fair. Pumpkins can also be coaxed into growing very large by culling many of the smaller ones. Bury the vine so the roots can reach into the soil close to where the pumpkin has been produced. The principle here applies as with the super big tomato — all the energy of the vine is directed at that single pumpkin, and it grows to be very large. You can have the Great Pumpkin, Charlie Brown!

I also like to grow carrots. Plant carrot seeds directly into a furrow in the soil garden bed. Once the seeds germinate and start to grow, you must give them room by doing some thinning. This gives the carrots you leave less competition with one another for space. Carrots can't mature when tightly seeded.

You can feed them the compost tea after thinning them out to at least two inches apart. The roots will double or triple in size with less competition from other plants for the soil's nutrients. By giving them the proper spacing, you can grow up to a two-pound carrot!

When it comes to garden beds in general, I plant tomatoes and eggplants in the full sun. They seem to do best without any competition or weeds. I save grass clippings to place around the plants or use mulch. This combination contains nitrogen that helps the plants grow lush and green, and produces a beautiful crop.

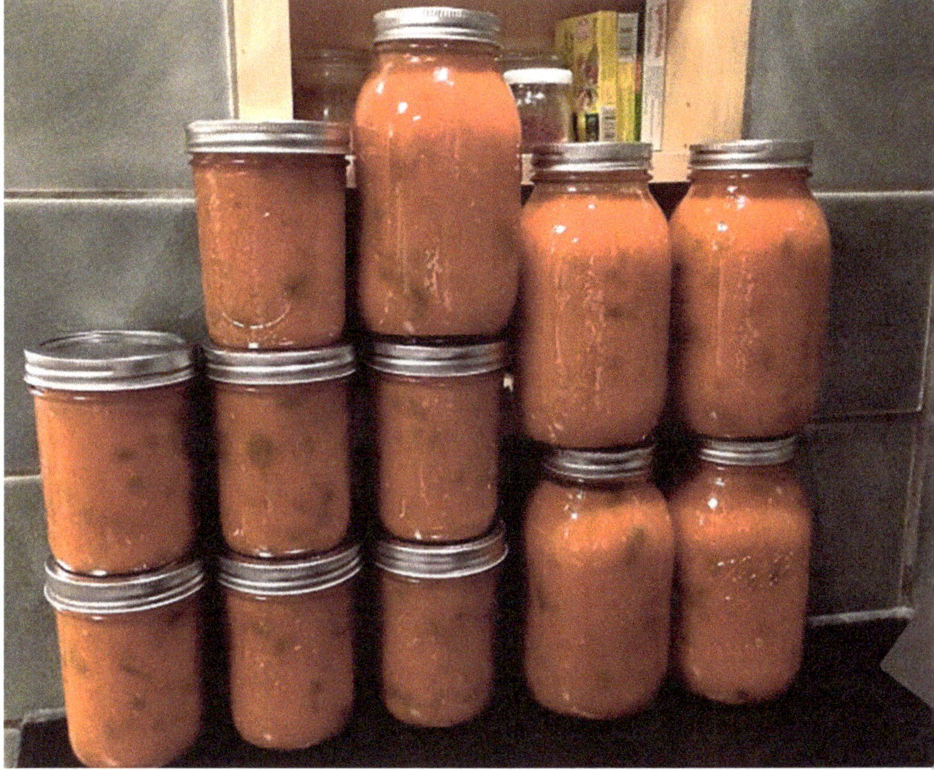

Gardening in raised beds allows you to plant a variety of vegetables, including plum tomatoes. Plum tomatoes, when grown in a row, can produce an abundance of fruit. The problem with plum tomatoes is they all tend to ripen at once, in late August. When this happens, you can pick all the tomatoes, blanch them, and put them in jars to make sauce. My family gets together every year at the family winery to make tomato sauce.

We all pitch in with our tomato harvests. We get a large pot of water boiling and then put in the tomatoes. As soon as we notice them cracking, we take them out and let them drain in a colander. We take the skins off the tomatoes and put them into the crusher to purée them. We then put them back in a pot and on the heat. After adding a little bit of salt, we bring them to a boil.

We put several basil leaves at the bottom of the mason jars we use for canning. When the sauce comes to a boil, we ladle it into the jars. We top off the jars, seal them, and return them to the hot water bath for 15 minutes on a steady boil. Then we remove the jars and let them rest on a table covered with a towel. Within a half hour or so, once the jars start to cool, it almost sounds like an orchestra when all the lids start to seal. They'll last for over a year and a half to two years once sealed. You can enjoy them throughout the winter months.

*Page 60: Large Chioggia beet and sweet potatoes.*

*Top: Tomato sauce recently jarred.*

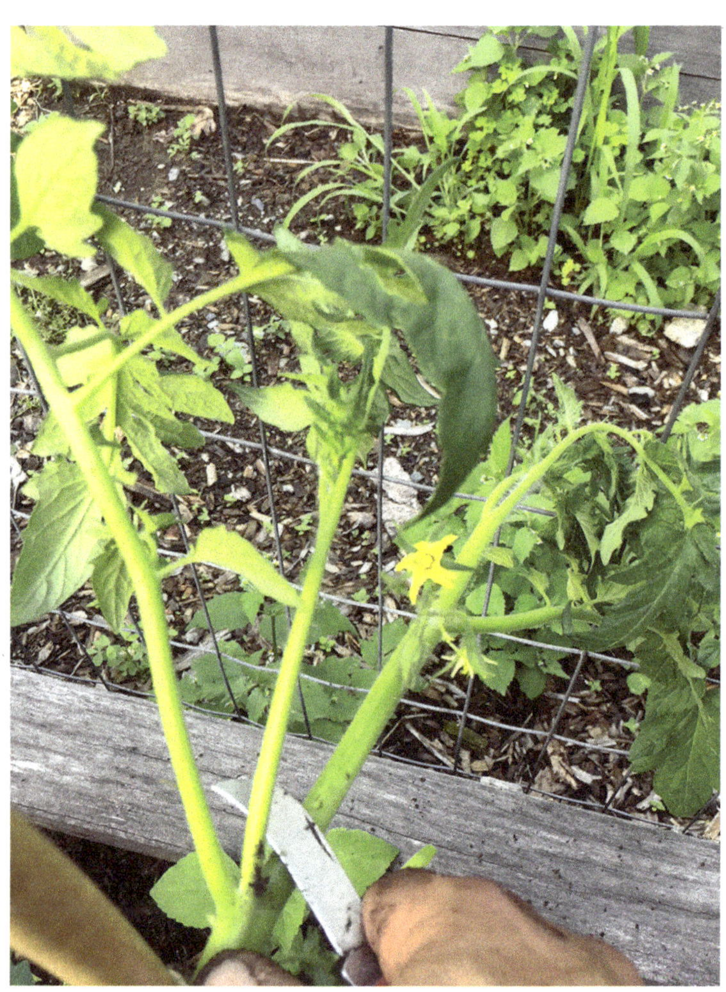
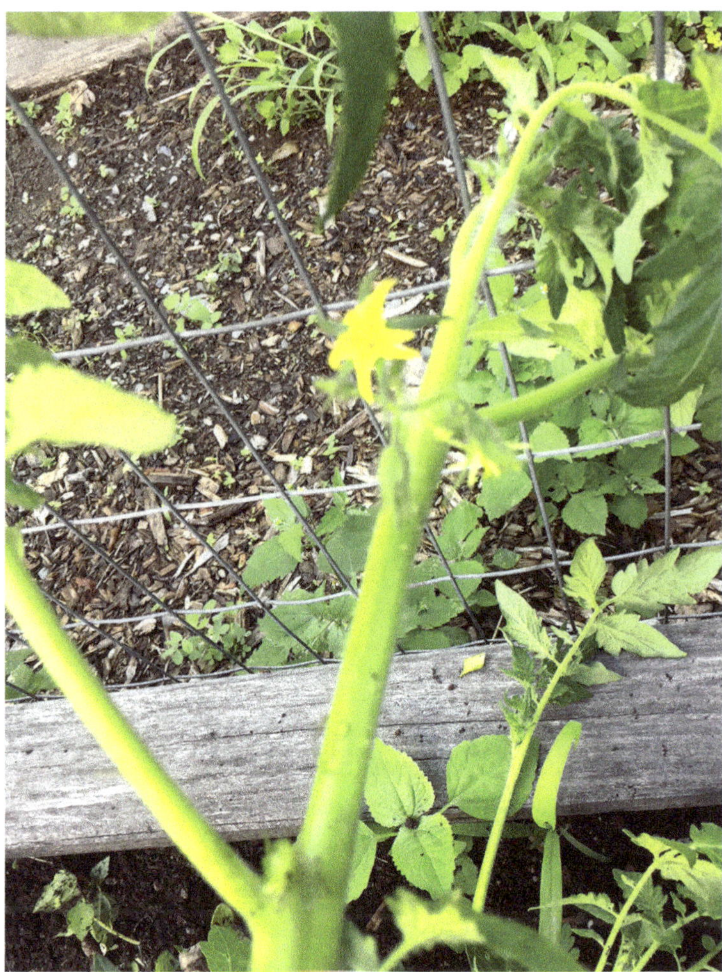

*Removing tomato sucker.*

You must guard against pests and critters in your garden beds. People often start a garden and then don't realize what shut down their plants. Zucchini or a cucumber plant — anything in the cucurbits family, including melons — are susceptible to squash borers. These insects enter the plant at the base, just above the root system in the soil line. They drill a small hole into the stem and burrow into it, working their way up it. They feed on the internal tissue of the plant, eventually killing it.

You won't know what happened, because the insect is inside. A good indication of this problem is a small hole at the bottom of the plant as it starts to wilt. When this happens, it's telling you that something is wrong. Something else people don't realize is that when a plant starts to wilt, you can save it quite easily.

When you notice the small hole at the base of the plant, and sawdust appears to come out of the hole, that's an indication that the squash borer has entered. Make an incision in the stem of the plant with a sharp paring knife, trying not to go through to the other side. Then look for the borer. You can remove it with tweezers or a small toothpick.

After removing the borer, close the wound of the stem. Wrap it with a piece of garden twine and then pile soil over the wound. Once you mound soil over it, create a well so that it holds water. The plant will drink up and create a new root system above that soil where you buried the stem.

There's a good way to prevent the squash borer from getting to the plant at all. Let's say you planted a bunch of zucchini. Cut up a few cloves of garlic and place them around the base of the plant. This will discourage and repel a lot of the passing squash borers. They'll decide to go the opposite way.

Another good way to repel insects from the bases of your plants, especially tomato hornworms or squash borers, is to make a circle of diatomaceous earth around each plant once they begin to sprout. Diatomaceous earth is a natural, organic product that comes from the ground. It's pulverized into very fine dust. Under a microscope, that tiny dust has very sharp edges that will bother insects and small microorganisms. Slugs, grubs, and pests that will attack your plants will not cross the path of the diatomaceous earth. This will repel many different insects that are looking to attack them.

I also place plants that are natural insecticides around vegetable beds. Marigolds have a very pungent smell that repels insects. Garlic, chives, thyme, and marjoram are herbs that keep pests away. Thyme contains thymol, which is a natural insecticide. Chrysanthemums also give off a fragrance that will repel insects.

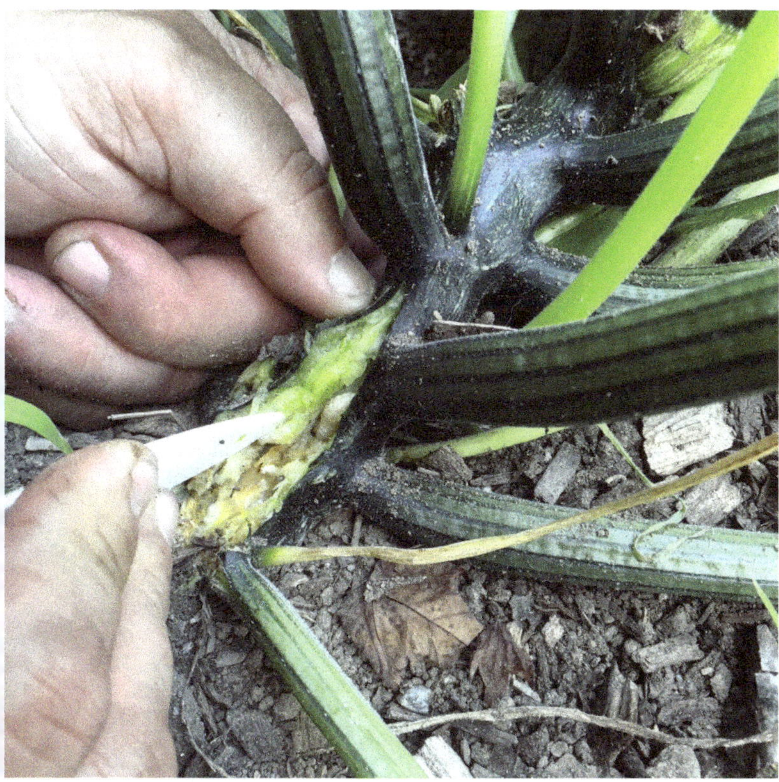

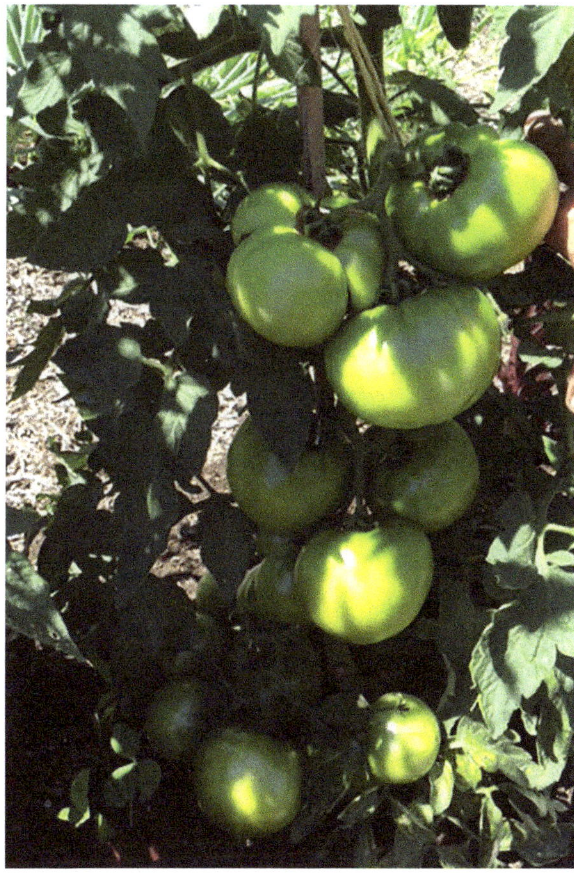

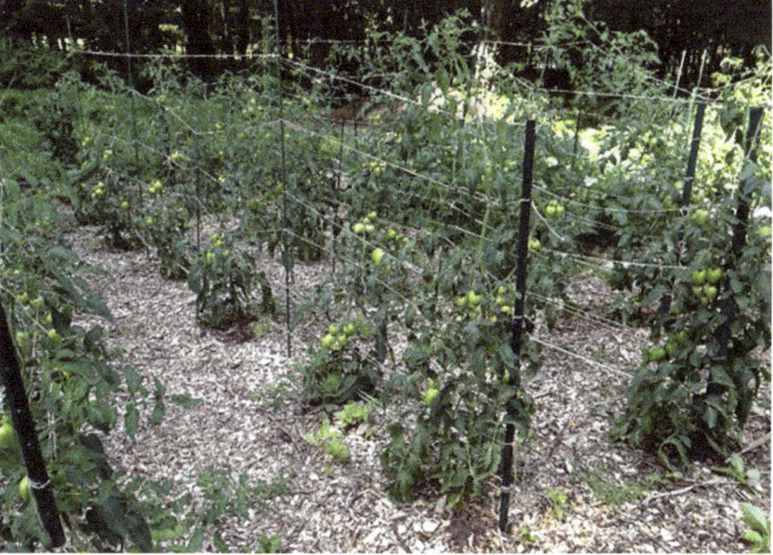

*Above: Well trained suckered tomato producing a larger crop.*

*Left: Removing squash borer.*

*Bottom: San Marzano tomatoes staked for sauce production.*

*Page 64: Belgium Giants.*

*Page 65: Heirloom cherry tomatoes.*

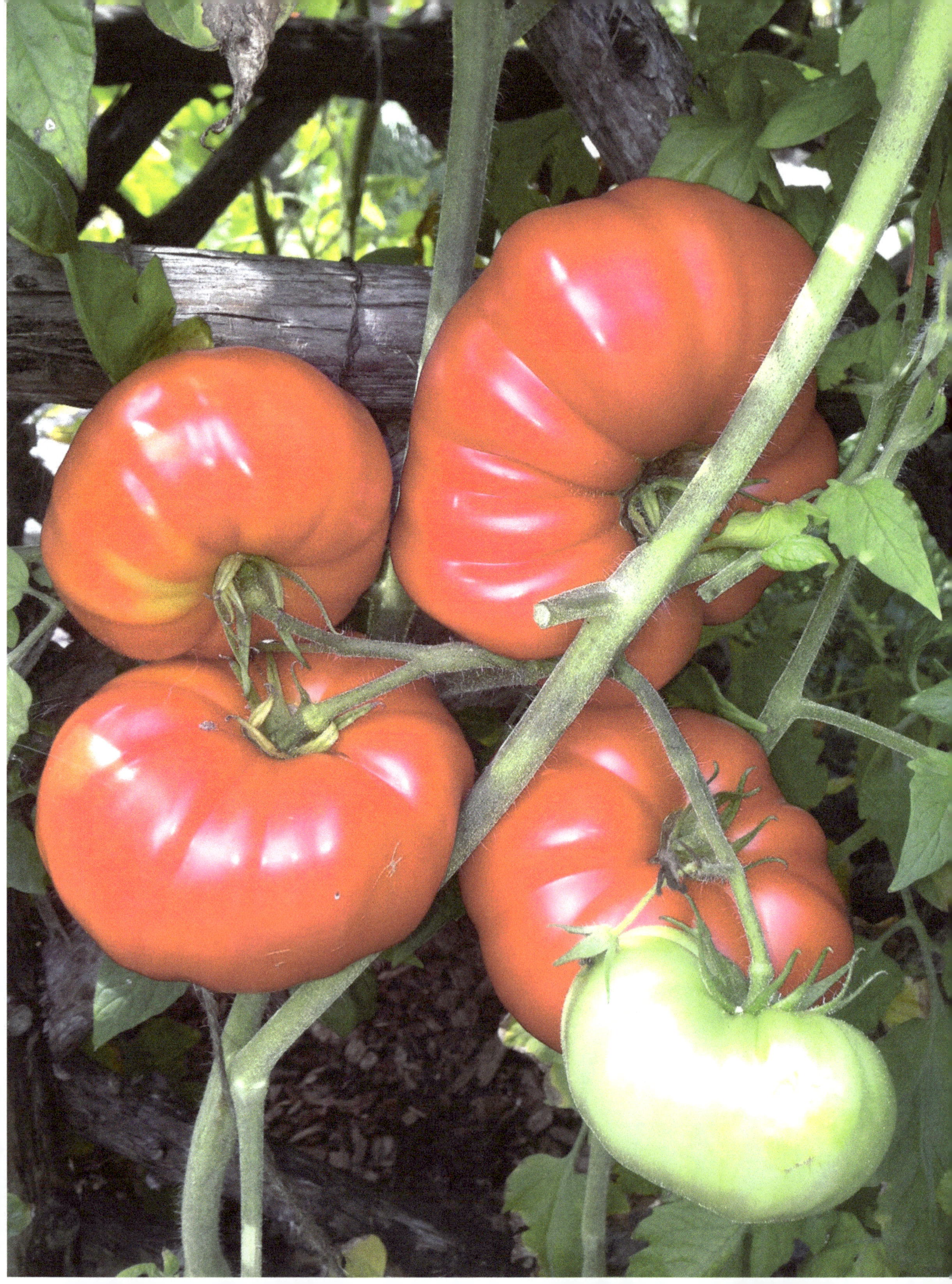

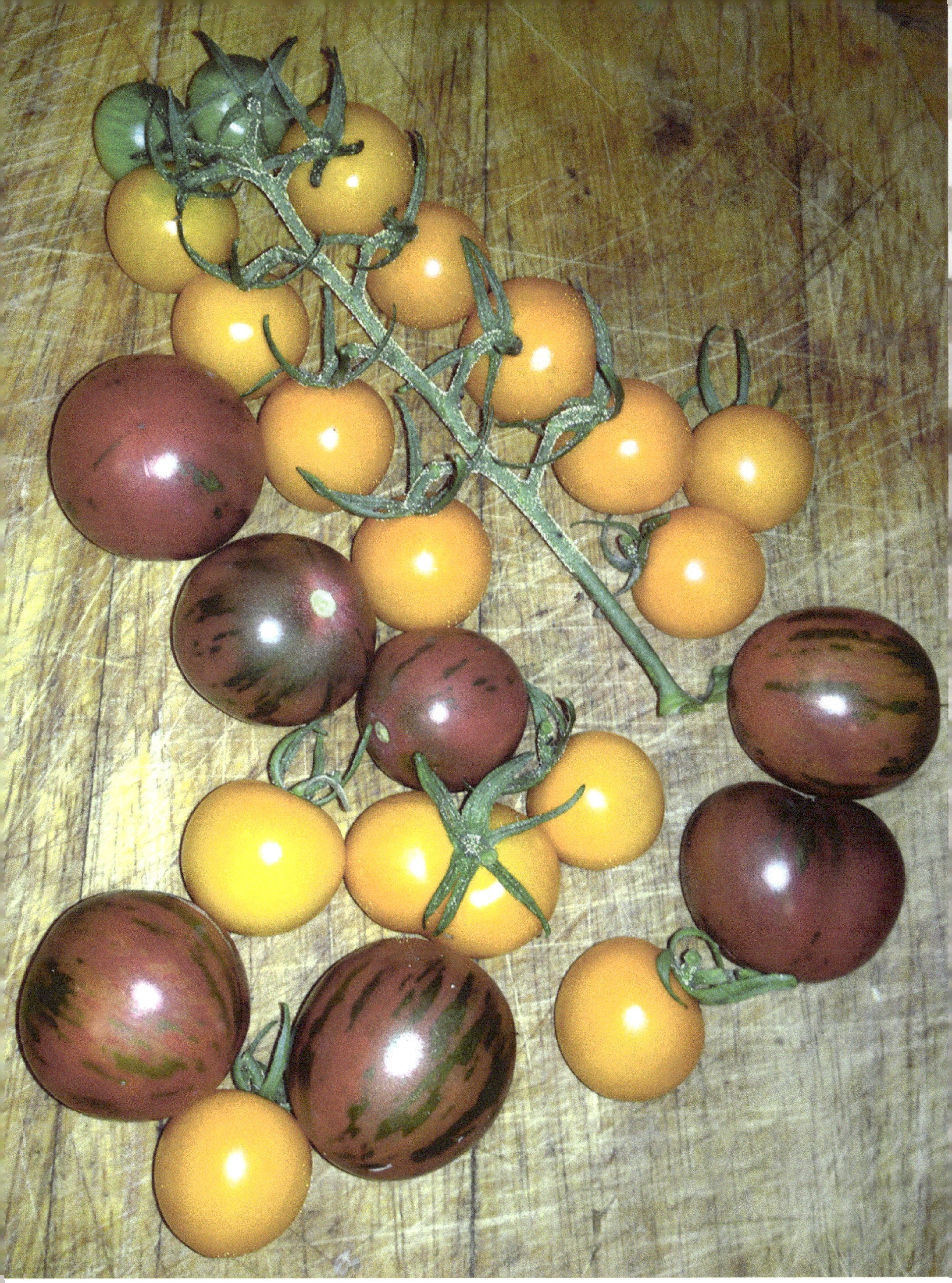

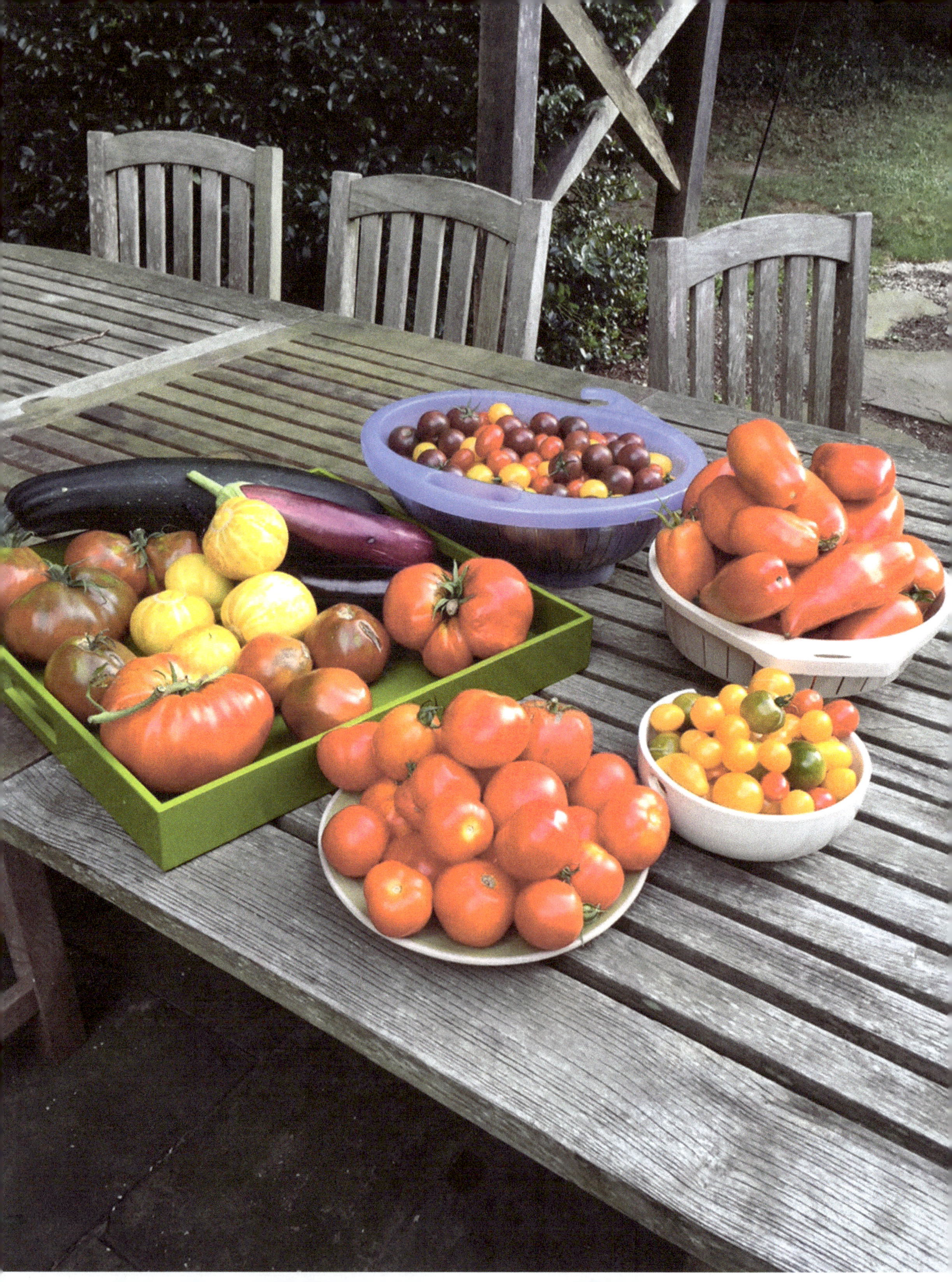

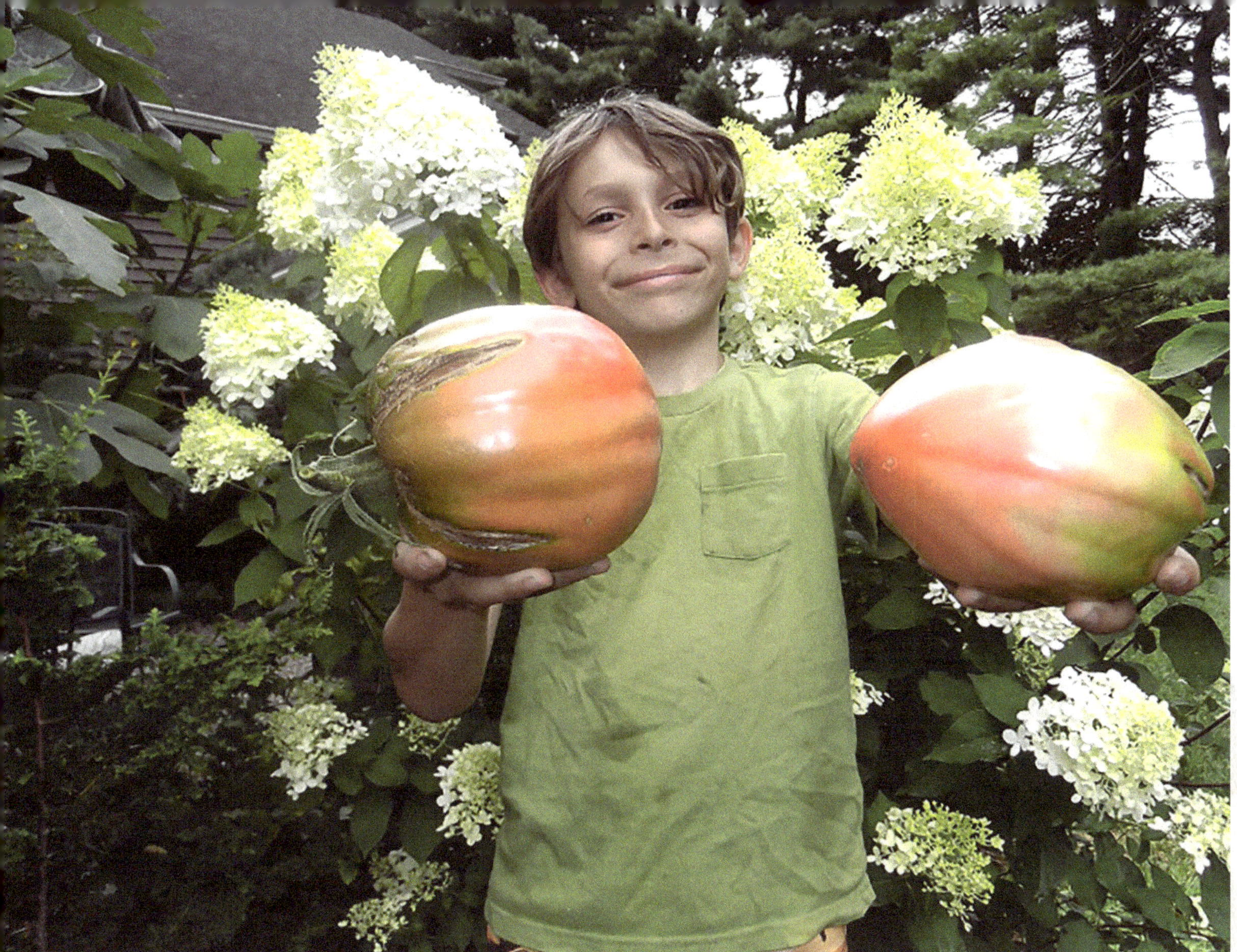

*Left: Just harvested veggies including lemon cucumbers, zucchini, eggplant, San Marzano and beefsteak tomatoes.*

*Above: Julian with giant Oxheart tomatoes.*

*Page 68: Freshly picked strawberries.*

*Page 69: Potato harvest.*

*Page 70: Blueberries, raspberries, and beets.*

*Page 71: Lucy with berries.*

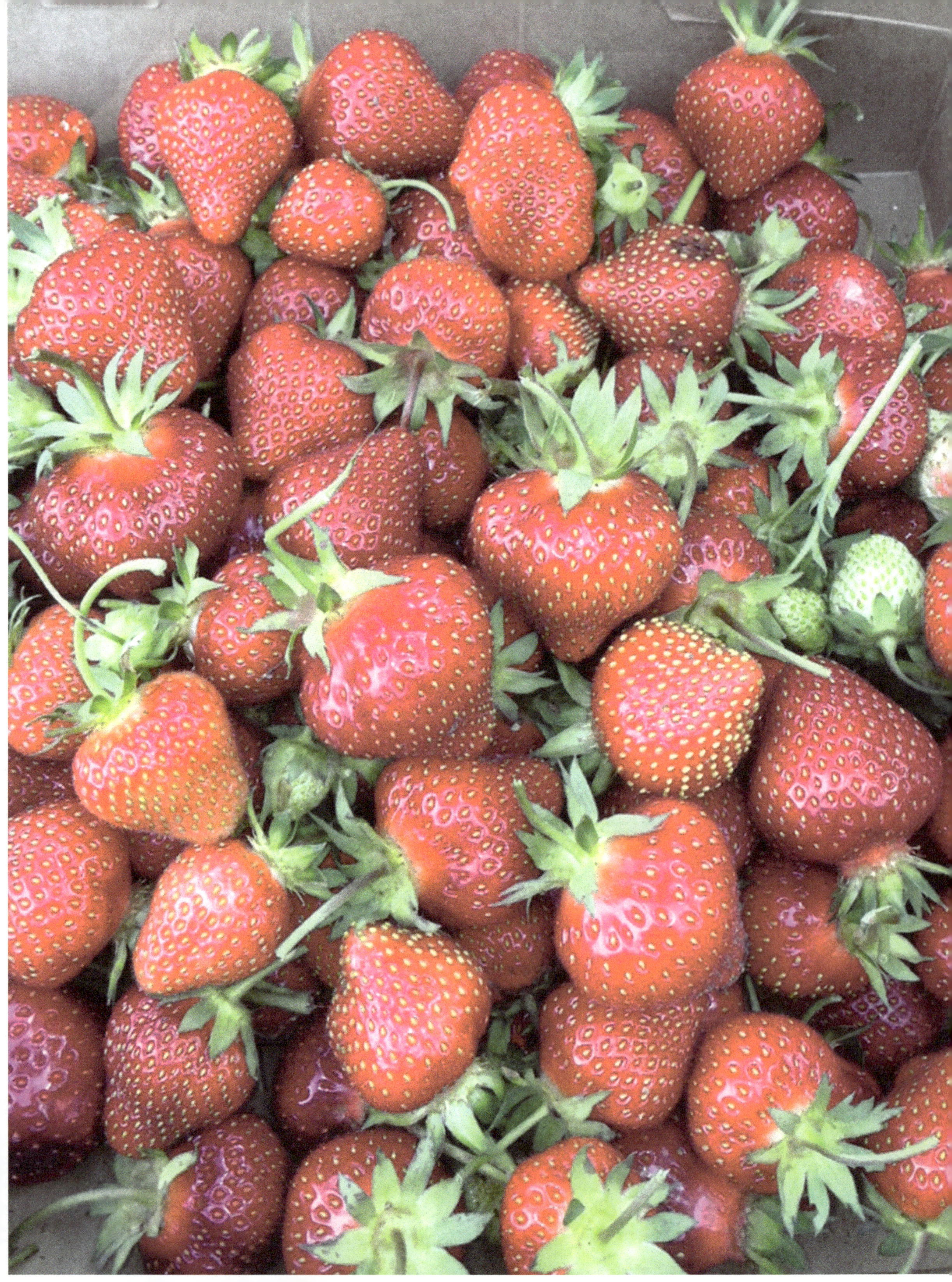

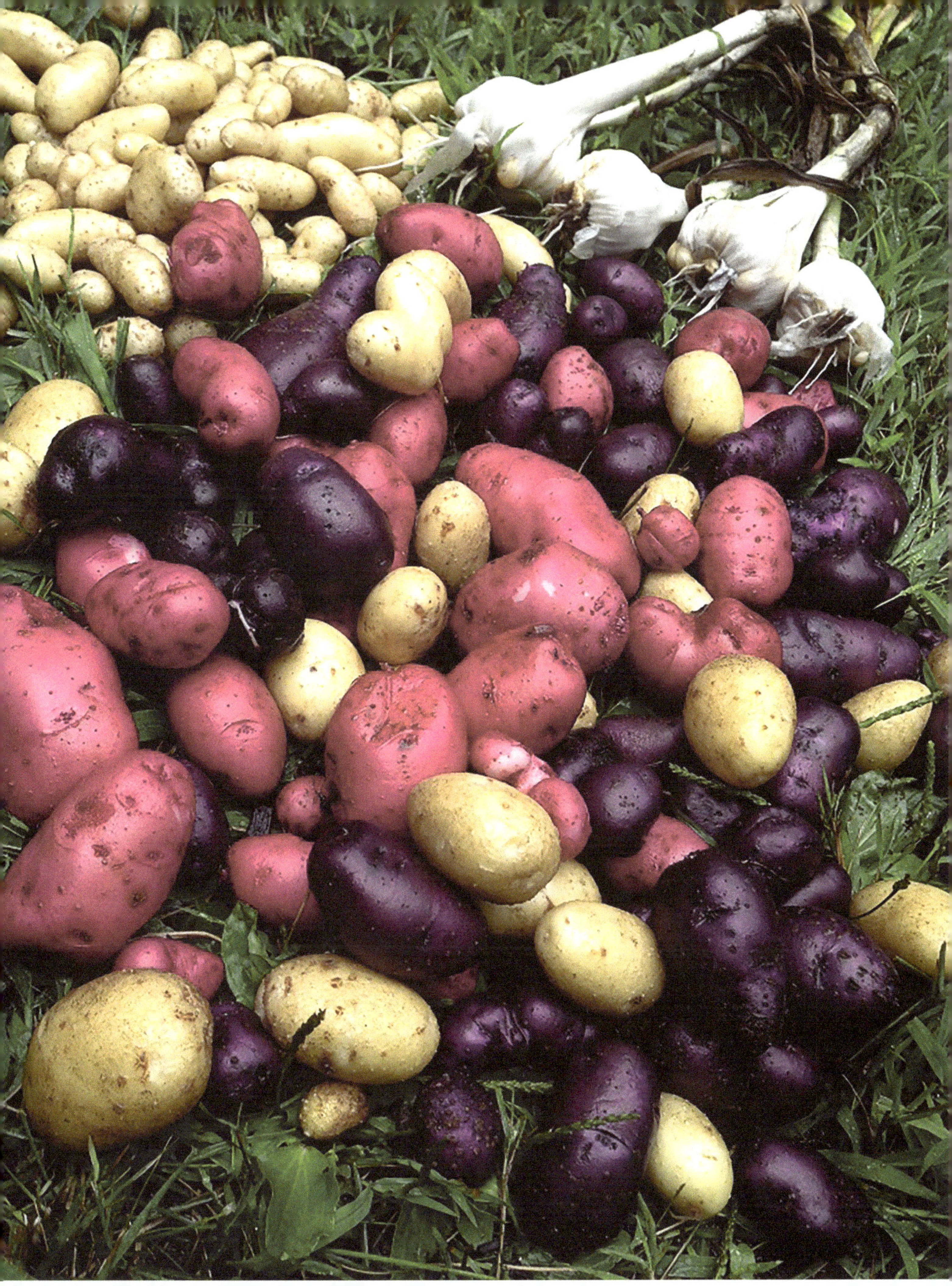

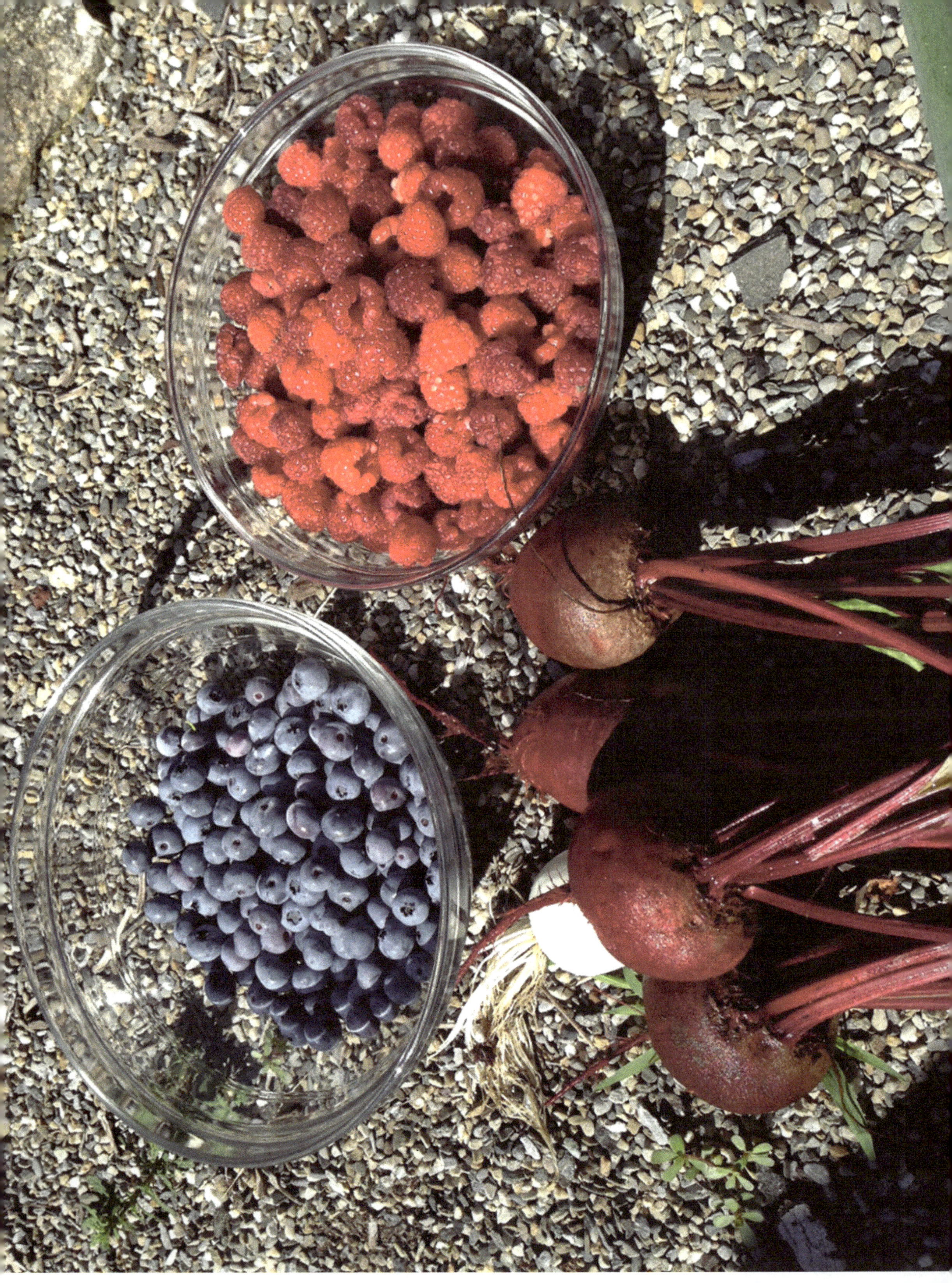

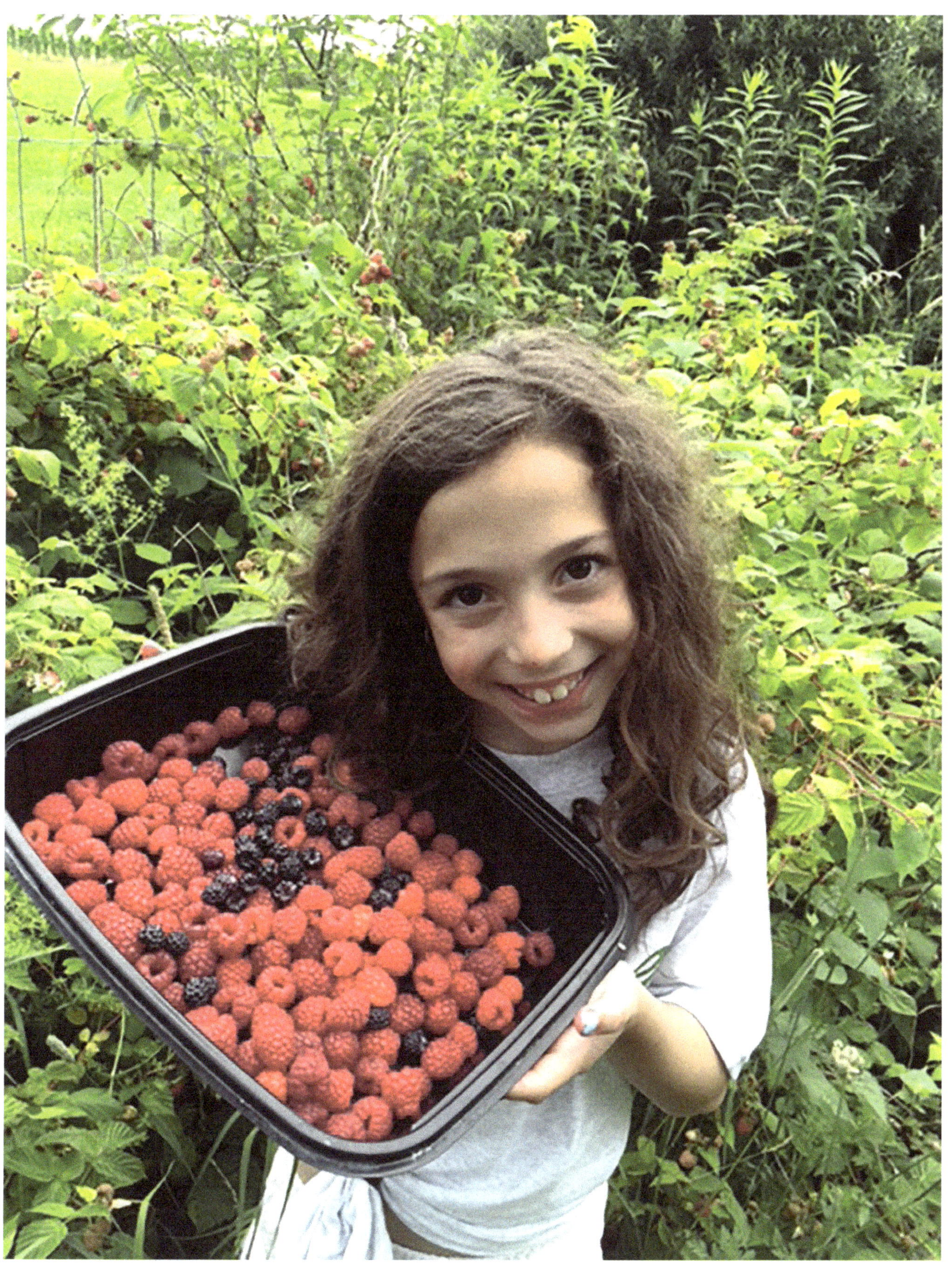

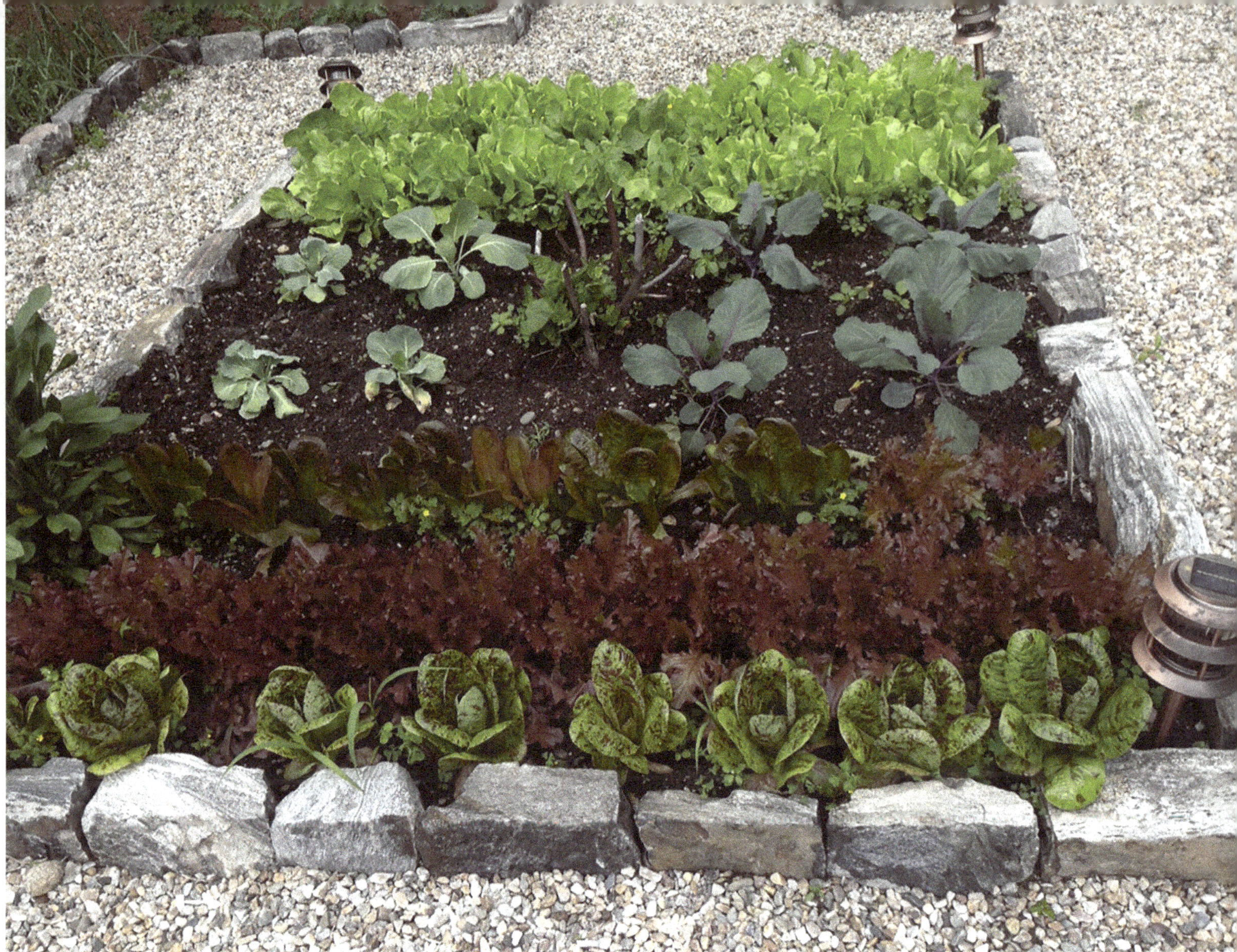

*Above: Cold crops in raised bed.*

*Page 73: Organized raised bed with broccoli, cabbage, and kale.*

*Page 74: Escarole in raised bed.*

*Page 75: Swiss chard in organized raised bed.*

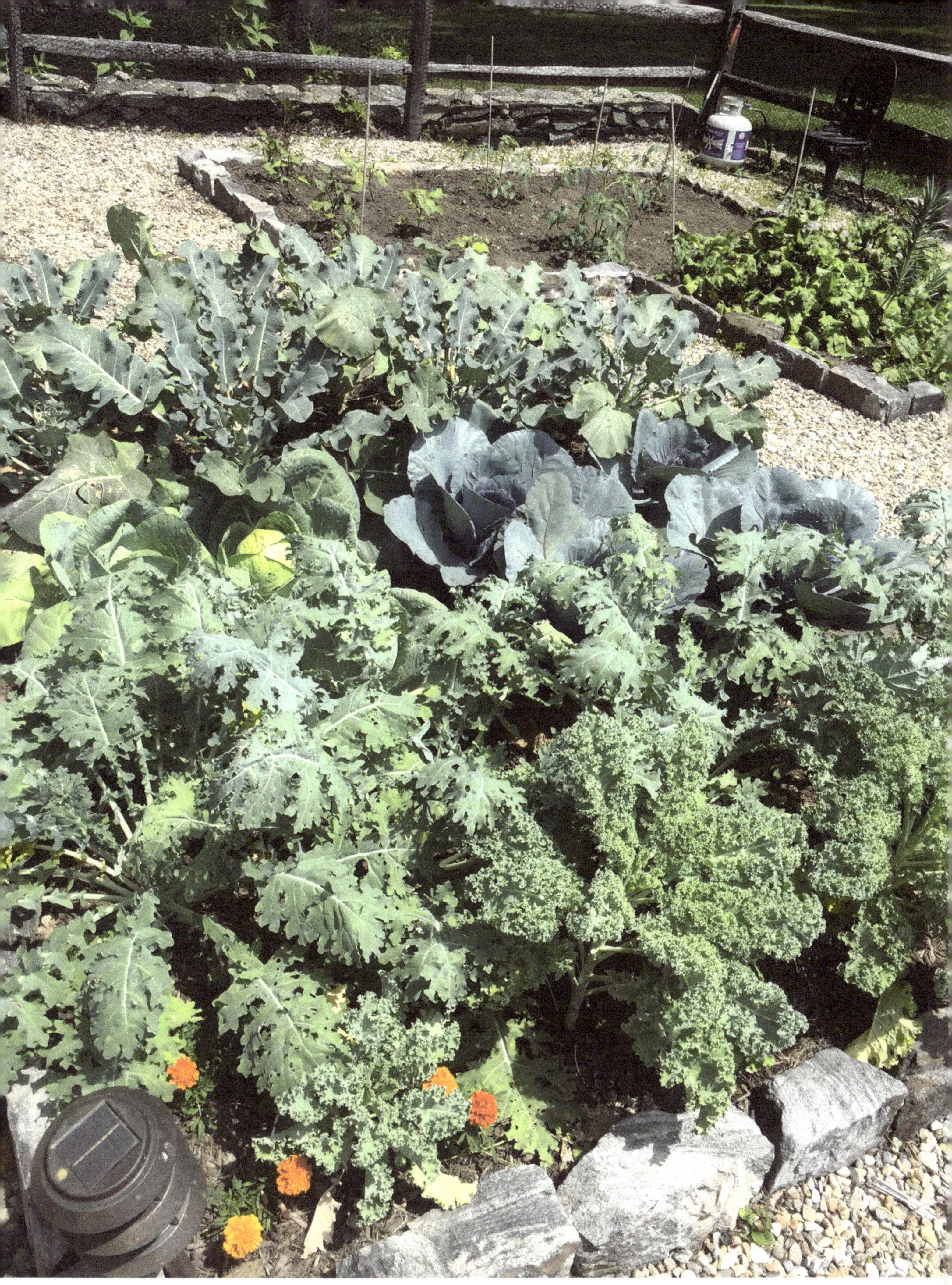

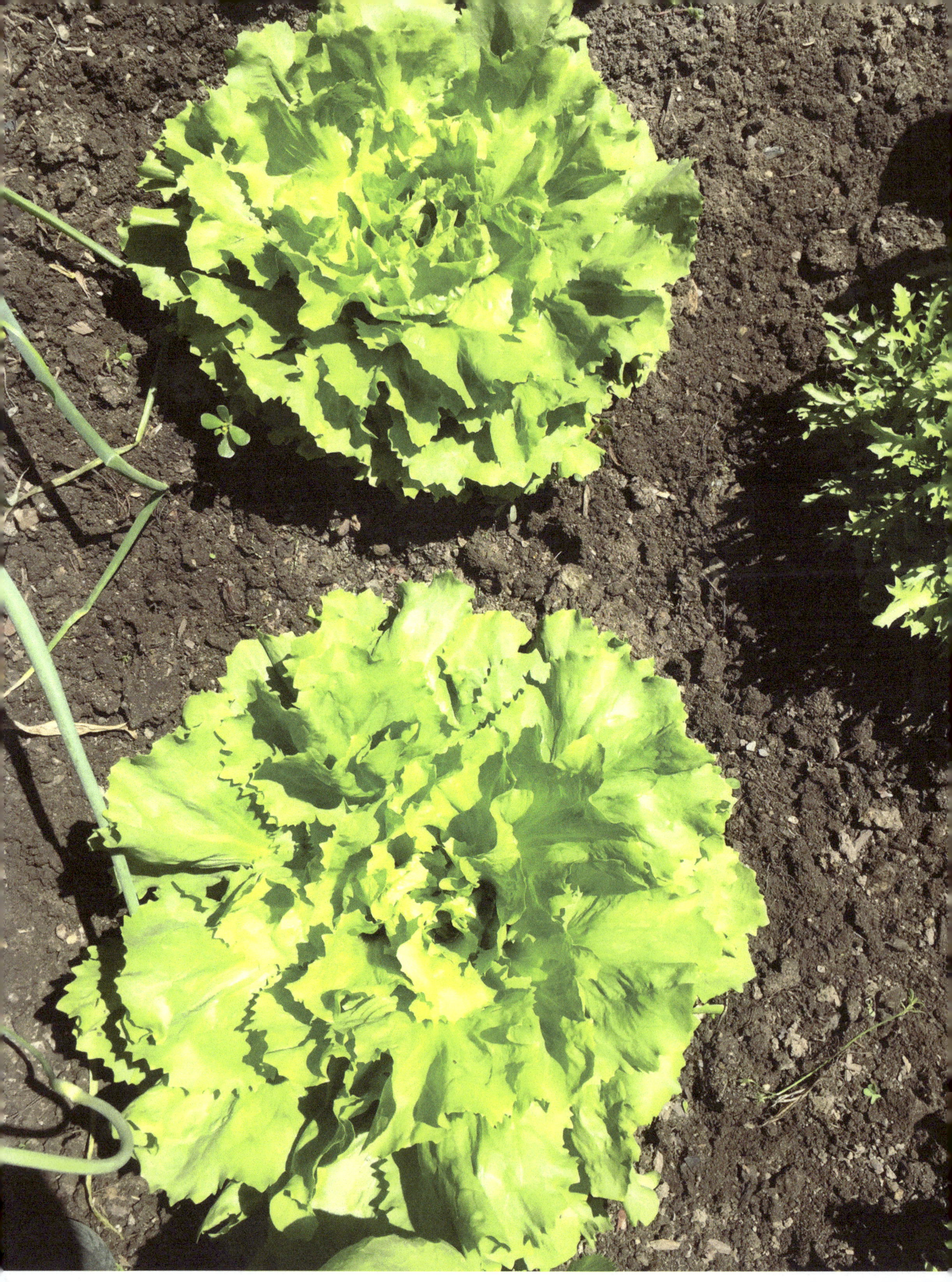

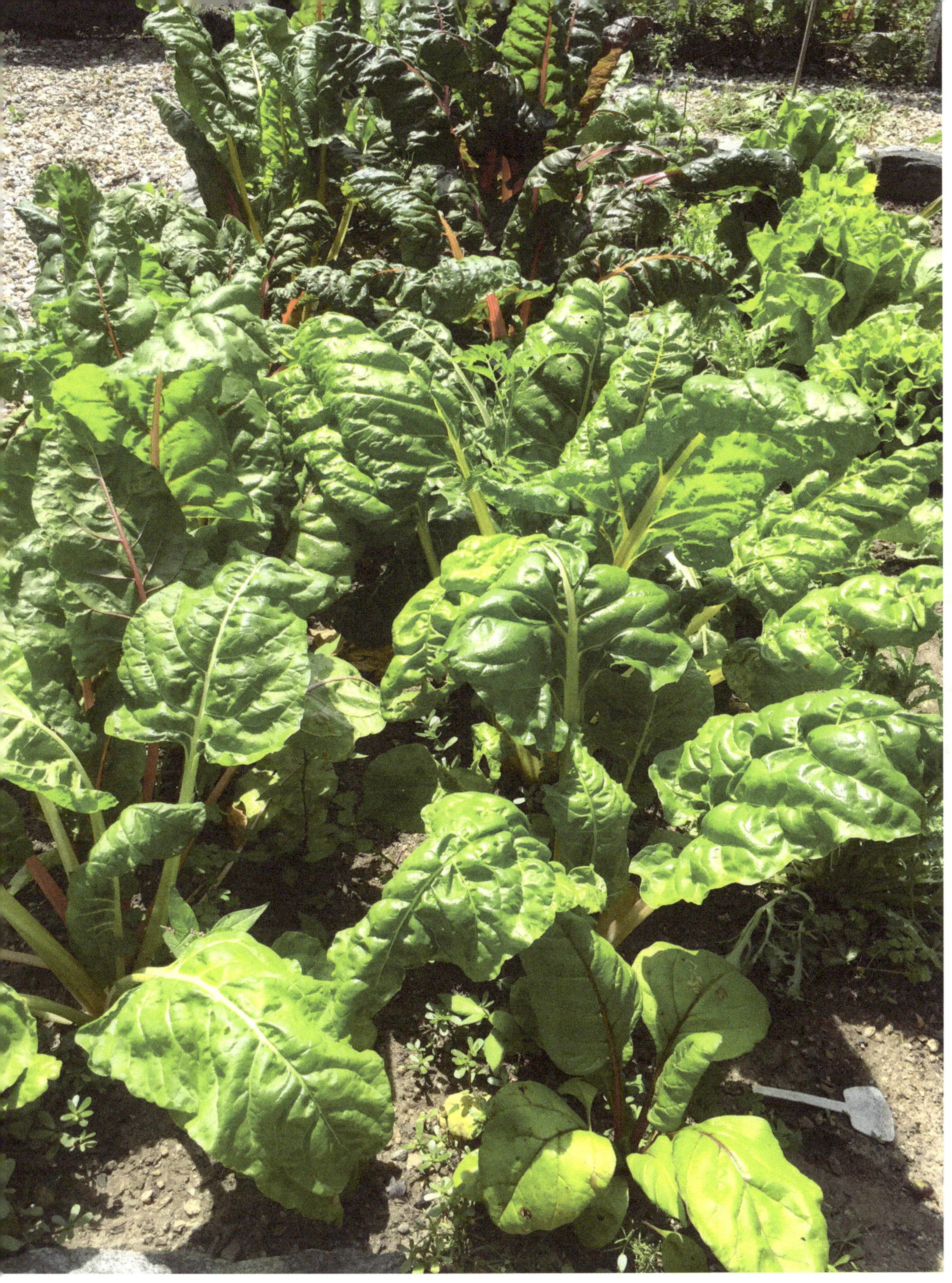

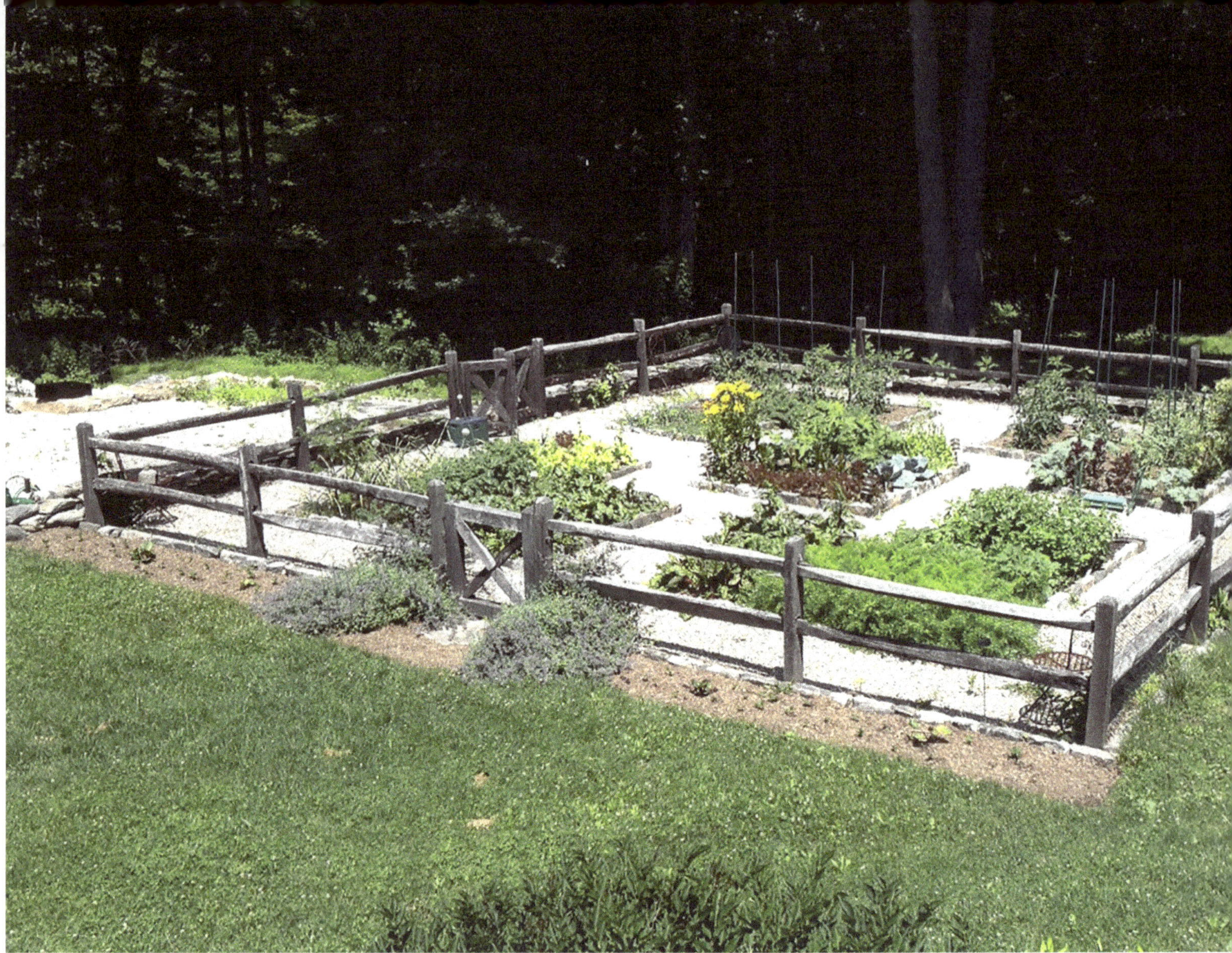

*Above: Well-organized garden.*

*Page 77: Raised bed cutting garden with zinnias.*

*Page 78: Honeybees forging on asclepias.*

*Page 79: Monarch caterpillar feeding on the butterfly weed.*

*Page 80: Nasturtium blossoms.*

*Page 81: Echinacea Carnival series.*

*Page 82: Hydrangeas.*

*Page 83: Dahlias.*

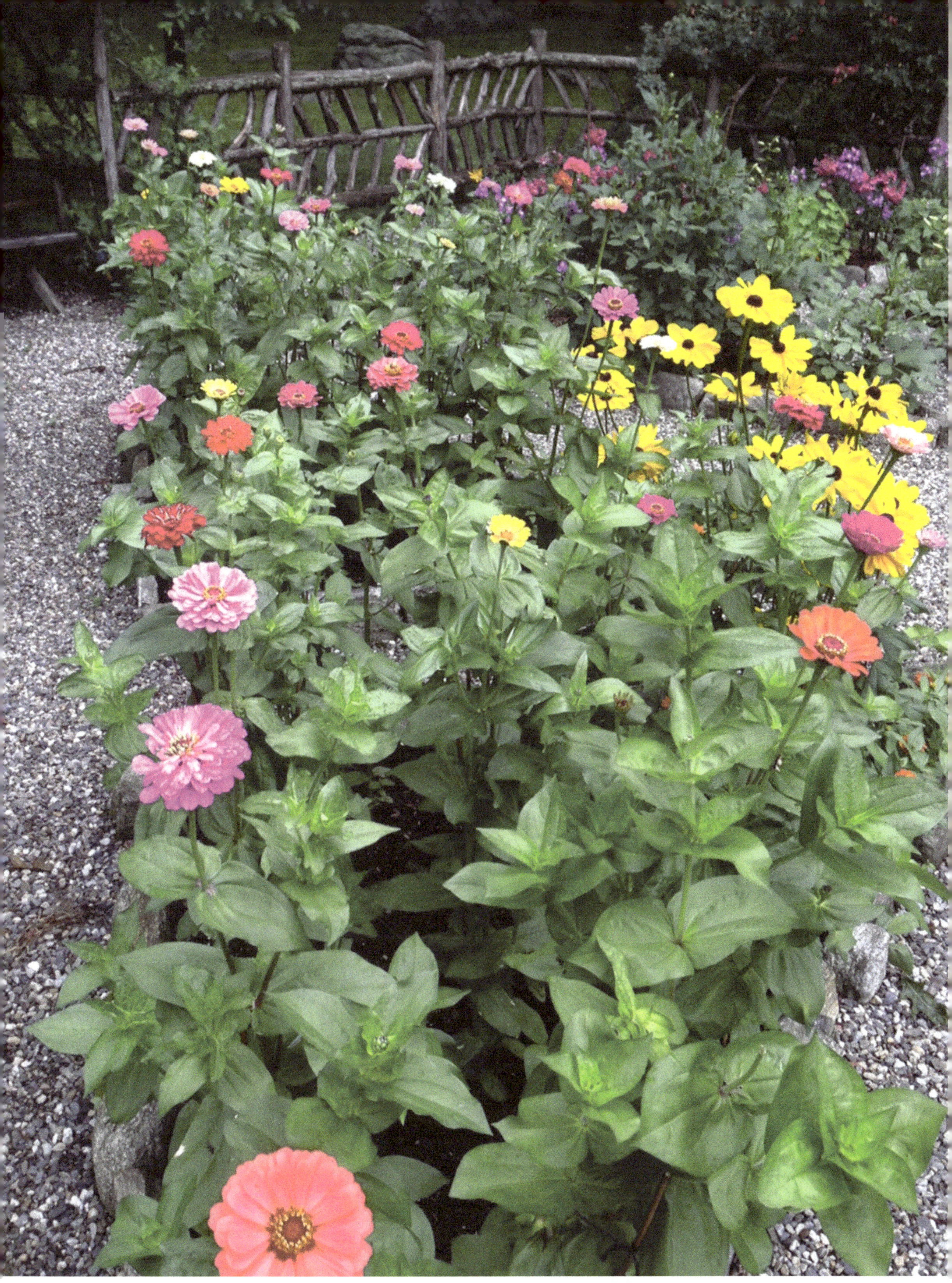

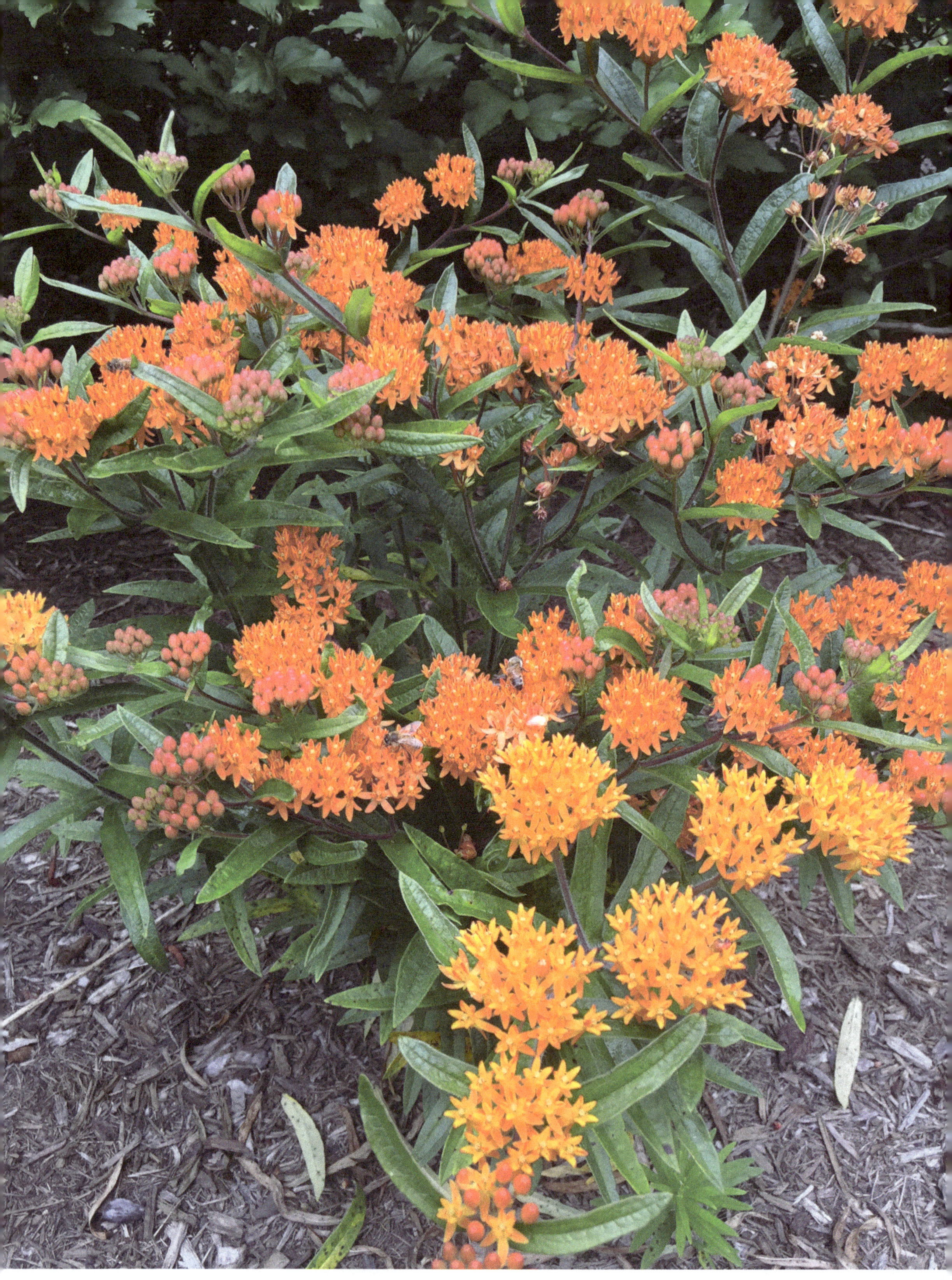

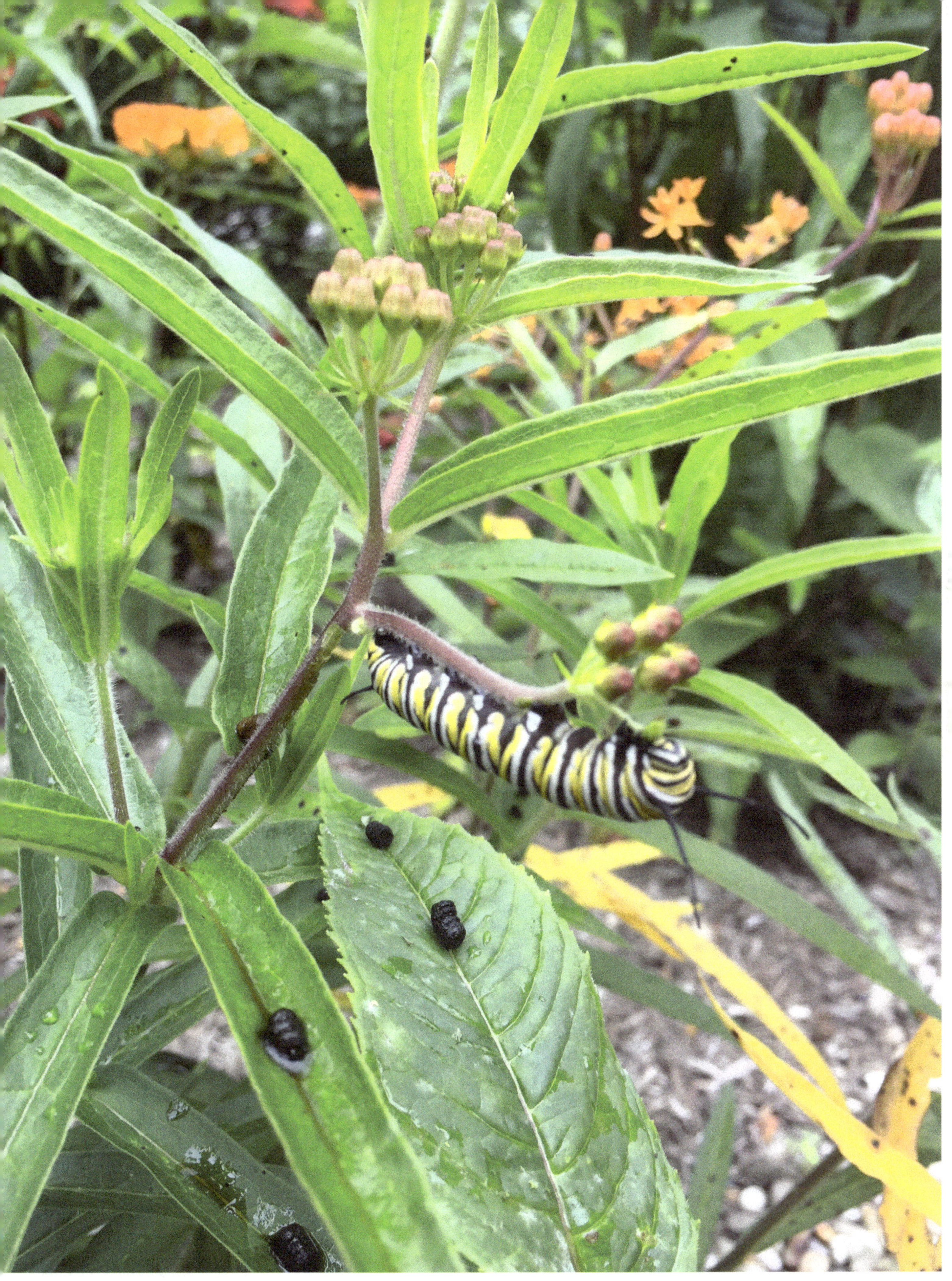

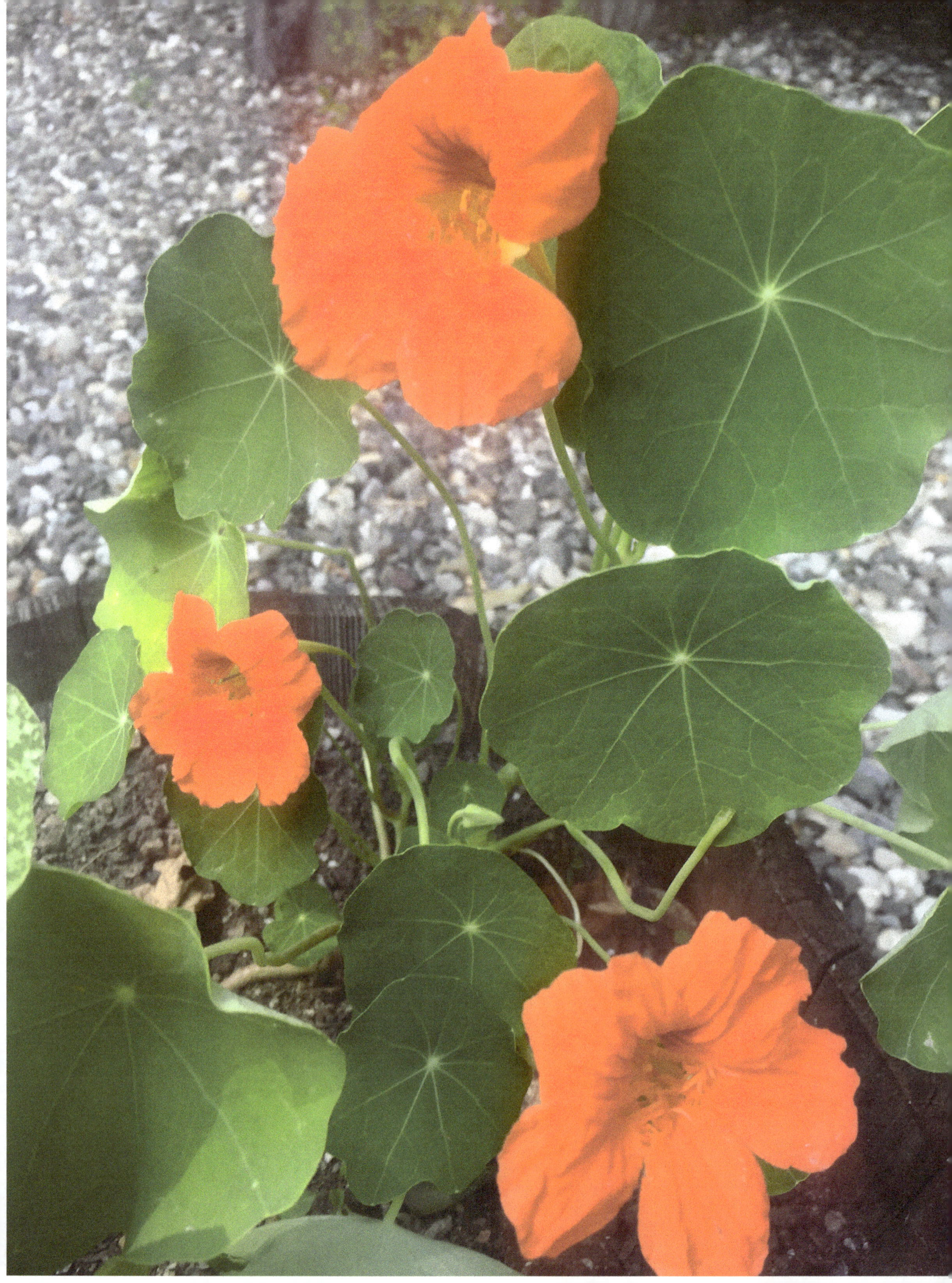

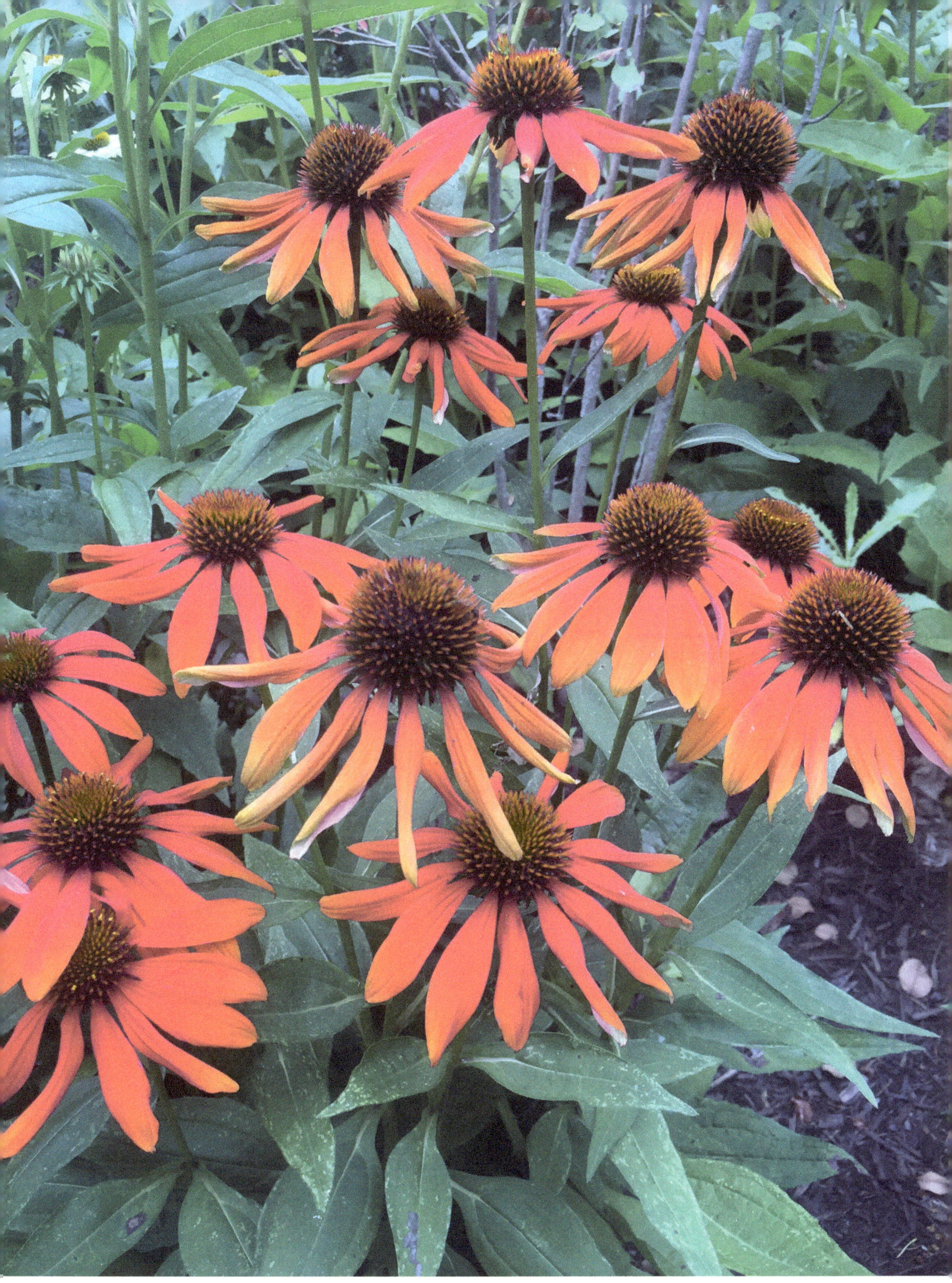

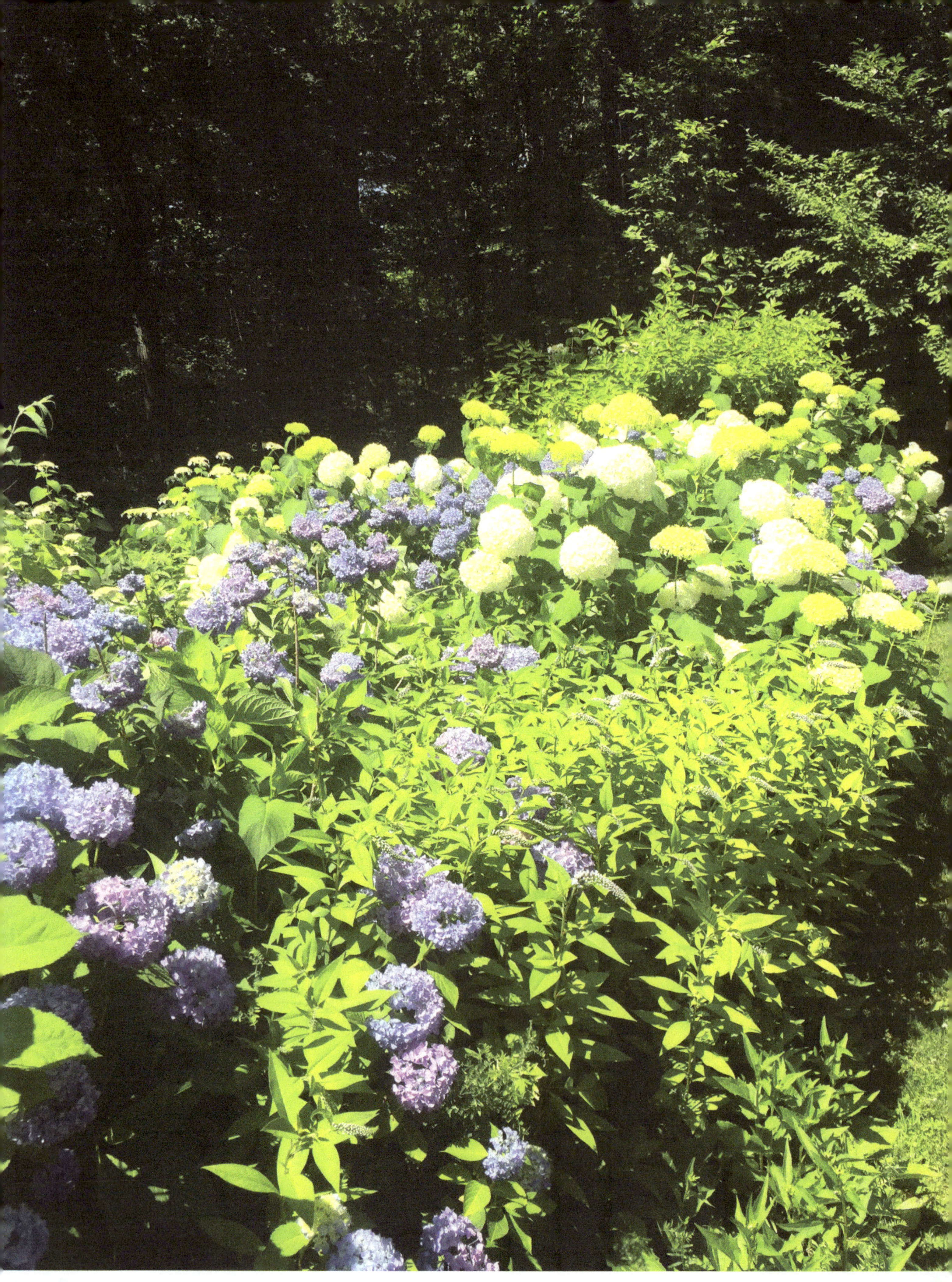

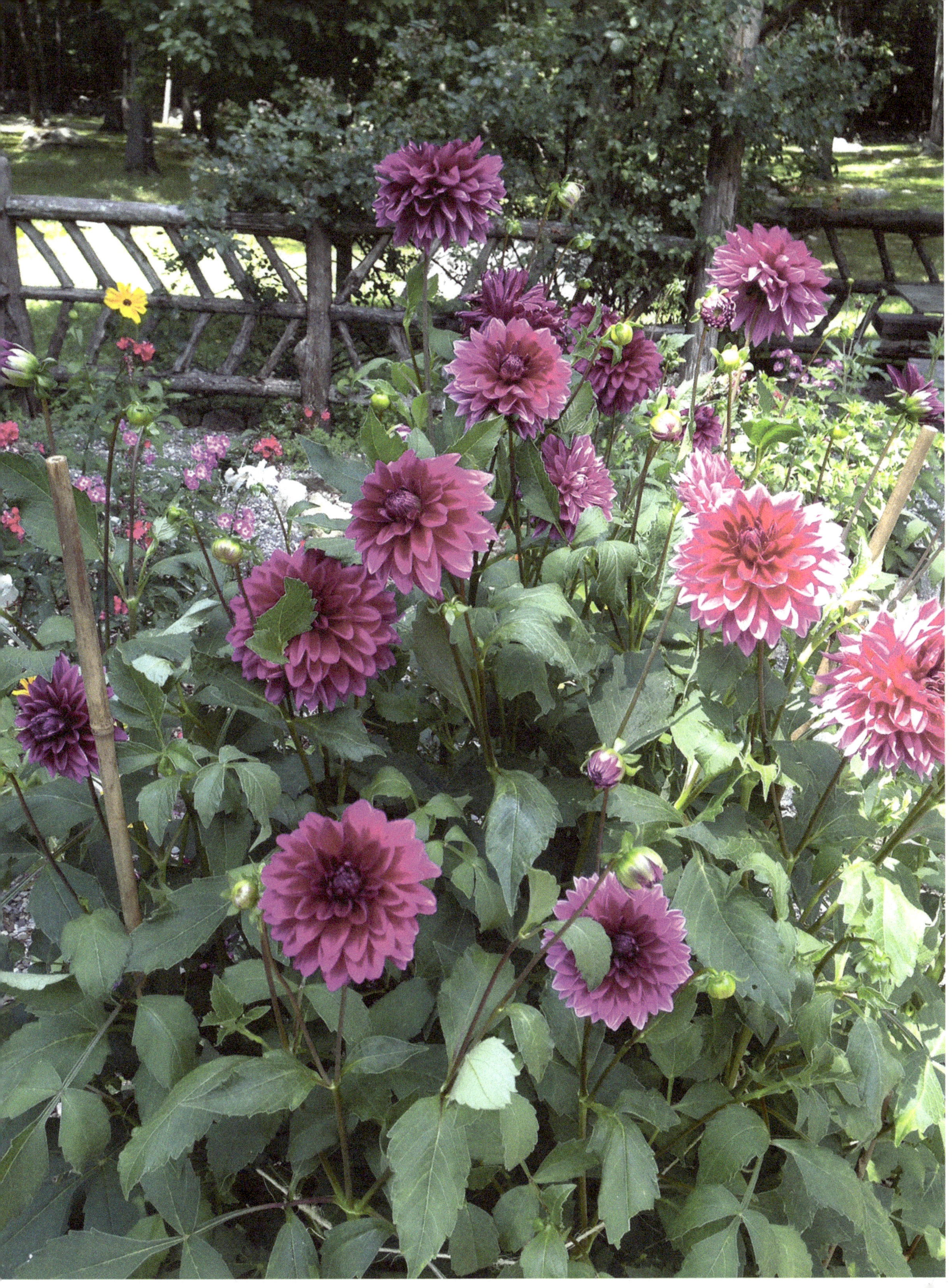

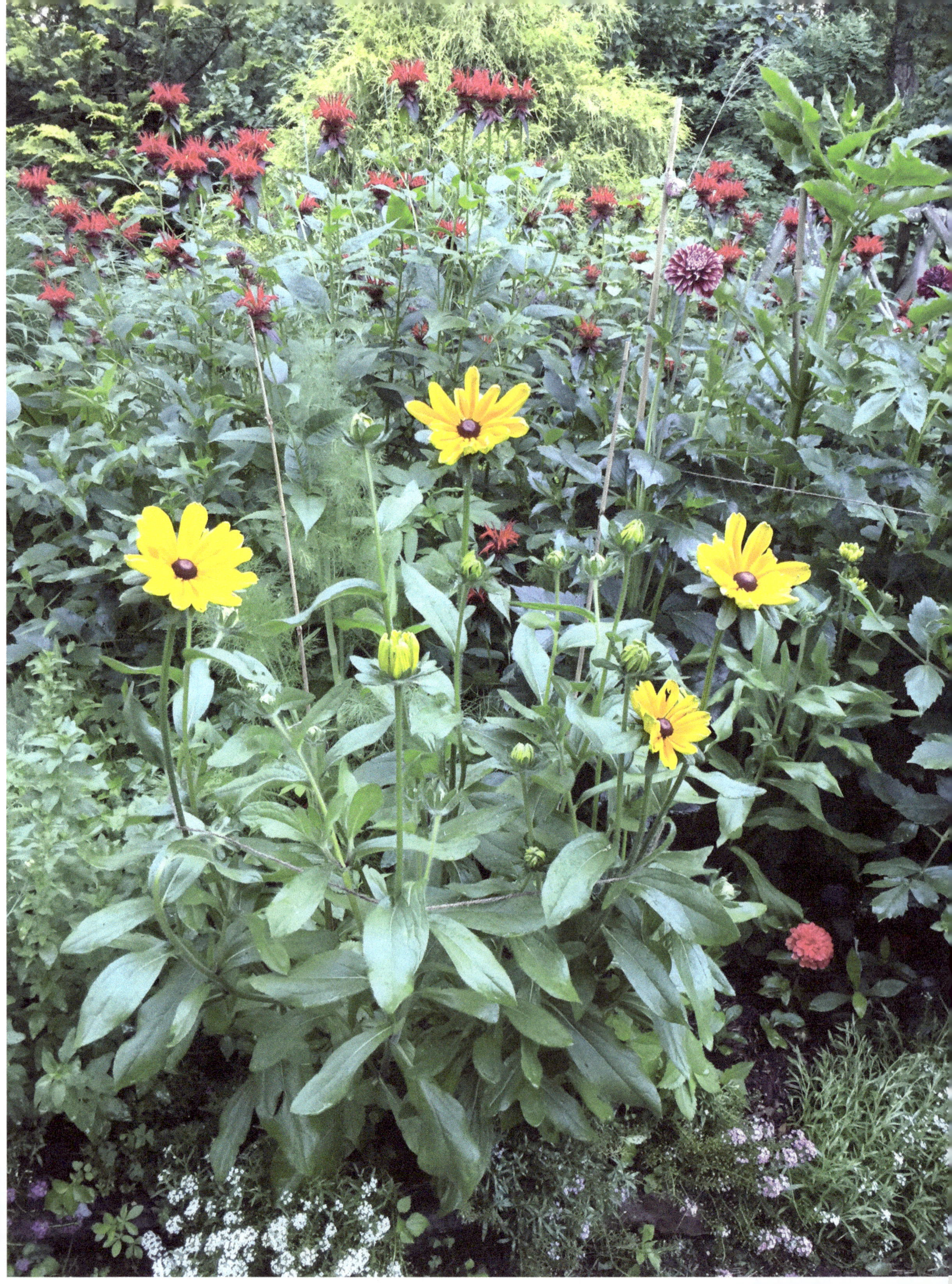

*Left: Indian Summer rudbeckia and bee balm. Also dahlias with an alyssum border.*

*Below: Early spring preparing the beds for the cutting garden.*

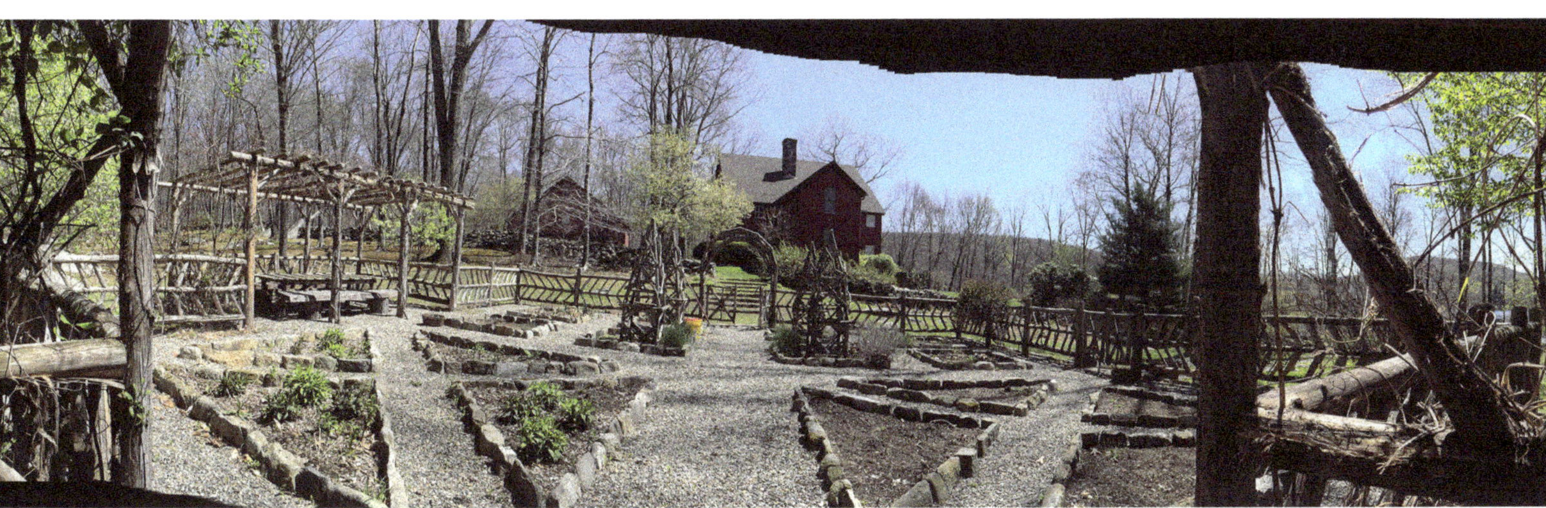

*Page 86: Beautiful mixed cutting flowers, including Indian Summer rudbeckia, zinnias, verbena, cosmos, and cleome.*

*Page 87: Blue Fortune agastache busy with bumblebees.*

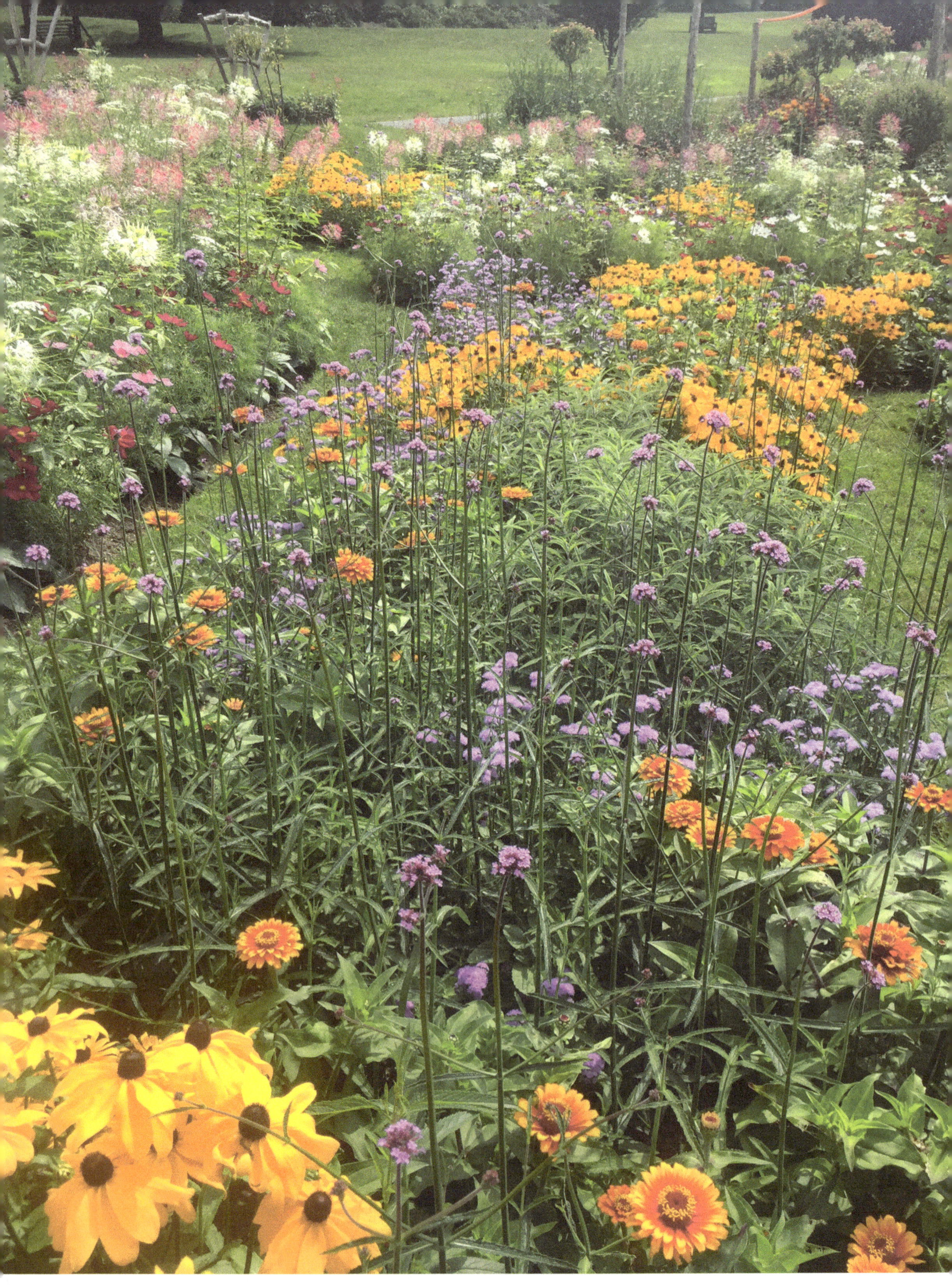

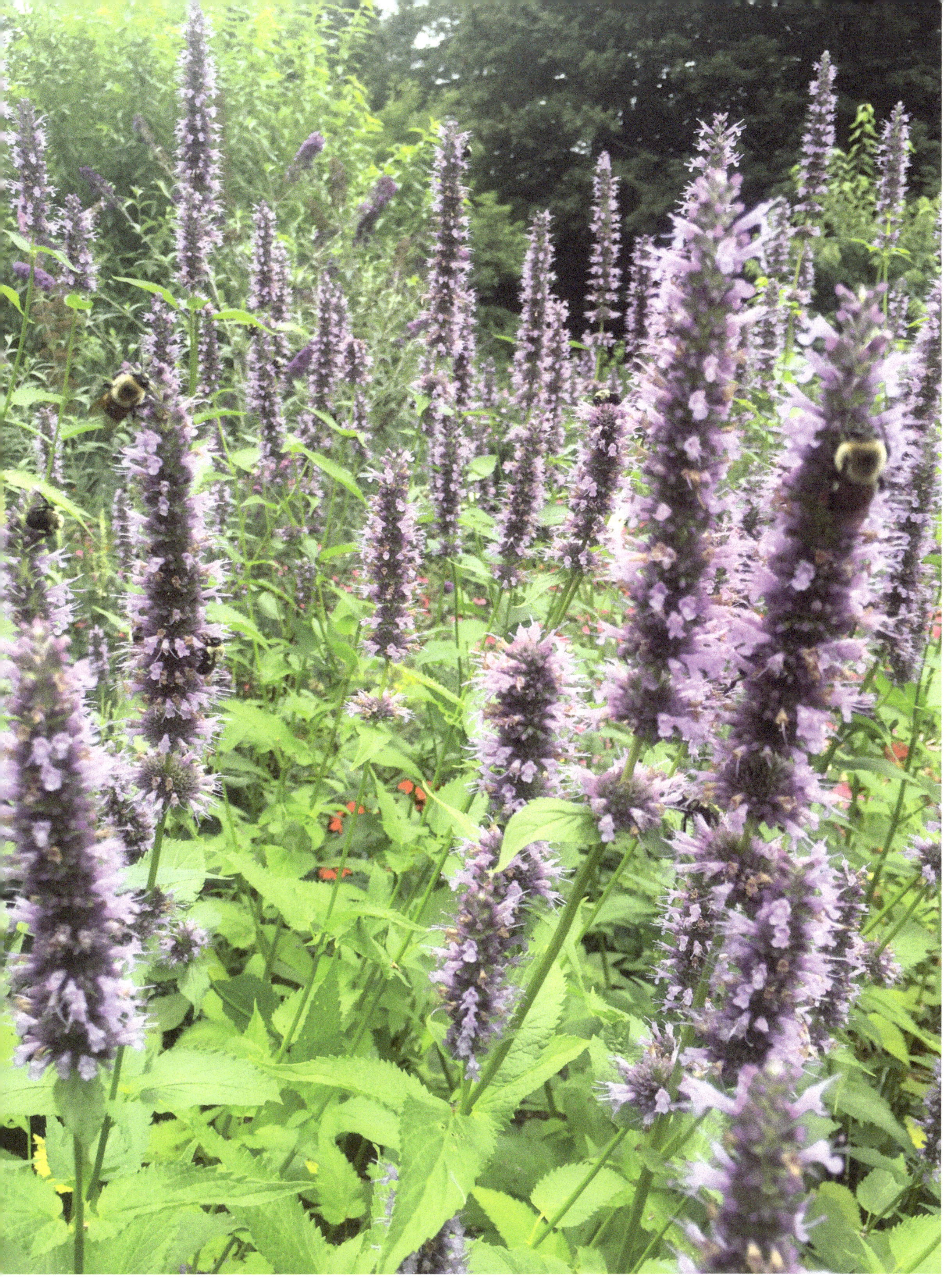

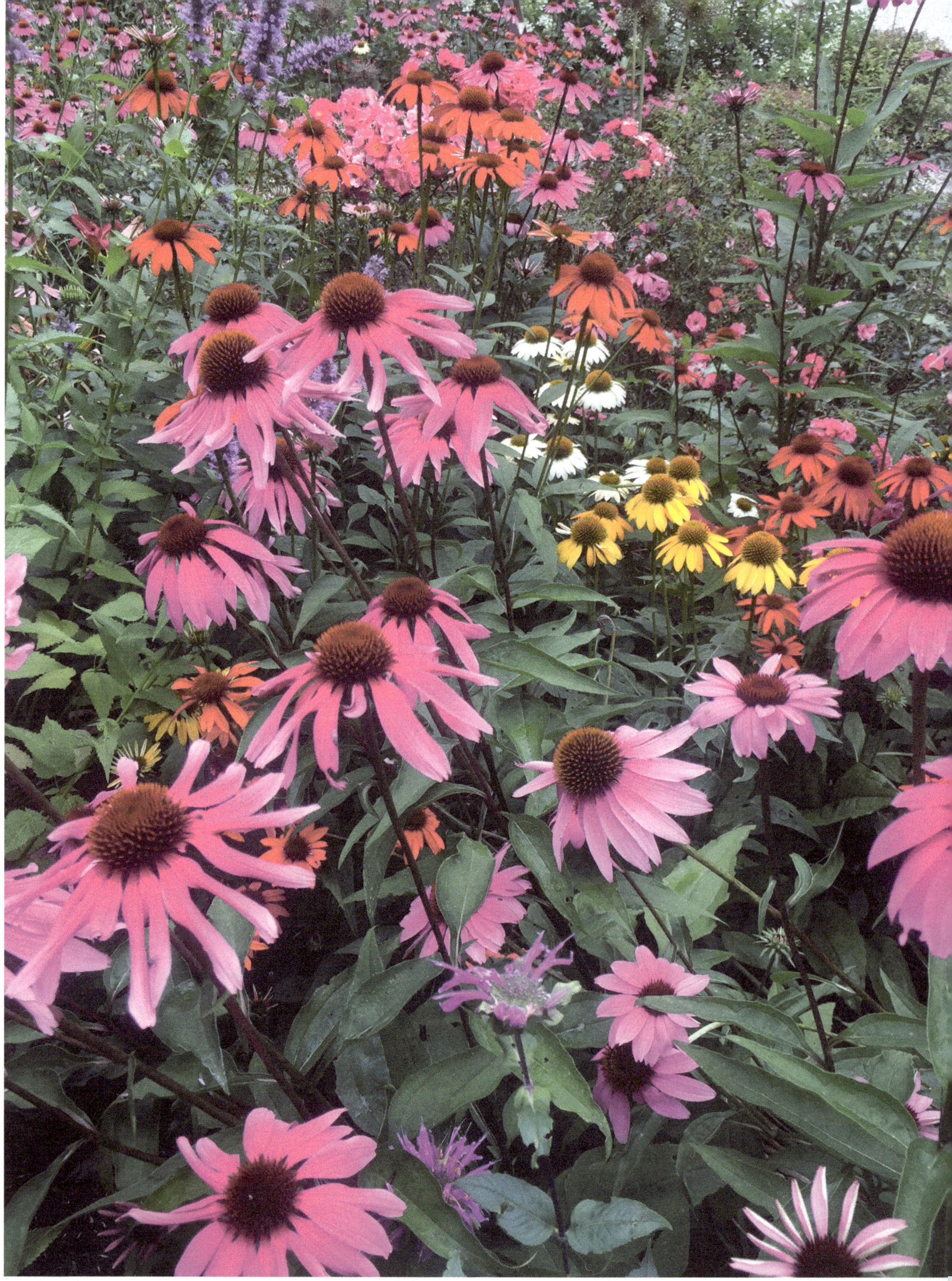

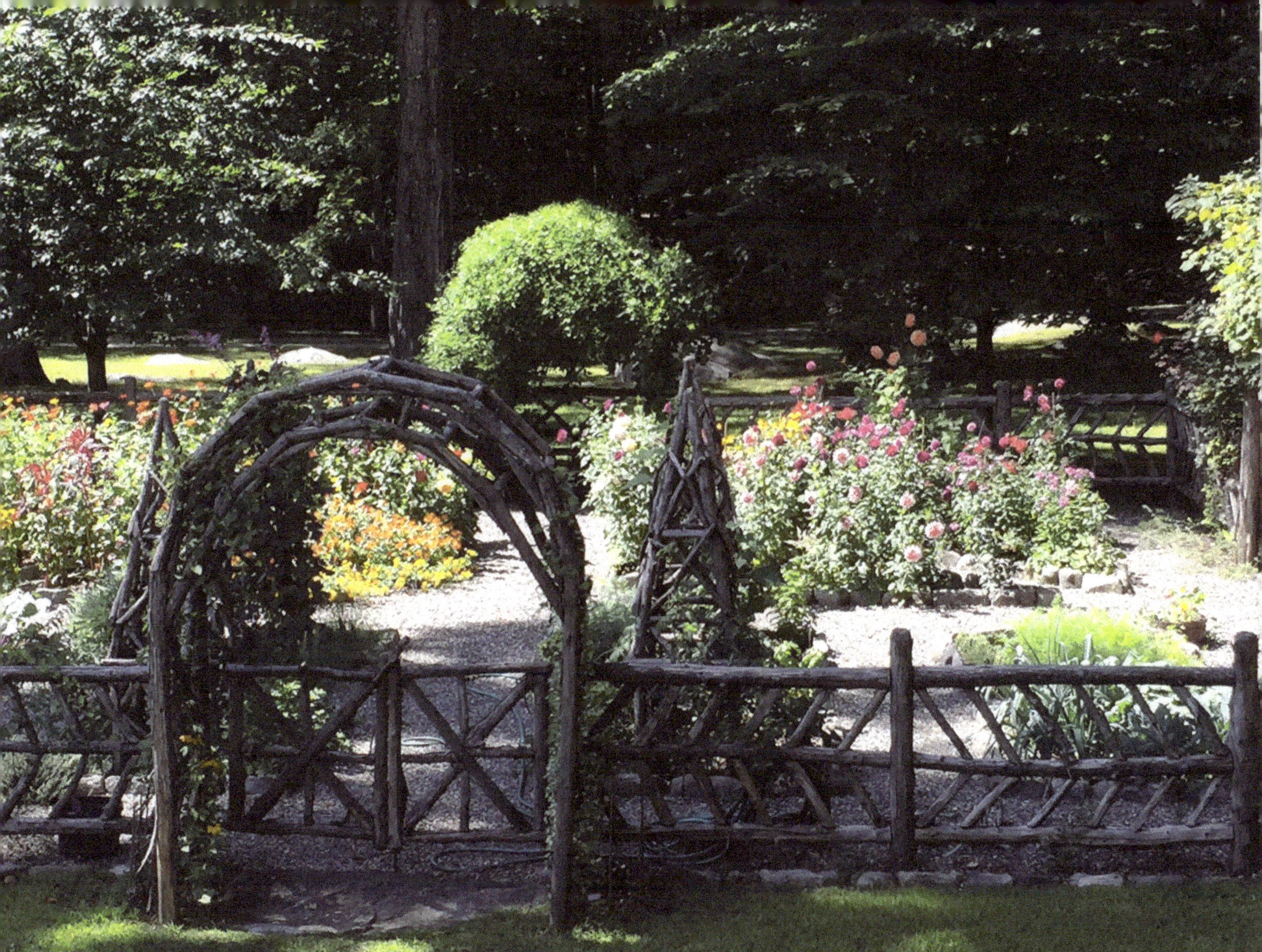

*Page 88: Echinacea and agastache.*

*Above: Cutting garden in full bloom in August consists of dahlias, zinnias, phlox,and sunflowers.*

*Page 90: Echinacea planted amongst allium; in the foreground, Elberta peach, blueberries, and nonstop roses.*

*Page 91: Echinacea growing with a peach tree.*

*Page 92: Colorful window boxes with begonias, euphorbia, petunias, geraniums, and lobelia.*

*Page 93: Echinacea, bee balm with an alyssum border.*

*Page 94: Non-stop tuberous begonias.*

*Page 95: Mother Nature can create some of the most beautiful colors that nature has to offer.*

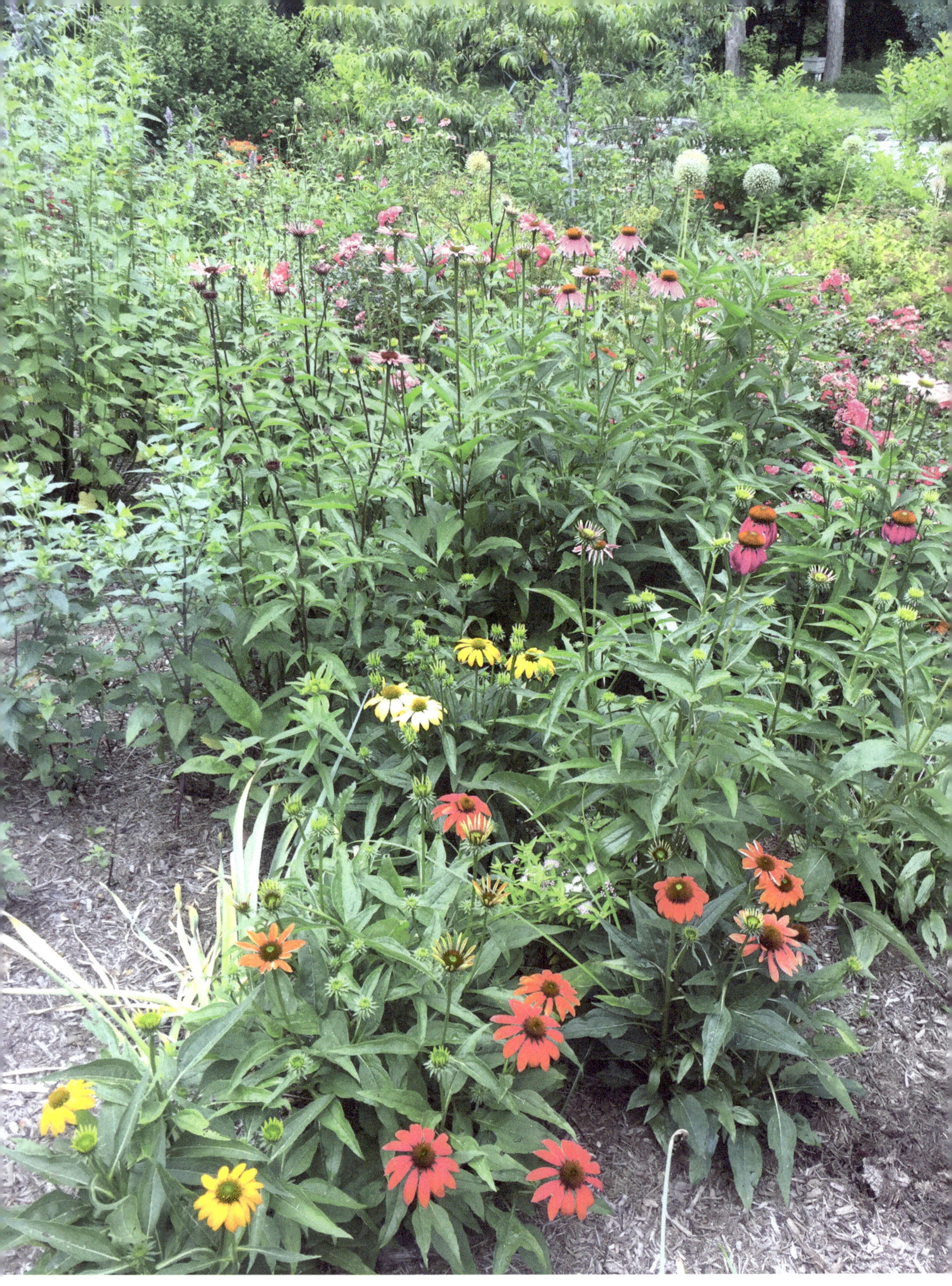

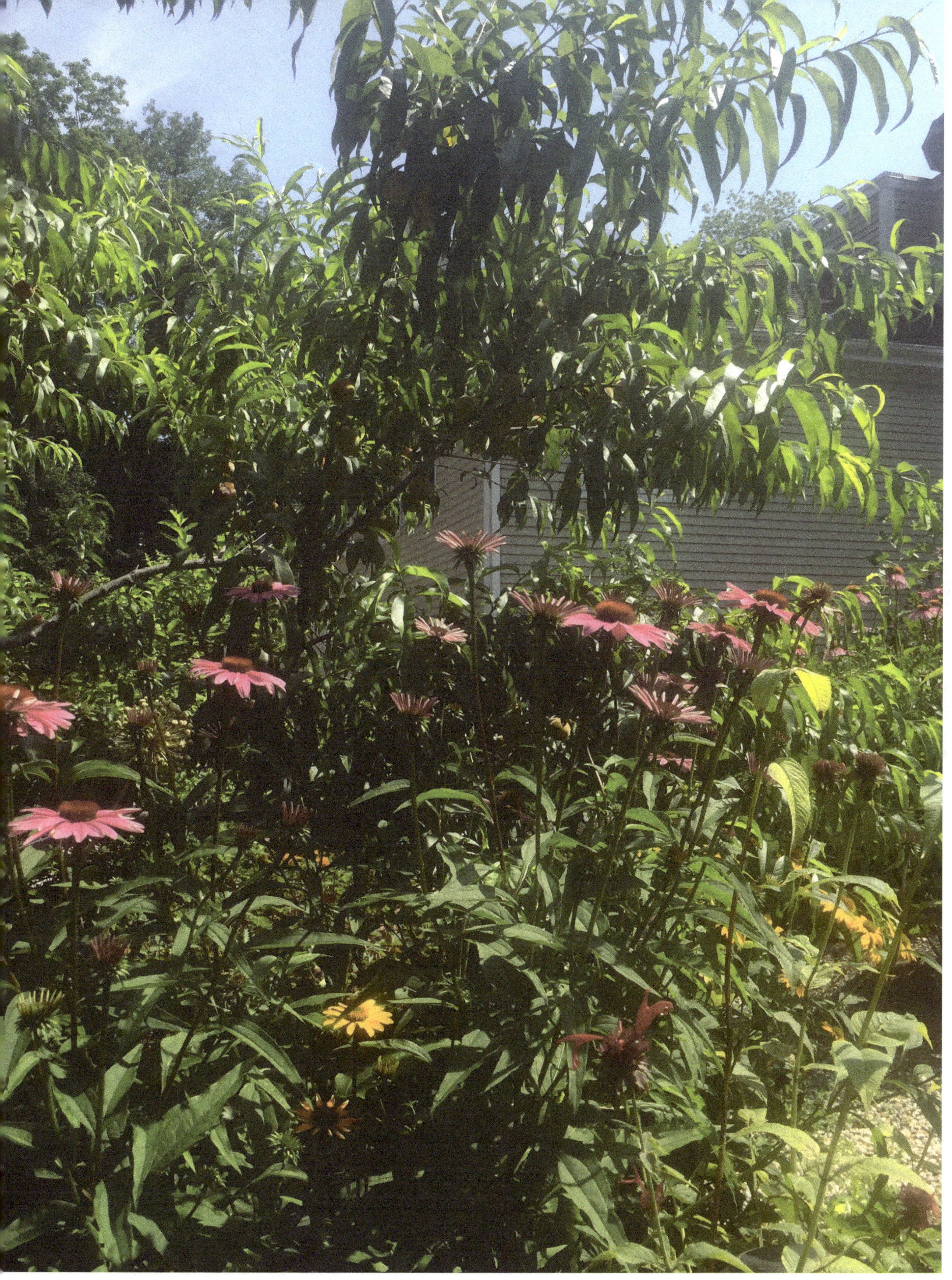

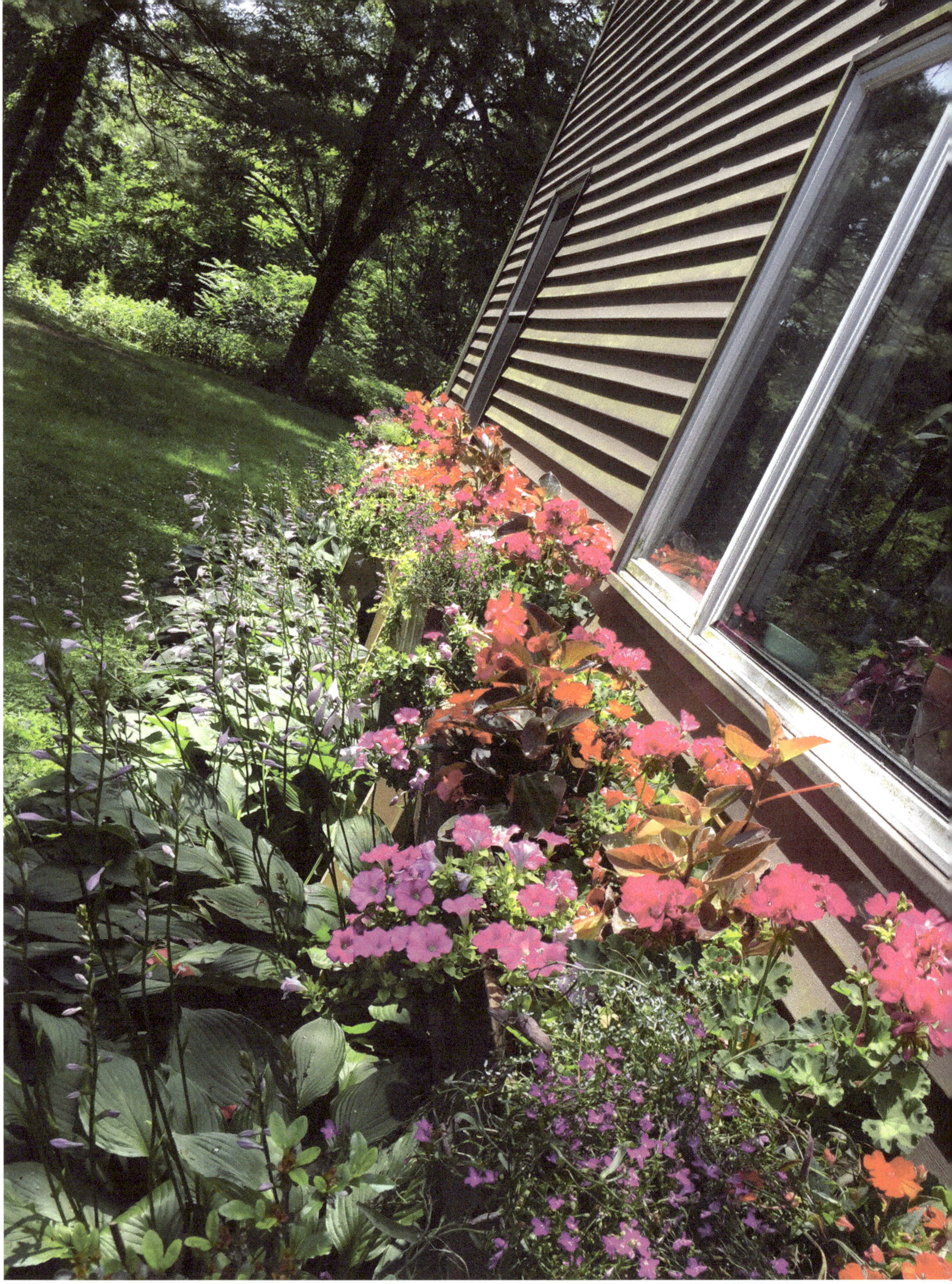

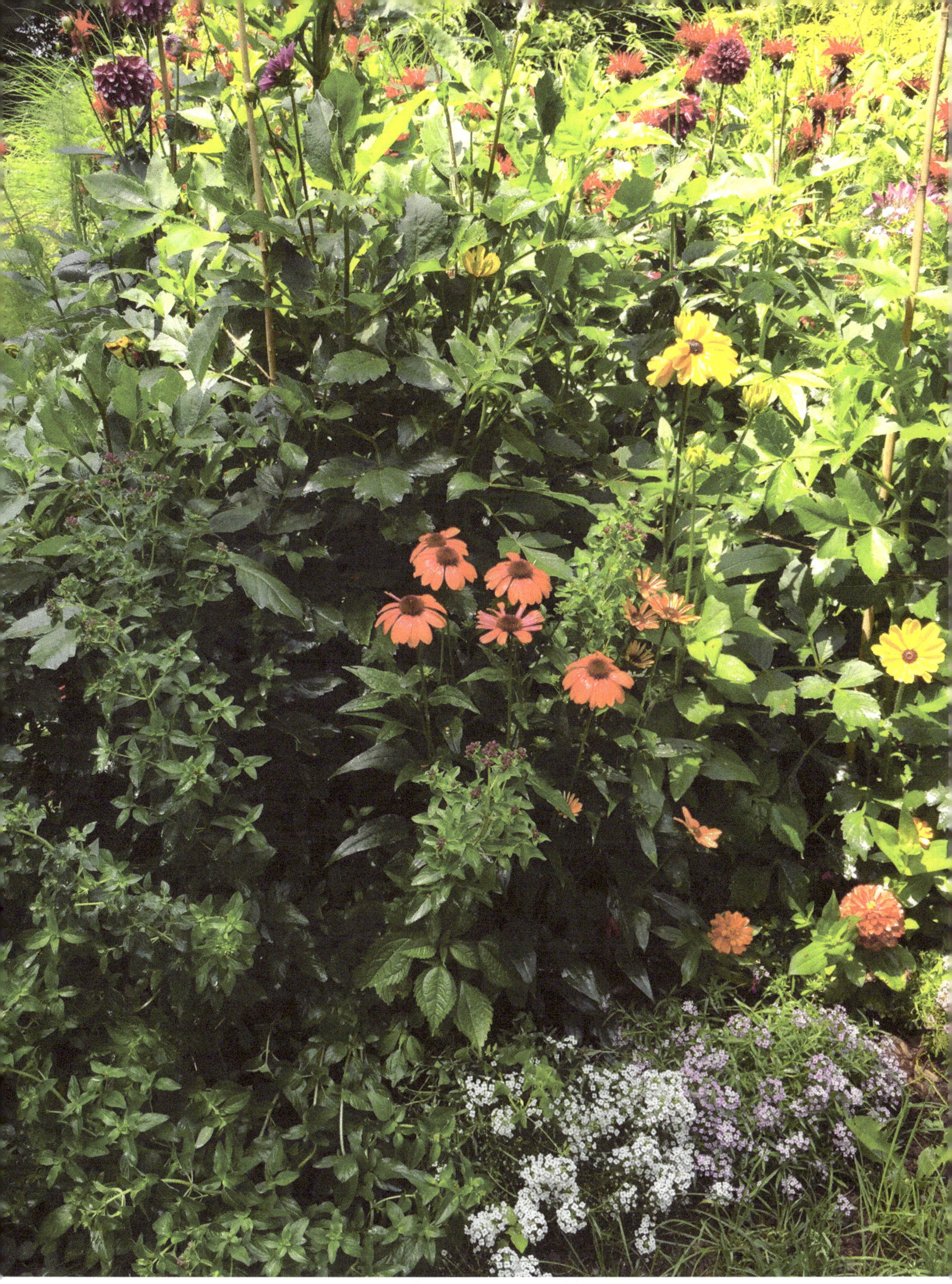

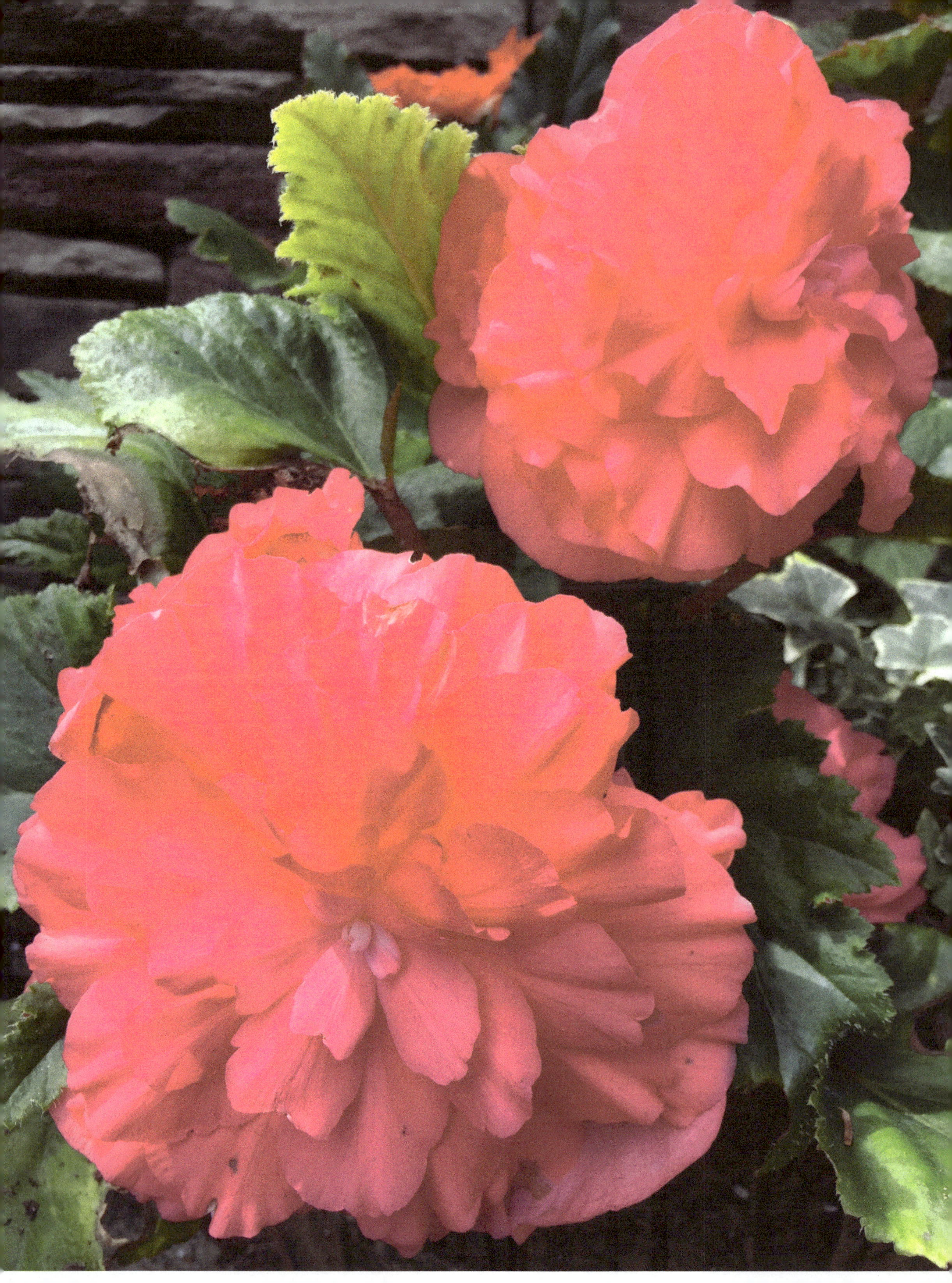

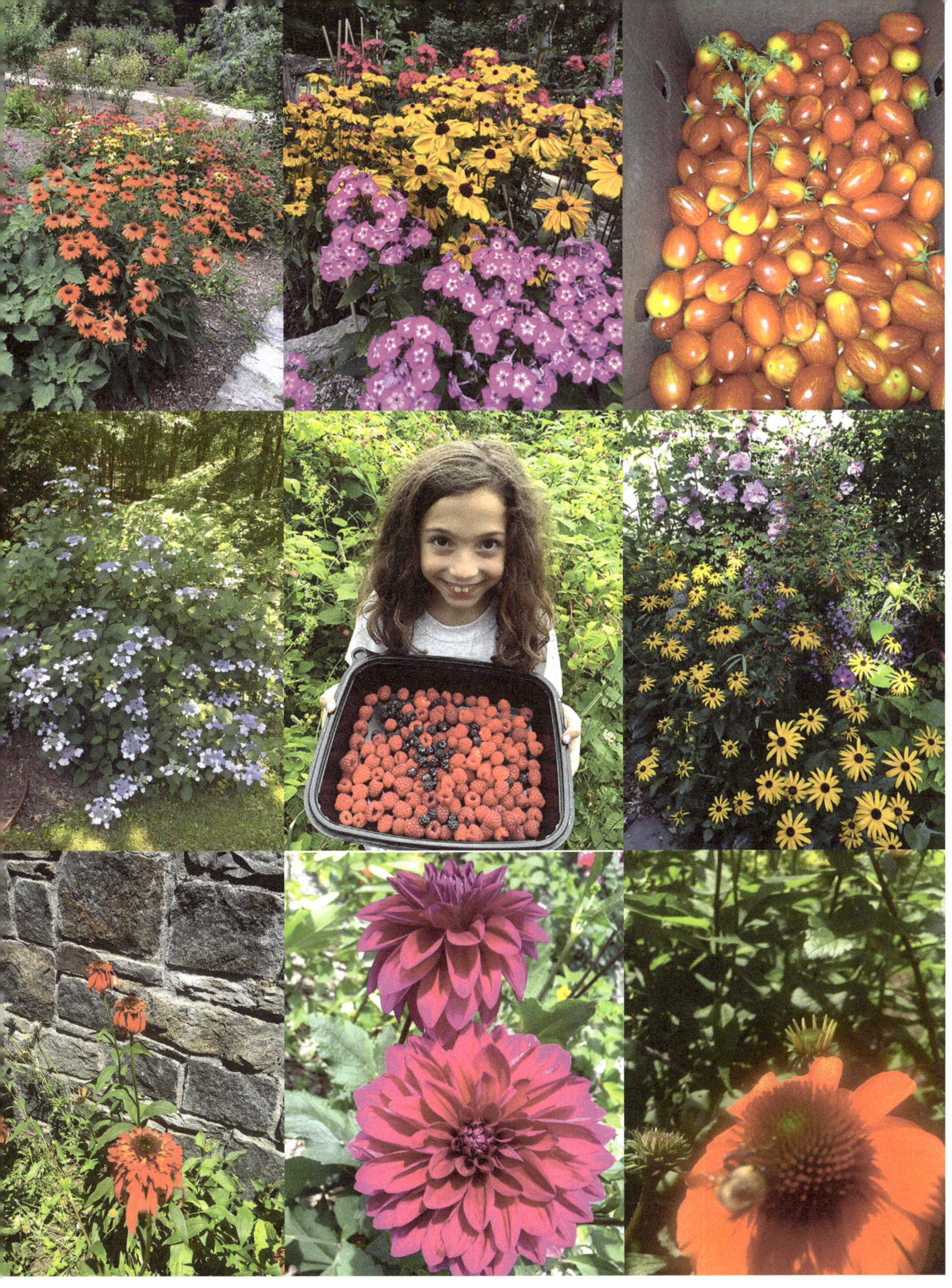

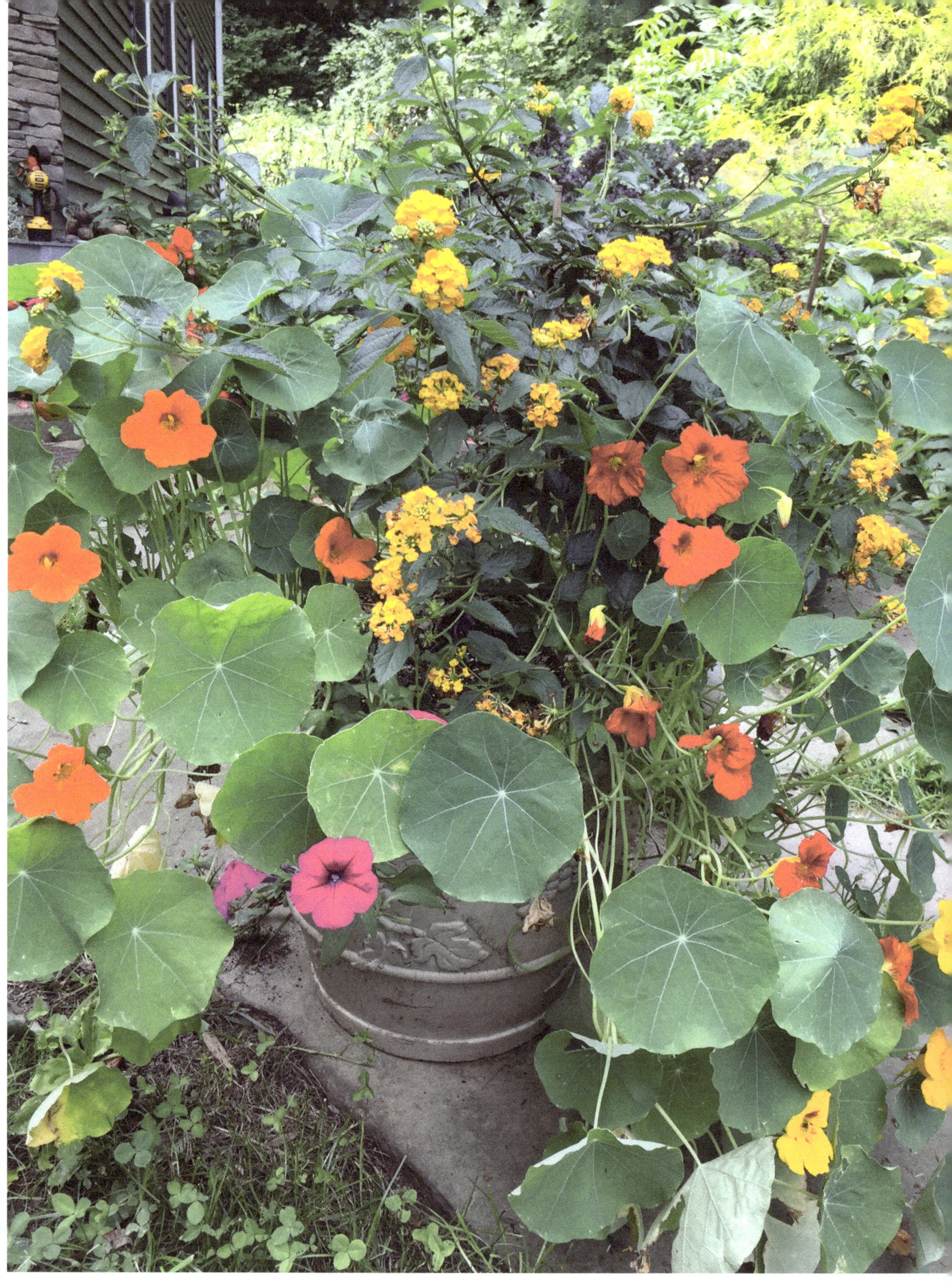

# Container Gardening

*"Every flower is a soul blossoming in nature."*

**John Muir**

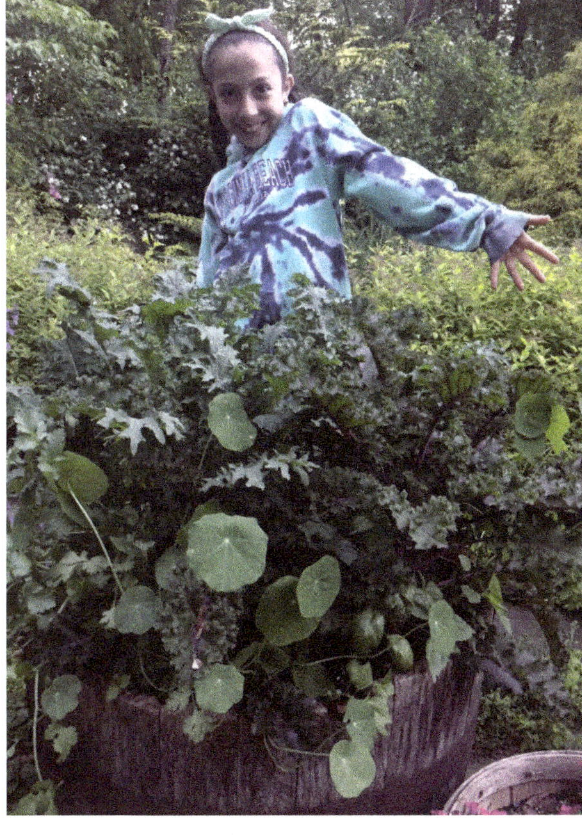

Container gardening is fun and very simple. It's a great way to grow herbs and vegetables if you don't have a lot of cultivated land to work with at your location. What I like to grow in the containers are different types of flowering plants in conjunction with herbs and edible greens.

A great thing about growing herbs in containers is they don't touch the ground, so they always stay clean and usually pest-free. It also provides quick access from the kitchen. You'll use them more often if they're located so close. You get used to stepping outside and plucking the herb you need for a dish. If you have to walk all the way out to a vegetable garden, you won't use them as much.

I like to use whiskey barrels as planters because they're constructed of wood, which holds moisture in and tends to not dry out as much. You can buy them at any garden center. They come cut in half, and they hold about 40 quarts of soil. They usually don't have drainage holes. I drill four holes a half inch in diameter into the base of each whiskey barrel.

Once I've drilled the holes, I put gravel on the bottom to support the drainage, as it will flow out of the holes. Then I fill the container with potting soil. I like to use Complete Planting Mix or Pro-Mix. It's a great blend of different humus, compost, and soil, along with perlite and vermiculite to hold moisture.

I choose my herbs after filling the containers with soil. I plant smaller growing herbs such as thyme, oregano, parsley, and cilantro in the front of the barrel. You can also plant basil and rosemary. Most herbs love full sun, and they thrive in those conditions, as do most vegetables.

The flower varieties I use in containers are zinnias, cosmos, dahlias, and marigolds, typically used for cutting gardens. The taller flowers, such as the zinnias, can support the taller plants, like basil, so put the flowers at the back of the container.

*Left: Nasturtiums potted with lantana. The edible blossoms have a peppery radish flavor and are great tossed in a salad.*

*Above: Lucy with her kale barrel garden.*

Peppers, eggplants, and patio tomatoes also do well in container gardens. Patio tomatoes are a wonderful addition to any garden pot. They are smaller, compact plants that don't require much staking or support. They also produce a heavy yield.

Growing herbs in containers is very fulfilling because what you don't use fresh can be cut and laid out to dry. You can use them during the winter when fresh herbs aren't available. I feed the herbs twice a month with Plant-tone, an organic, granular fertilizer you can purchase at any garden center. It keeps the herbs fed and helps them continue to produce highly throughout the summer.

Any time you notice some of the herbs starting to go into bloom, it's always good to pinch the blooms off to encourage new growth and bushiness. For instance, basil is one of the first to flower. It's a foliage herb, and you want to harvest the leaves. Its flowers won't produce leaves, so you'll want to pinch back the small blossoms once they protrude out of the center of the plant.

Other perennial herbs you can grow in containers are mint, tarragon, and sage. Once these plants are in the containers, they'll be back year after year. Other types of plants I like to grow this way are in the Brassica family, including kale, collards, Brussels sprouts, and broccoli. They do well in containers, and they can be harvested right up until the first hard frost.

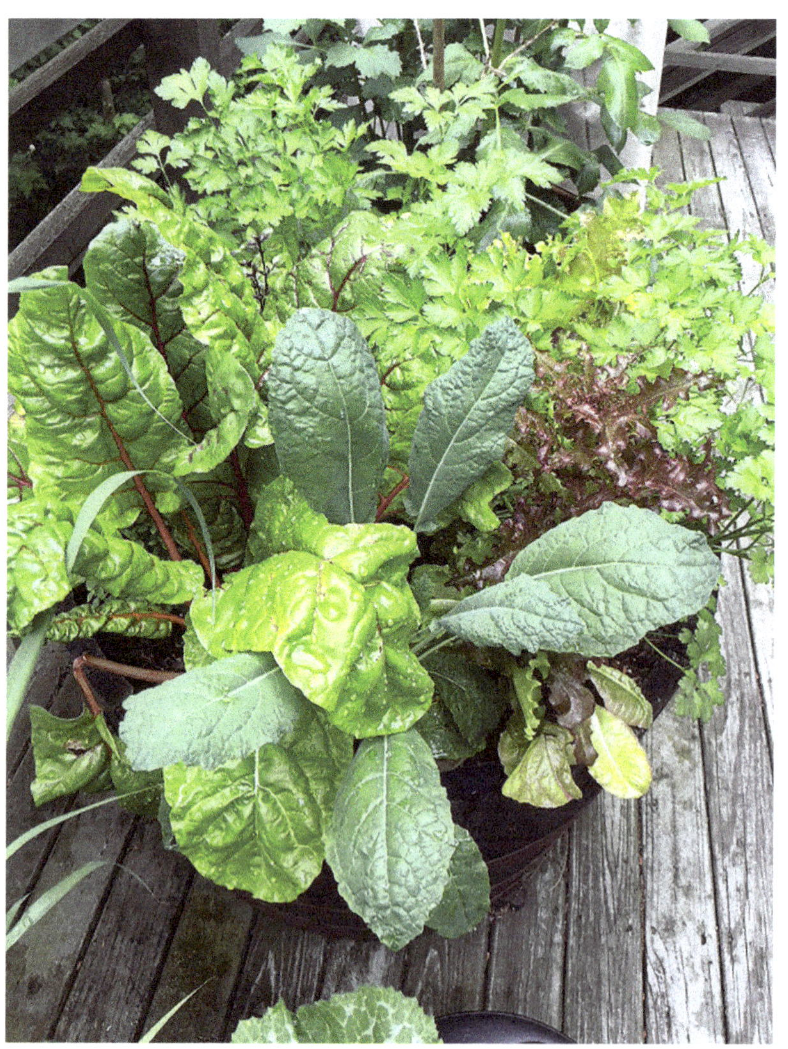

*Left: Container with Swiss chard, cilantro, kale, lettuce, and parsley.*

*Page 99: Whiskey barrel with electric blue petunias, and barrel teeming with lettuce.*

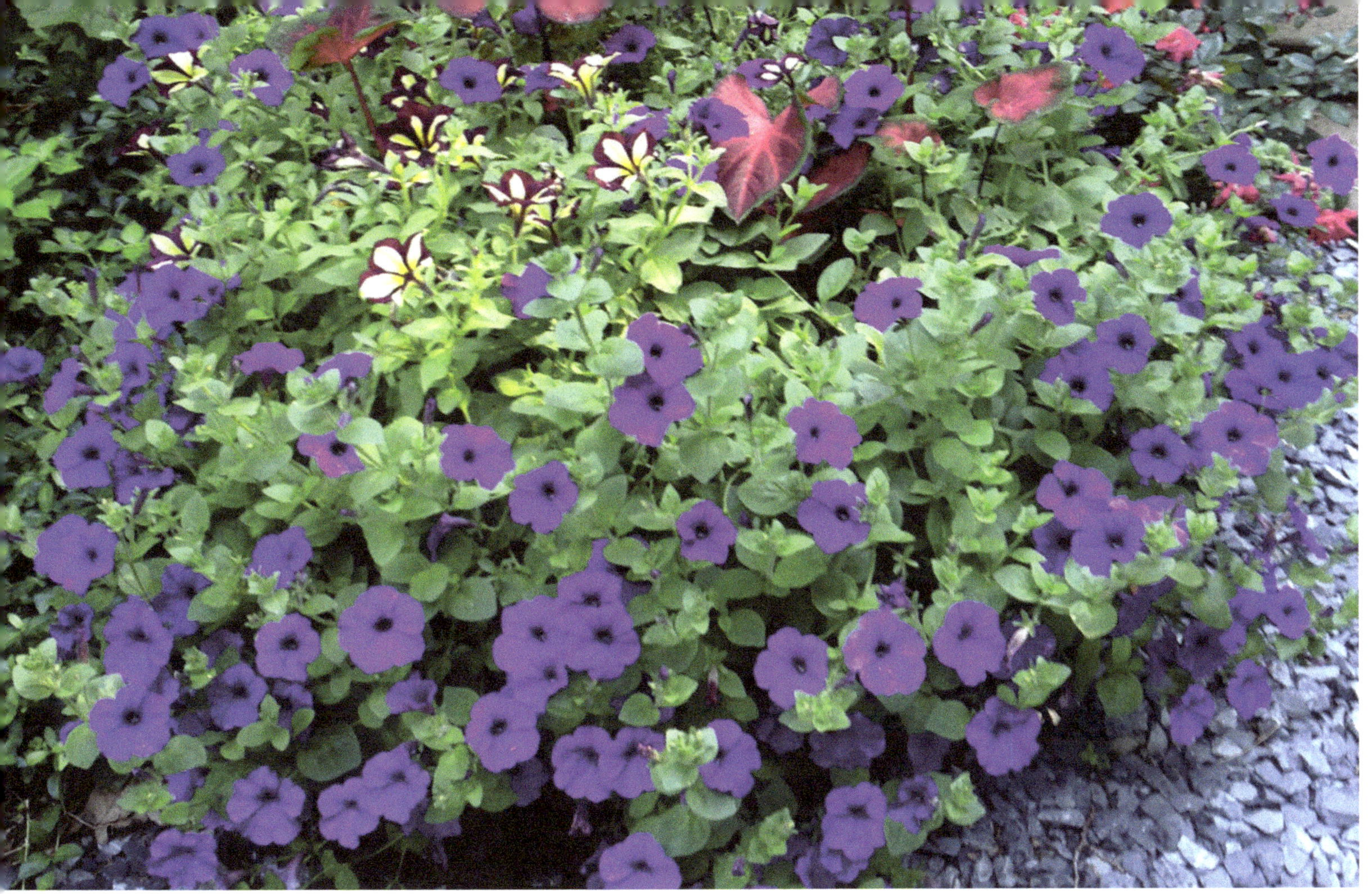

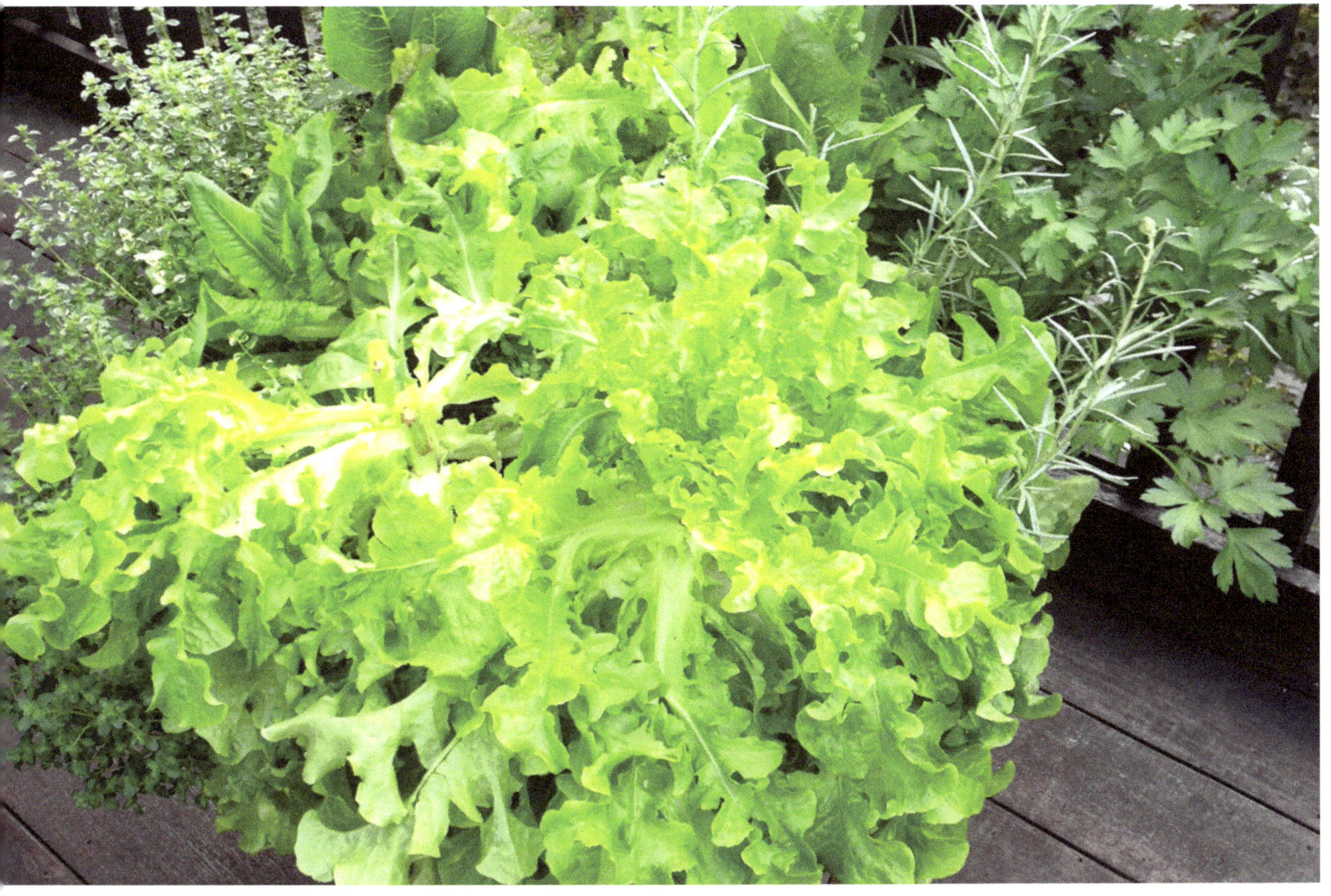

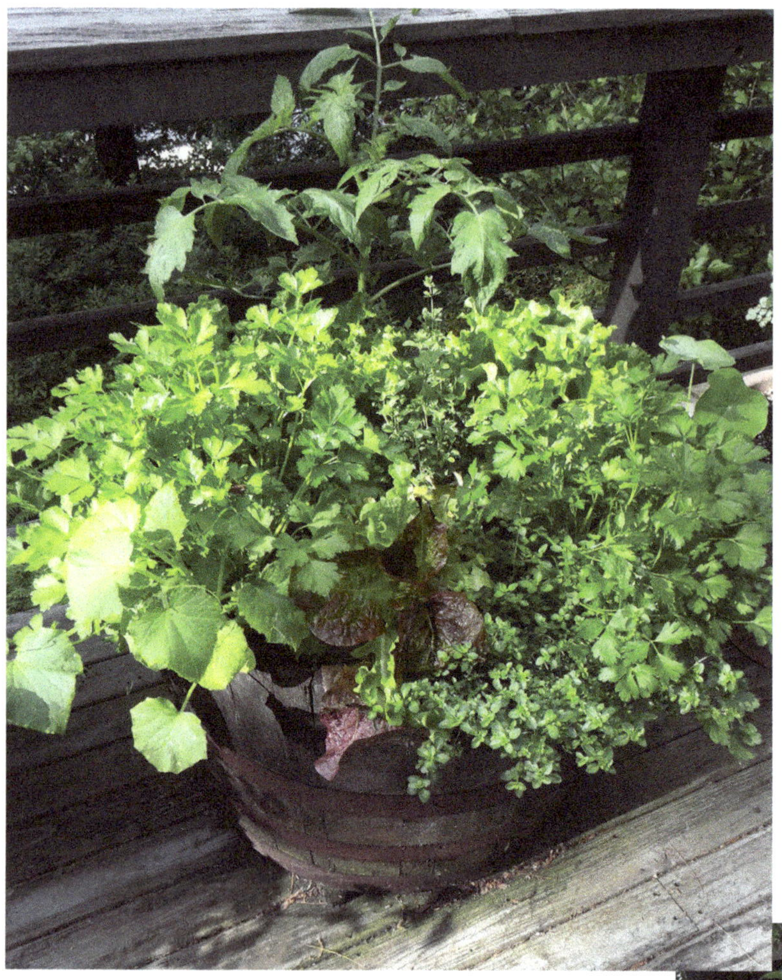

*Above: Whiskey barrel planter.*

*Right: Blueberries in container.*

*Page 101: Assorted begonias in a full wine barrel.*

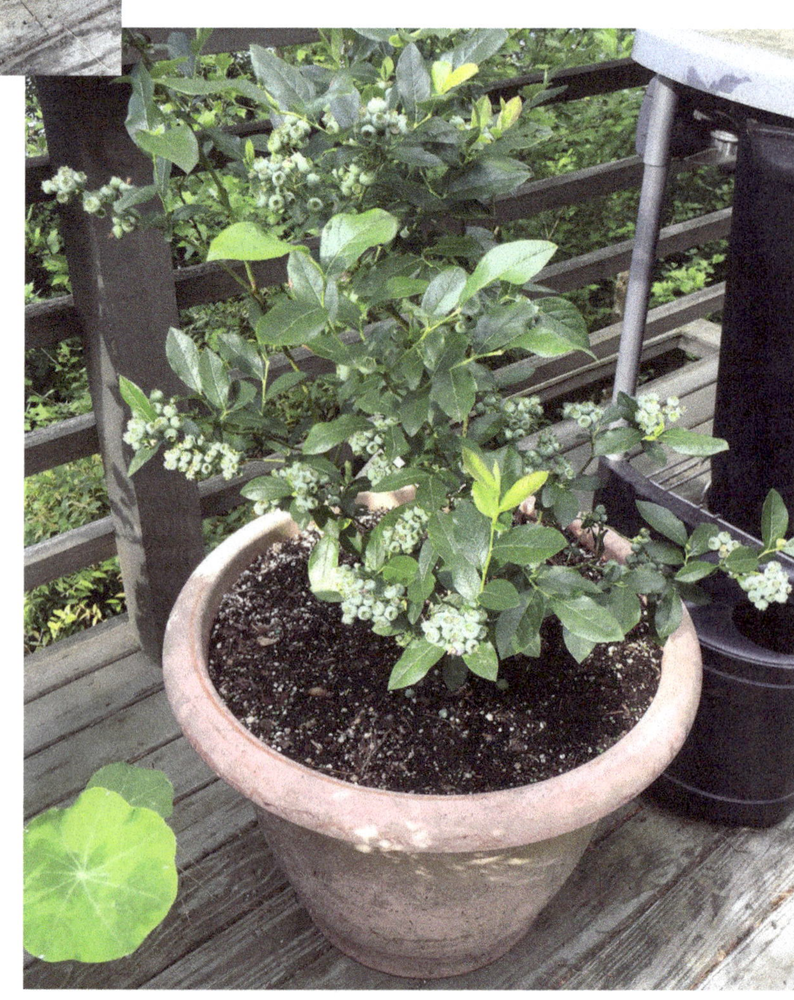

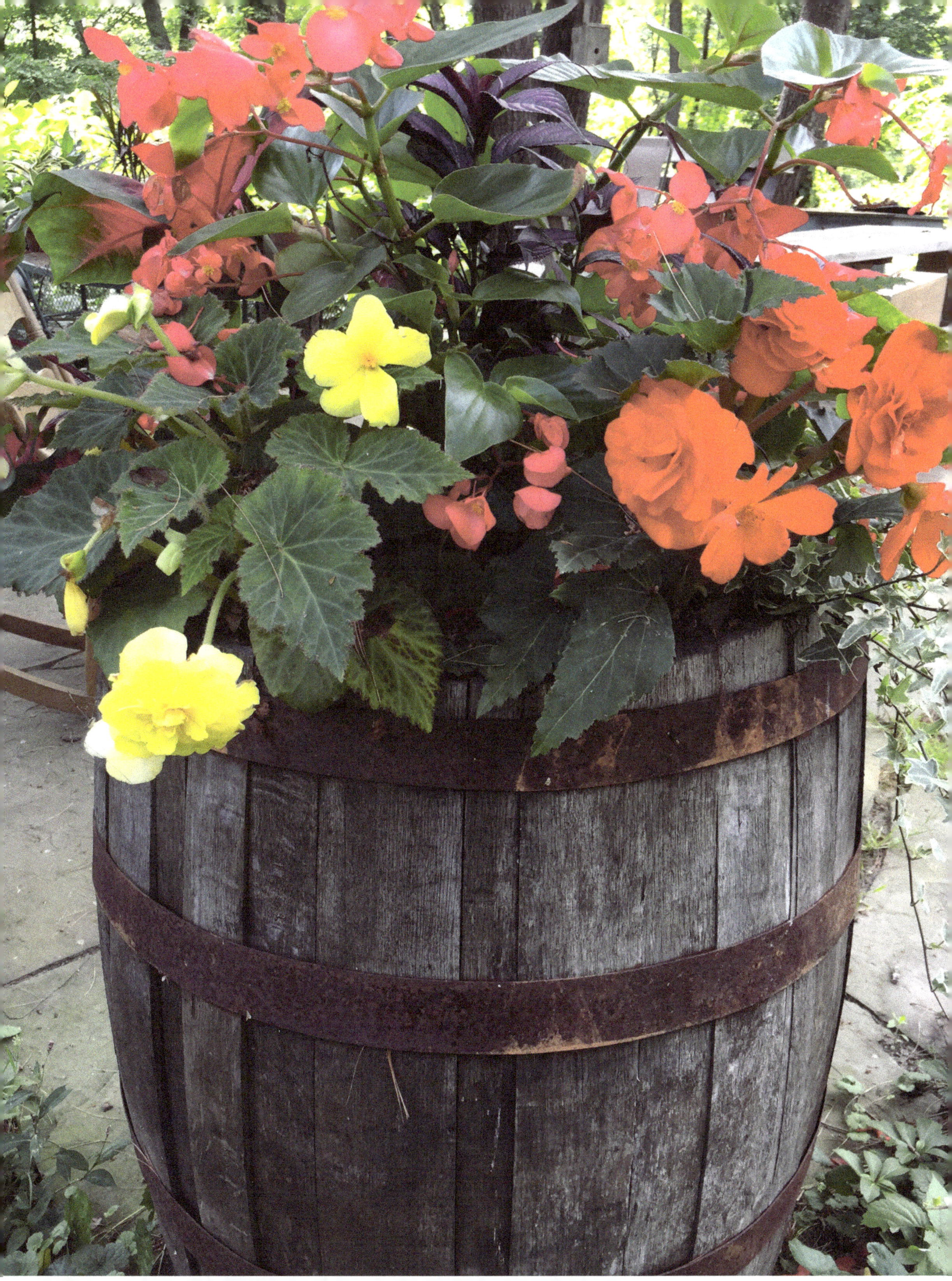

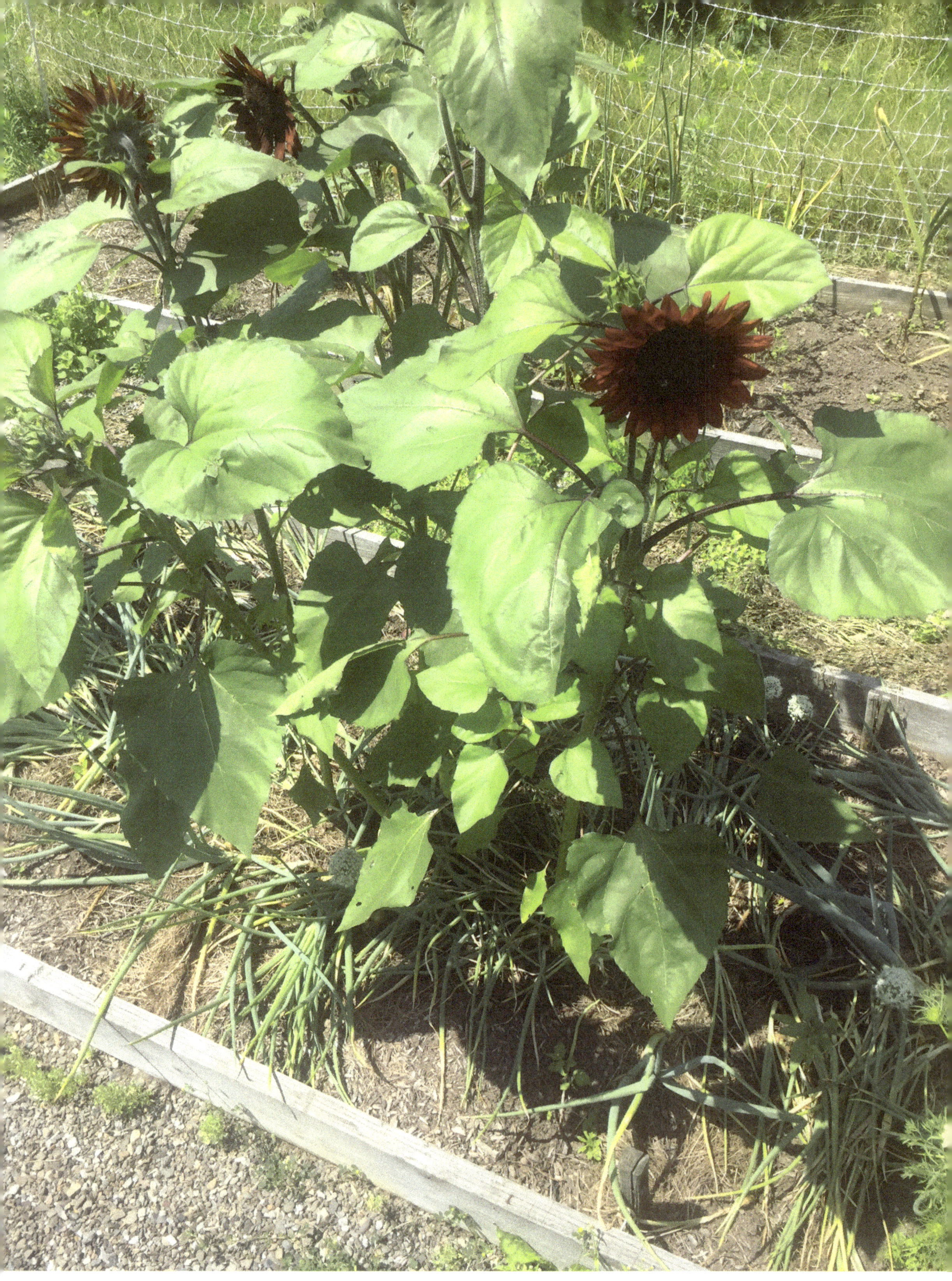

# Permaculture

*"The plants we've chosen will collect and cycle Earth's minerals, water, and air; shade the soil and renew it with leafy mulch; and yield fruits and greens for people and wildlife."*

**Toby Hemenway**

Permaculture is a way of gardening and growing fruit so that everything is compatible with each other in small places. Its beauty is in its plain old simplicity. I practice permaculture in many ways. I've designed and developed orchards using the permaculture system. There have been many circumstances where I've planted vegetables among fruit trees, corn along with cucumbers, and squash along with beans.

To illustrate the concept, say that you have a small area to grow vegetables and/or fruit. You plant some corn, and instead of finding a new place to grow your cucumbers, you let the cucumbers run up the corn plants. The cucumbers cling to the corn, but the corn will ripen later in the season. The cucumbers will bear fruit earlier in the year, and they'll be easy to reach for harvest since they're climbing up the corn.

Permaculture is a great concept for gardening, and there are many ways to utilize it. In relation to landscaping an area, I like to grow different fruiting berries, instead of azaleas and rhododendrons. For example, when deciding what to put into foundation borders and garden beds, I like to incorporate blueberries. They produce a pretty white flower in the spring, a delicious, edible fruit in the summer, and strikingly red foliage in the fall. They're an acidic-loving plant, so they do very well among ground cover.

Another example is that when it comes to ground cover, why use English ivy or pachysandra? Why not use strawberries? Strawberries are acidic-lovers, also. During the growing season as I install the blueberry bushes, I plant strawberries among them. The strawberries act as a dense ground cover, keeping the soil cool and moist, which the blueberries like. You're now also producing a wonderful crop of strawberries throughout the season.

Most people aren't familiar with another good foundation plant that produces wonderful fruit. Gooseberries are beautiful, taste great, and are disease-resistant. They don't require much care and are very productive. I like to plant rhubarb with them. Rhubarb is a perennial plant. Unlike an annual plant, which is killed by frost and must be replaced in the spring, perennial plants come back year after year. Rhubarb plants have big, showy leaves and bright, red canes. As food, rhubarb goes hand in hand with strawberries. Strawberry rhubarb pie is one of my favorites. Once you throw in a handful of gooseberries, you have something that's simply amazing.

As you can see, using compatible landscaping is much more than just a decorative look. Why not have something that looks beautiful and can be deliciously enjoyed with your family! Another option instead of planting perennial flowers is to plant vegetables. Put in a couple of eggplants. Eggplants do well in full sun, look beautiful as part of the landscape, and produce delicious vegetables.

*Sunflowers planted amongst the onions to protect them from the scalding sun.*

I also like to use cherry tomatoes. I plant them at the front of evergreens, and I train them to grow up and over the trees for the growing season, since they're annuals. The trees give them a nice cushion and lots of support. I can also certainly see the cherry tomatoes against the green background of the evergreens. You'll have beautiful tomatoes all summer long.

Kale is another option. I plant it towards the front of the area I'm landscaping, as it's very showy and easy to pick. You can usually harvest it right up until winter begins to set in.

*Page 105: Tomato plant sharing space with a young pawpaw. They are both watered together and sharing nutrients. Once the frost arrives, the tomato will be pulled and the pawpaw will be established.*

*Page 106: Some beautiful kale growing and supporting snapdragons and painted daisies.*

*Page 108: Winterbor kale along with painted daises, calendula, and campanula in the background.*

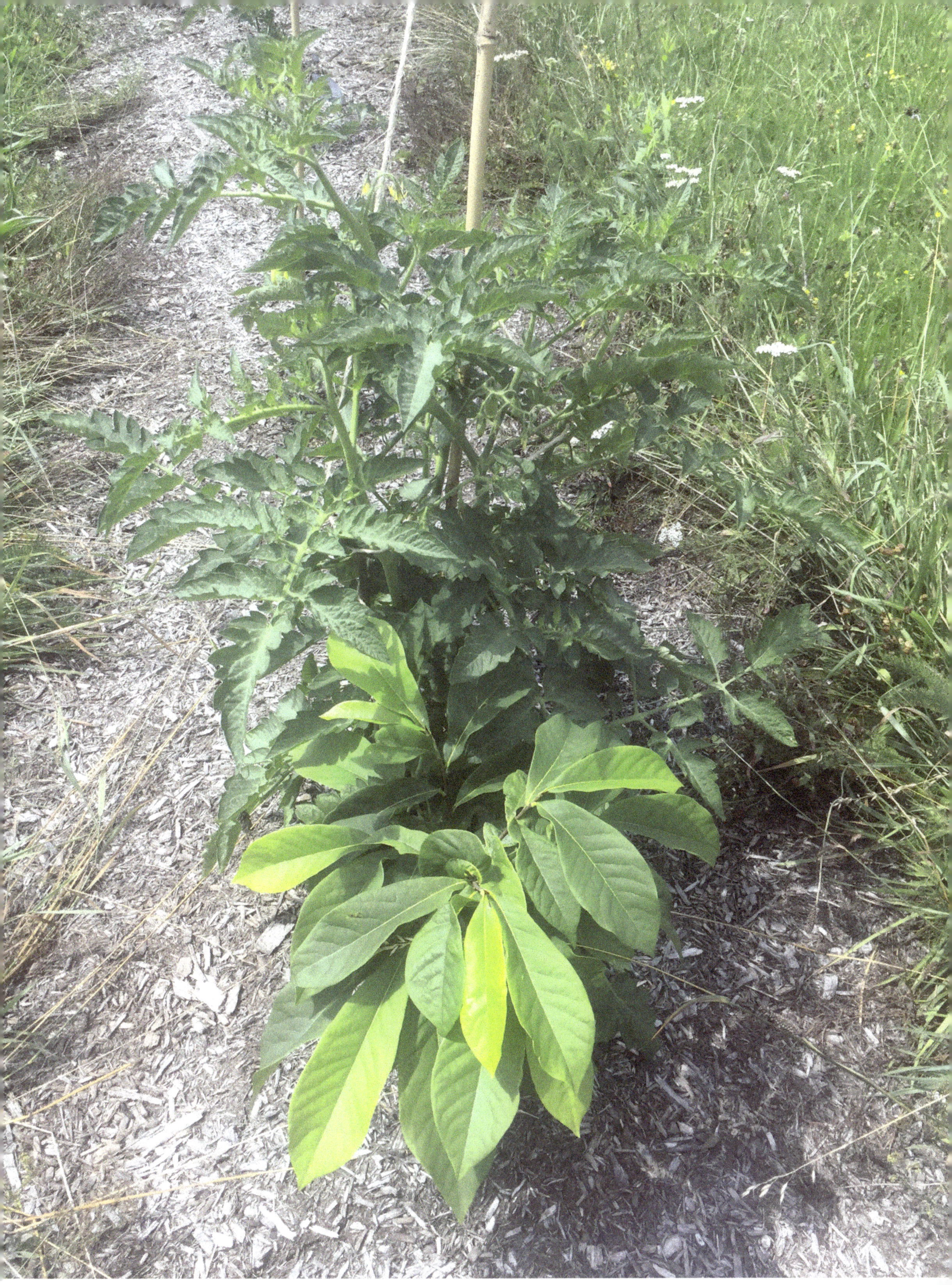

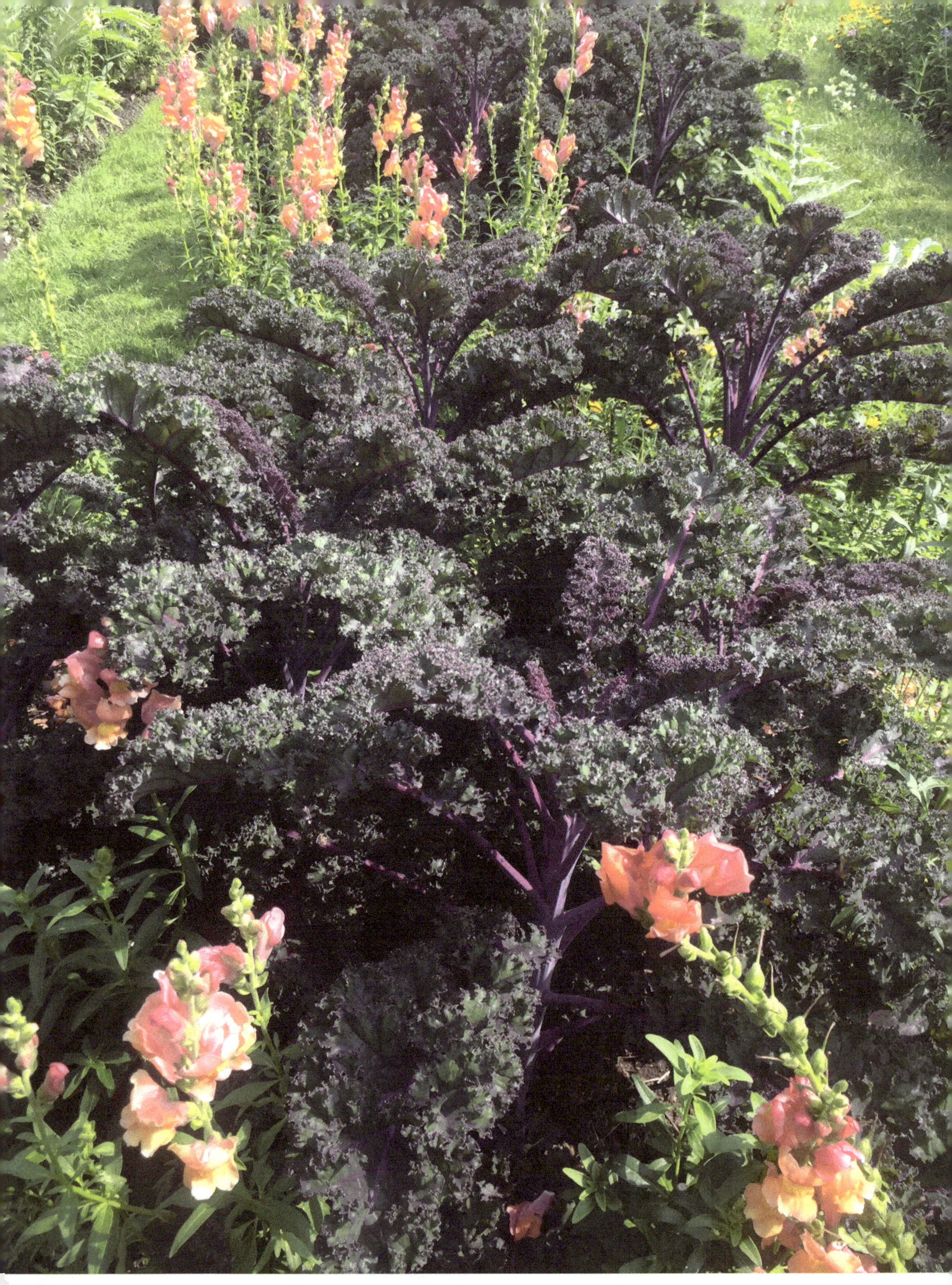

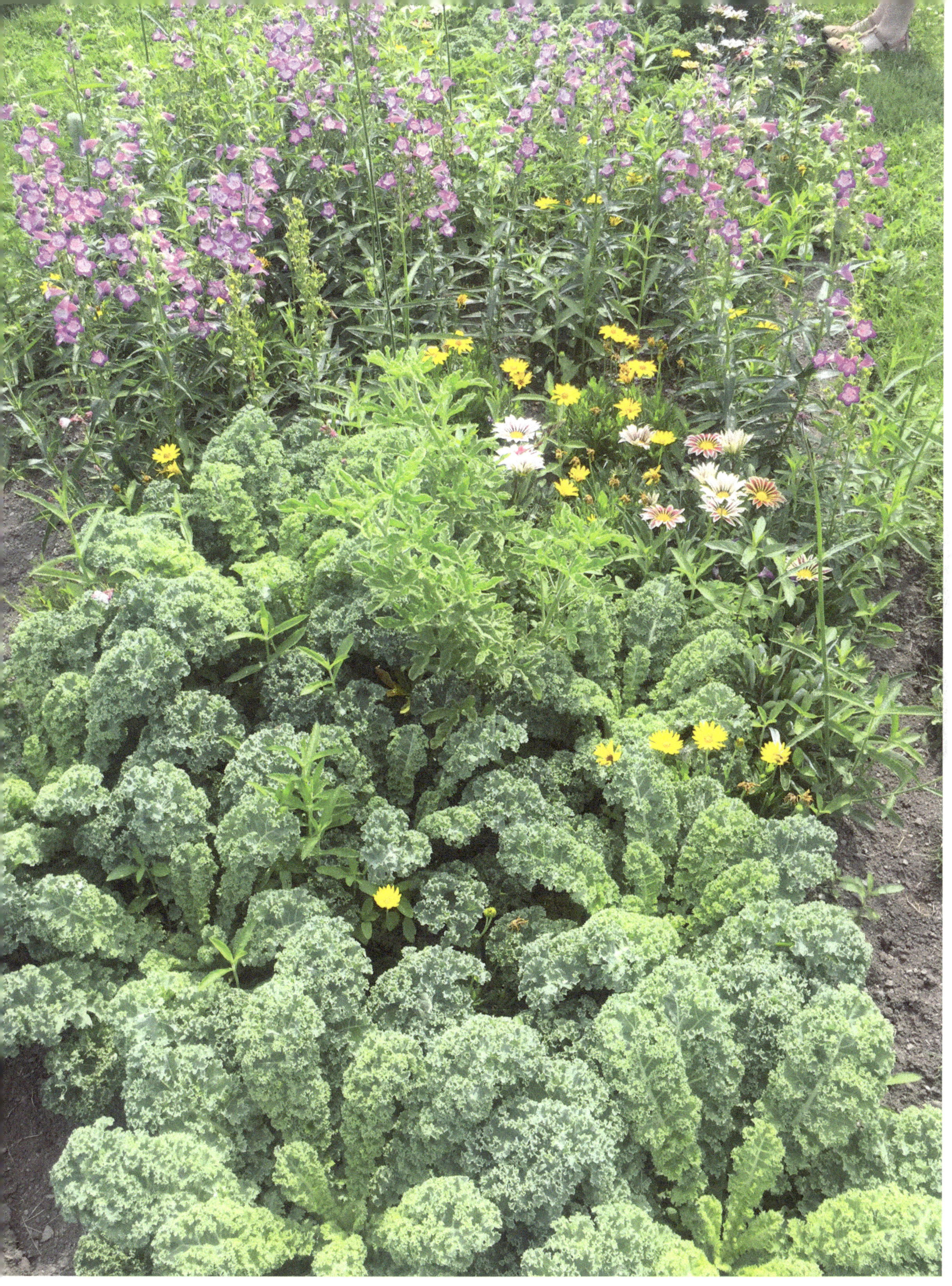

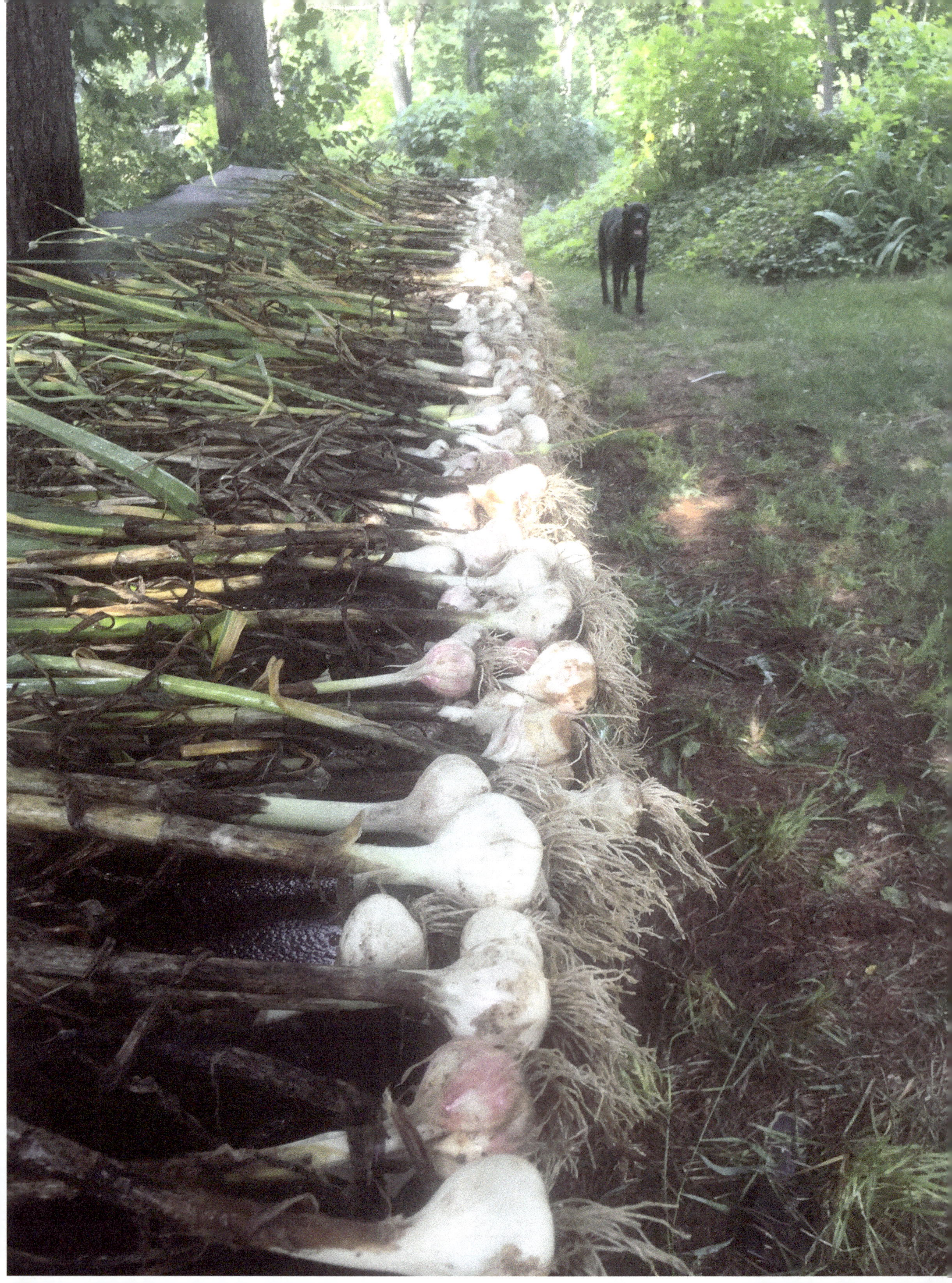

# Garlic

*"Garlic is divine. Few food items can taste so many distinct ways, handled correctly. Misuse of garlic is a crime...Please, treat your garlic with respect..."*

**— Anthony Bourdain**

One thing I love to do come autumn is grow my own crop of garlic. Growing garlic is quite easy. For one thing, it doesn't have any predators. After all, it even drives vampires away!

Garlic needs a sunny, well-drained area. Purchase a good garlic that's known to grow in your climate. You can usually buy garlic cloves from online distributors or the local garden store. The varieties I like to grow are Music and German White. These varieties are stiff-neck garlic.

To get started in the fall, cultivate your selected area by raking it over and then flattening it out. Now you're ready for planting. Separate the cloves from the bulb. Place each clove into the ground about two inches deep and six inches apart. Space the rows about a foot apart, enabling you to pass through them to harvest your crop later in the season.

I sprinkle some good compost over my garlic and use a well-balanced fertilizer. Garlic loves nitrogen. I use straw as a mulch to spread over the garlic. The straw acts as a blanket and protects the tender cloves during the winter months. When springtime approaches, you'll notice the garlic starting to push through the straw. The straw also helps eliminate weeds.

I cultivate around each of the plants when the garlic is about six inches. I also water them as needed. This enables the soil around them to remain loose and allows the bulbs to grow quite large. The center of the plant starts to emerge as a seed head when the garlic is about a foot tall. The seed head is attached to a long stem, called a scape, that comes out of the center of the plant. Remove the scapes so the plant can devote all its energy to producing a larger bulb. The scapes are delicious sautéed or mixed in with an omelet.

As the season progresses, the garlic will continue to grow until harvest time, in the month of August. When the garlic starts to yellow and show signs of stress, it's starting to shut down anymore growing, and the plant has reached its maturity. To harvest your garlic, pull it from the base using a small trowel or a pitchfork. Leave the garlic in the sun to dry for about three or four days so it can cure. You can also hang the garlic up in an old barn or a shed, so it has some air circulation and dries consistently.

*Bruno inspects just harvested Spanish Roja and German White garlic.*

Once the garlic seems dried, you can keep it hanging for a few more days, just to be sure. Then trim the roots and brush off any soil. You can now snip your garlic off at the neck. Garlic will keep in a bag over a long period of time in your pantry. Homegrown garlic has a longer shelf life than what you usually buy in the store. That garlic might be more than six months old by the time you purchase it.

I usually save 10 to 15 heads of garlic to repeat the planting again in the fall. Garlic is one of the most rewarding, enjoyable crops that I grow. I not only plant it in the garden, but I incorporate it throughout my landscape as well. It's great at repelling insects from attacking my fruits and vegetables. I also let some go right into flower because the bees love to forage on its nectar. I also add the edible flowers to my salads.

As a health tip, chopped up garlic mixed with honey and eaten in the morning with a glass of water for seven days is a way to cleanse your body. It also helps with weight loss.

*Page 111: Garlic ready to plant.*

*Page 112: Garlic starting to form scapes. They'll be removed so the garlic heads will mature and develop larger. If not, all the energy will go to the blossom and the heads wouldn't develop and remain small.*

*Page 113: Lucy picking garlic scapes.*

*Page 114: Garlic scapes.*

*Page 115: Garlic recently harvested and hung up to cure for a few weeks.*

*Page 116: Cured garlic.*

*Page 117: Garlic harvest.*

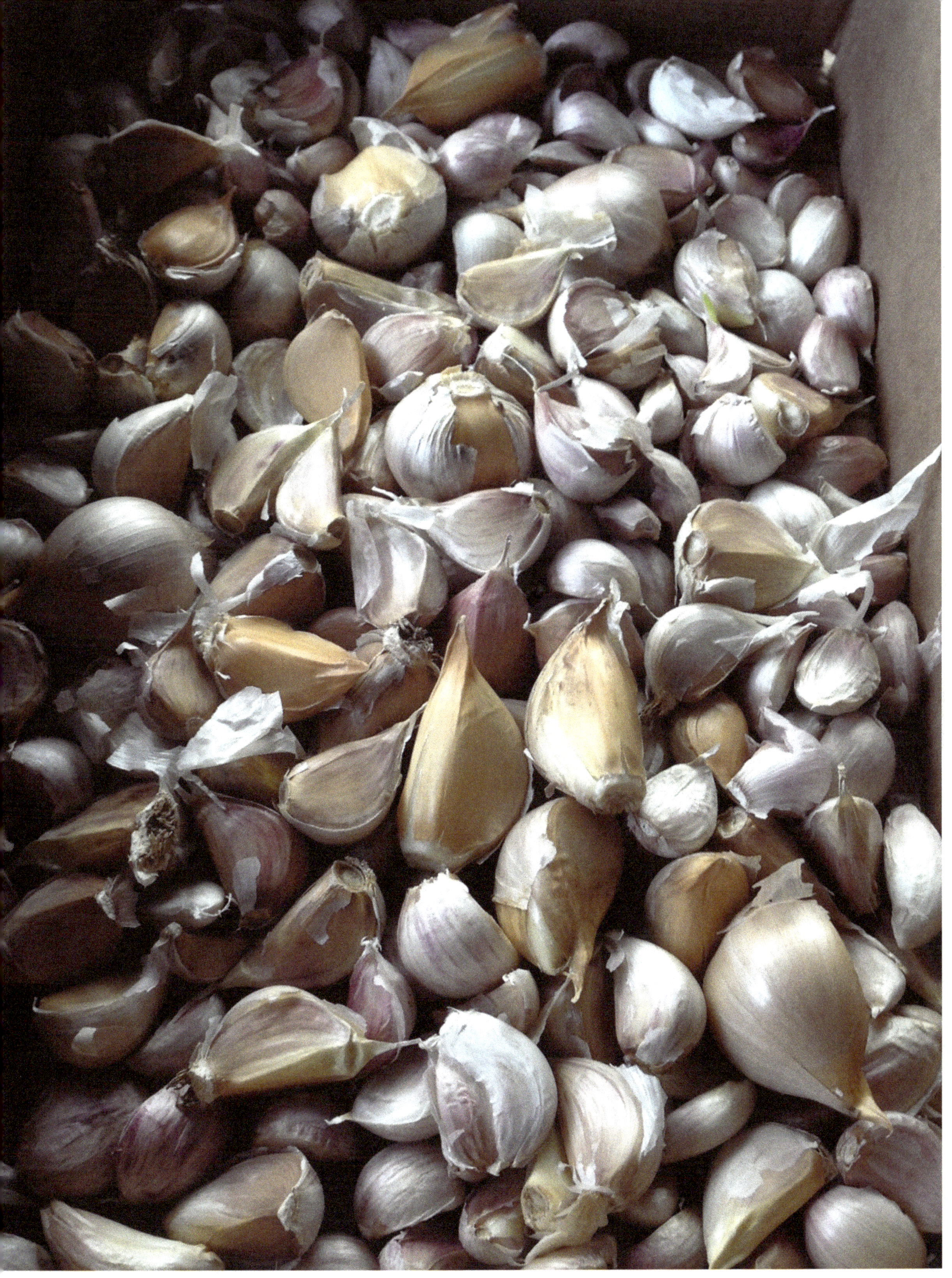

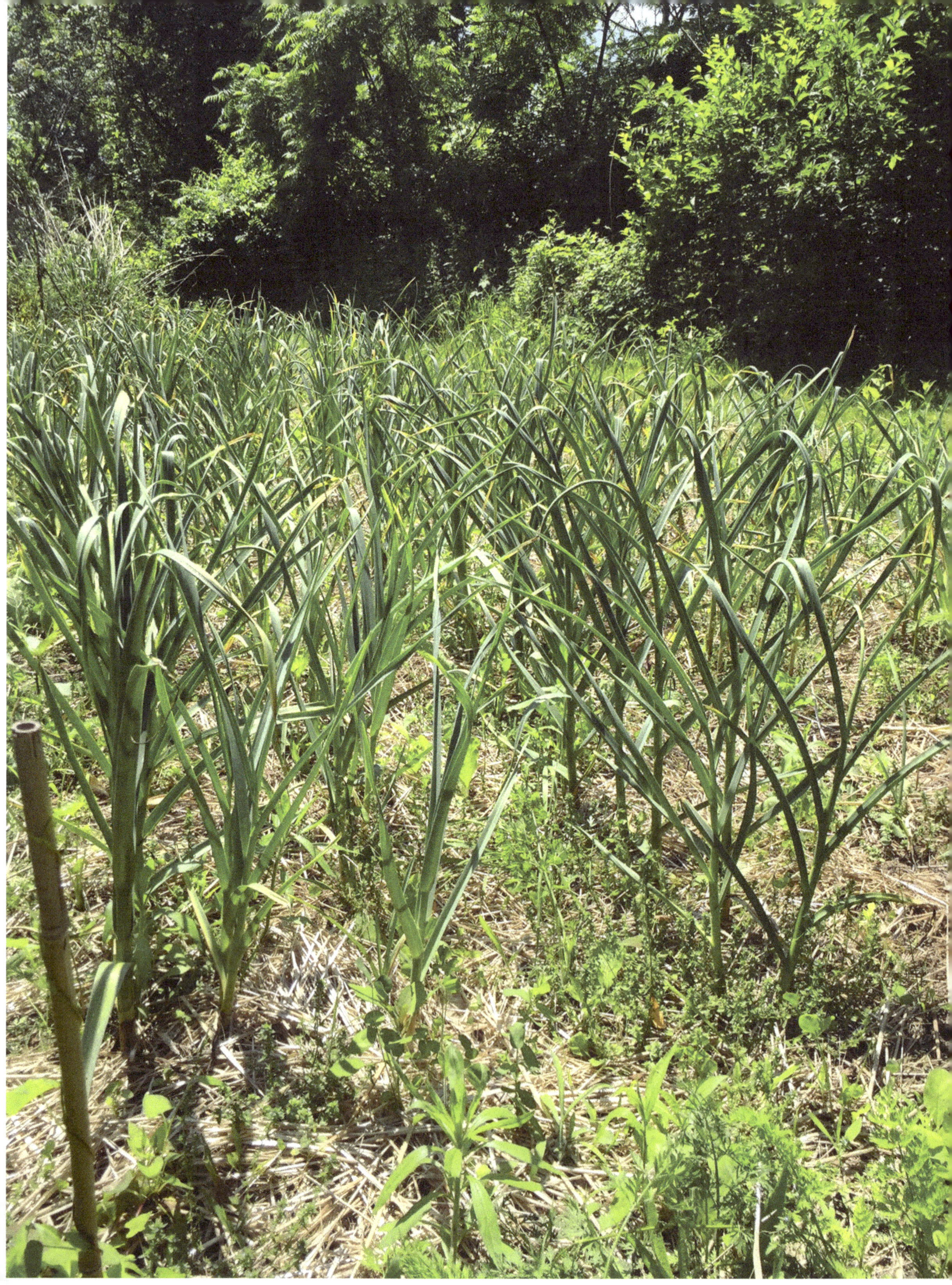

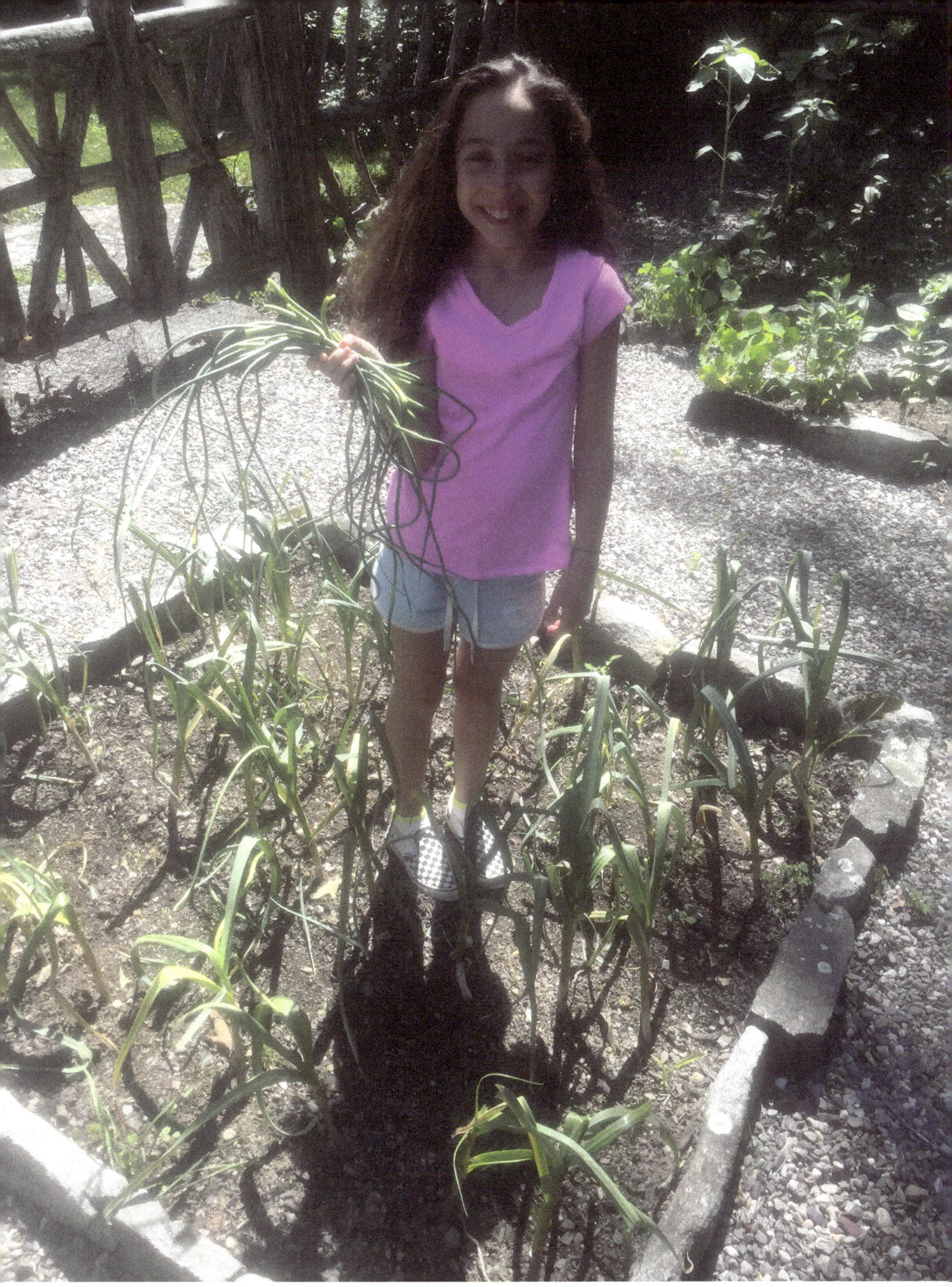

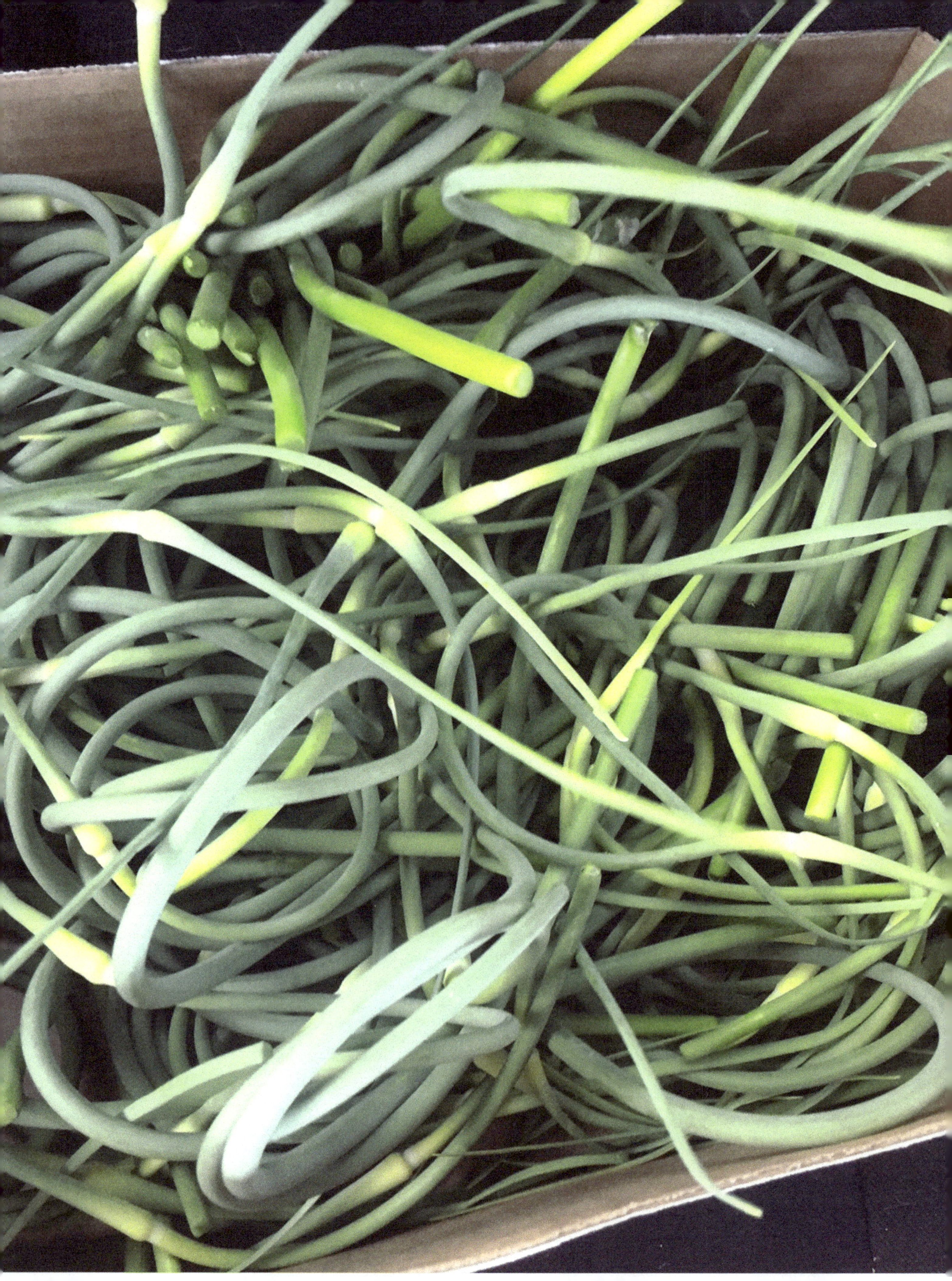

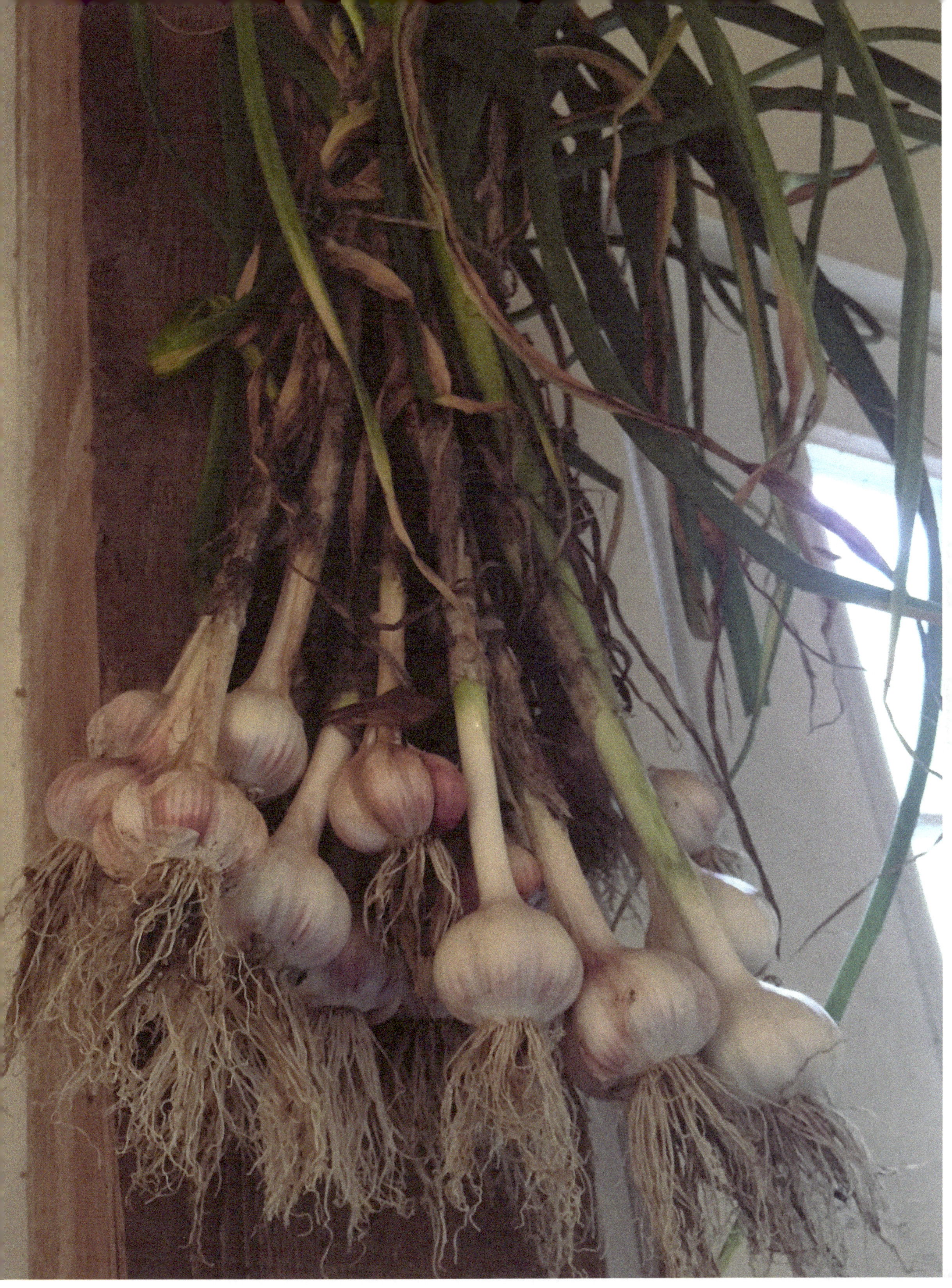

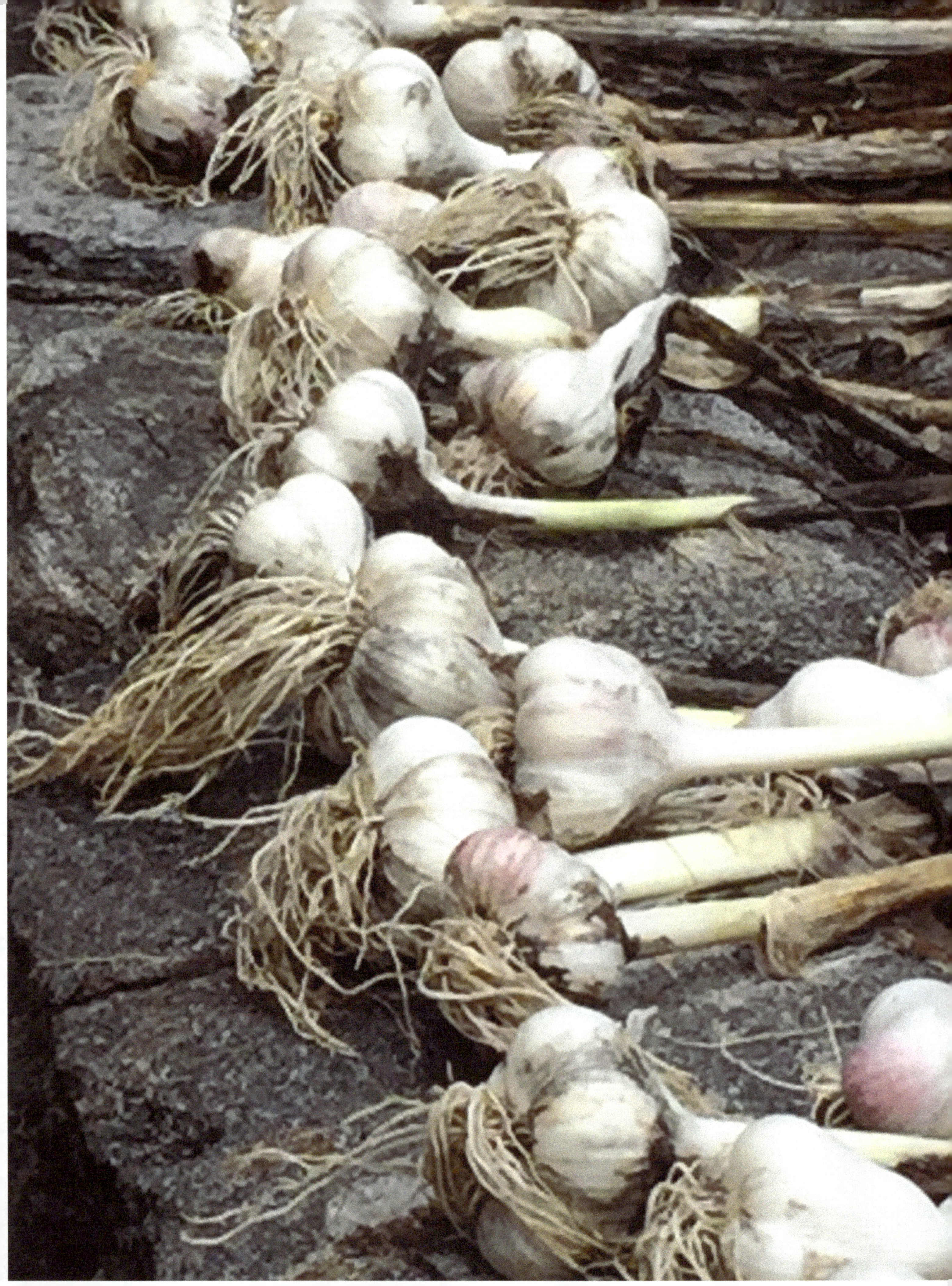

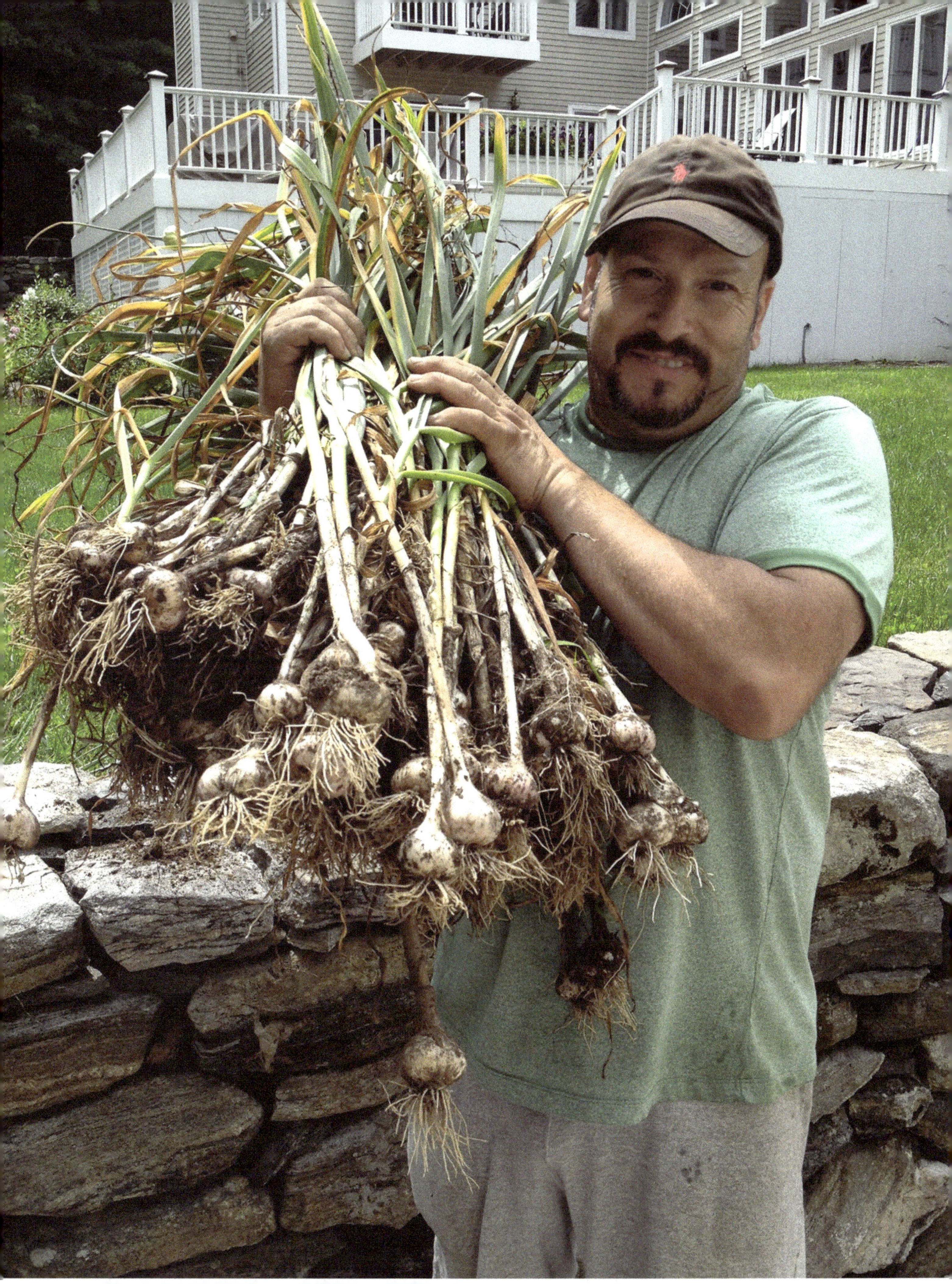

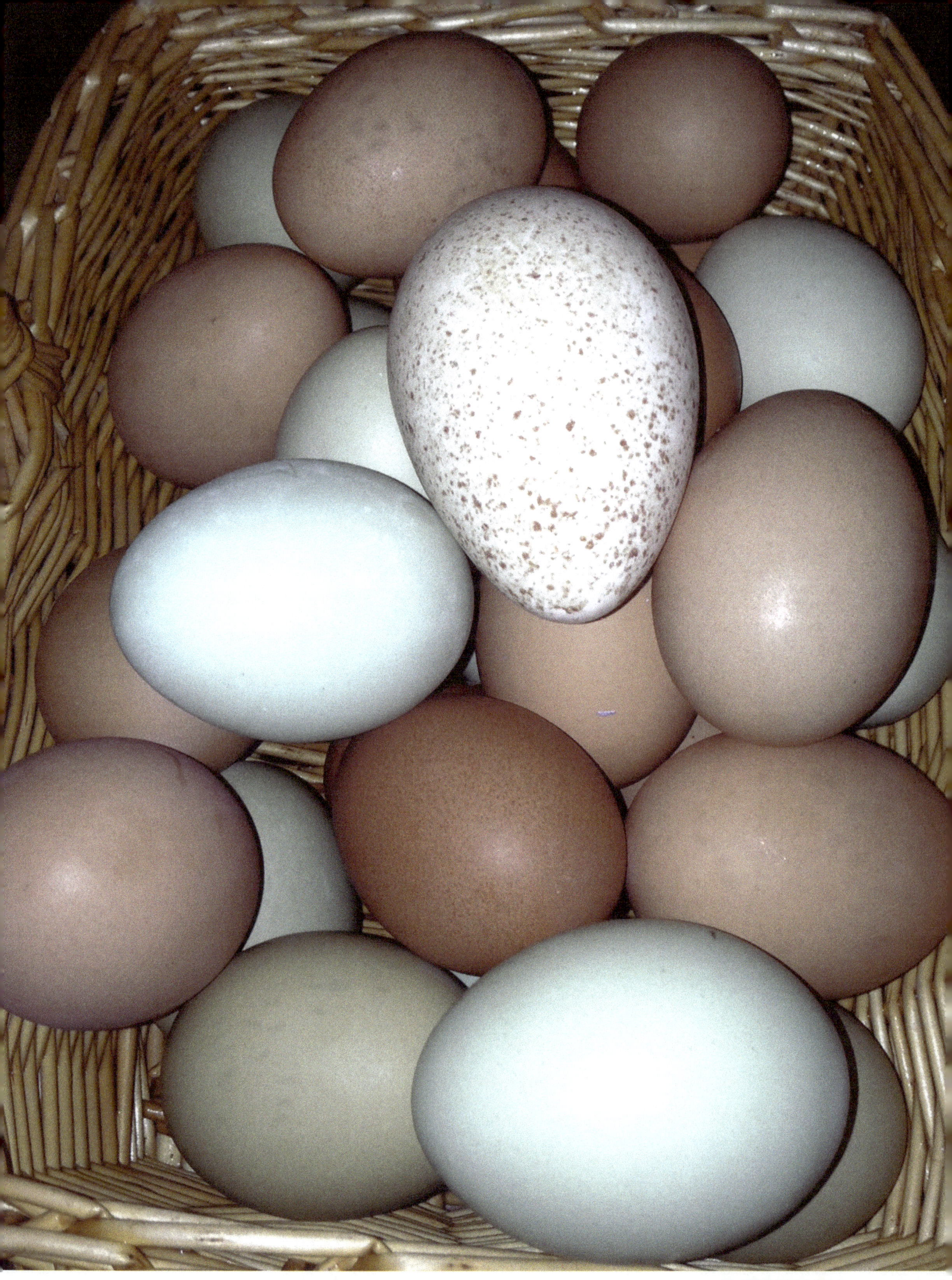

# Eggs

*"Love and eggs are best when they are fresh."*

**Russian Proverb**

Nothing is better than having fresh eggs. Chickens are fairly easy to raise and are a nice addition to any homestead, small property, or big farm. Some towns have ordinances regulating where you can keep them. If you live in an area where you can have chickens, it's best to let them out in free-range conditions, where they'll pick at the ground, eat bugs, and keep themselves clean. They're low-maintenance. You don't need a rooster to have chickens produce eggs.

There are many different breeds including bantams, standard-size chickens, meat chickens, and laying hens, also called egg layers. I like to have Barred Rocks or Rhode Island Reds. They produce a large, brown egg. The white eggs you buy in the supermarket come from a chicken called a White Leghorn.

Laying hens provide an egg a day and are easy to keep. If you decide to hatch your own, they take 21 days. You can buy the eggs and incubate them. Set the incubator to 99.9 degrees. After they've hatched, you can raise them in a brooder. If you don't want to do that, simply buy them from Agway or a hatchery. I usually get them as day-old chicks at Murray McMurray Hatchery.

Once you get them, raise them in a small box with a heat lamp on them. As the chicks start to produce feathers, you can graduate them up into a bigger box with no light. Feed them chick starter until they become pullets, at six to eight months old. They start to lay eggs between nine and twelve months. Then you can keep them in a coop. They can stay in a six-by-eight area with a four-by-eight screen section, where they can go outside and pick on the grass, or you can let them out to free range.

I mentioned before that I use chicken manure to make my Kickaba Juice to grow giant vegetables. Their manure is high in nitrogen, which provides an incredible fertilizer for the garden. Chickens are also good for eating ticks on the property. Once you let them out in the morning, all they do is pick bugs and scratch. They'll eat many different types of insects.

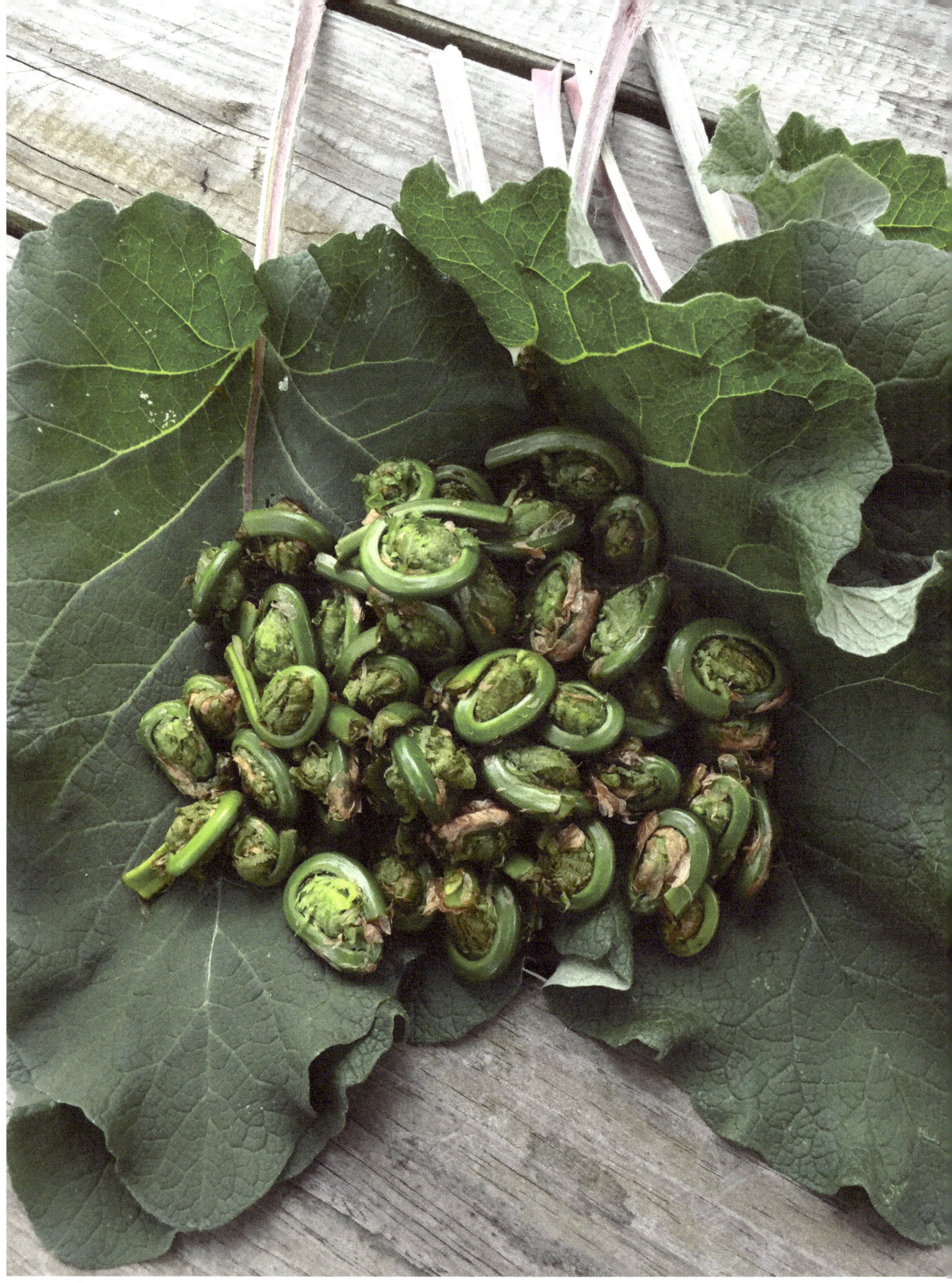

# Foraging

*"If you want to go foraging into the wilds of Canada without proper gear, you deserve what you get, even if that happens to include being attacked by an undead moose."*

**Mira Grant**

Going out into nature and gathering in its bounty is a terrific way to learn about our world. Foraging is how our earliest ancestors survived. The ability to live off the land has been the difference between life and death for many people, right up to the settlement of our own country. Today, it might not quite be a life-and-death situation, but you can greatly add to the nutrition and flavors you bring to your dinner table by walking through the woods and wetlands near where you live and finding wild foods that appeal to you.

When you gather food from the wild, you'll often find healthier alternatives than you would in the world of processed foods in the grocery store. Foods you forage for are usually richer in the vitamins and minerals that our bodies need. Also, you're embarking on a unique combination of hiking and gardening in your life. This is a healthy lifestyle for anyone. You're finding good food to eat and getting the exercise we all need more of these days.

I give some more general tips at the end of this chapter, but I do want you to think of a few basic concepts if you're new to foraging.

First, don't be afraid to find a mentor to help you get started. Foraging alongside someone who knows your area and the native plants is the quickest way to learn and avoid things that do not taste good or are bad for you.

Nothing can replace a mentor, but finding a good field guide comes close. A reference book illustrating plants and their pros and cons is something you should acquire and carry with you. You can use it for identifying plants in your area, and to show you nearby plants you haven't yet discovered. It can give you that motivation to seek out the natural edibles that you have yet to find.

As you decide on a field guide, make sure you use one with a wide variety of plants in your area. It should have clear photos so that you can identify a plant you find as well as information on when and where it grows. It should also be clear on just how "edible" a plant is. Unless you're foraging for pure survival, you aren't going to be interested in plants that taste like stale tree bark. You want what's delicious and a treat to the palate.

There seems to be an app for any subject. Plant apps will tell you a lot about a plant, including if it's edible. However, remember that if you're foraging out in the wilderness, or at least far enough from a cell tower, the app might be worthless to you. Good, old-fashioned books with photos aren't a bad thing.

*Left: Burdock and fiddleheads.*

*Page 122: Foraging for alpine strawberries on the sunny meadows; they're small but very flavorful!*

*Page 123: Wild asparagus with shiitakes in upper right-hand corner and morels.*

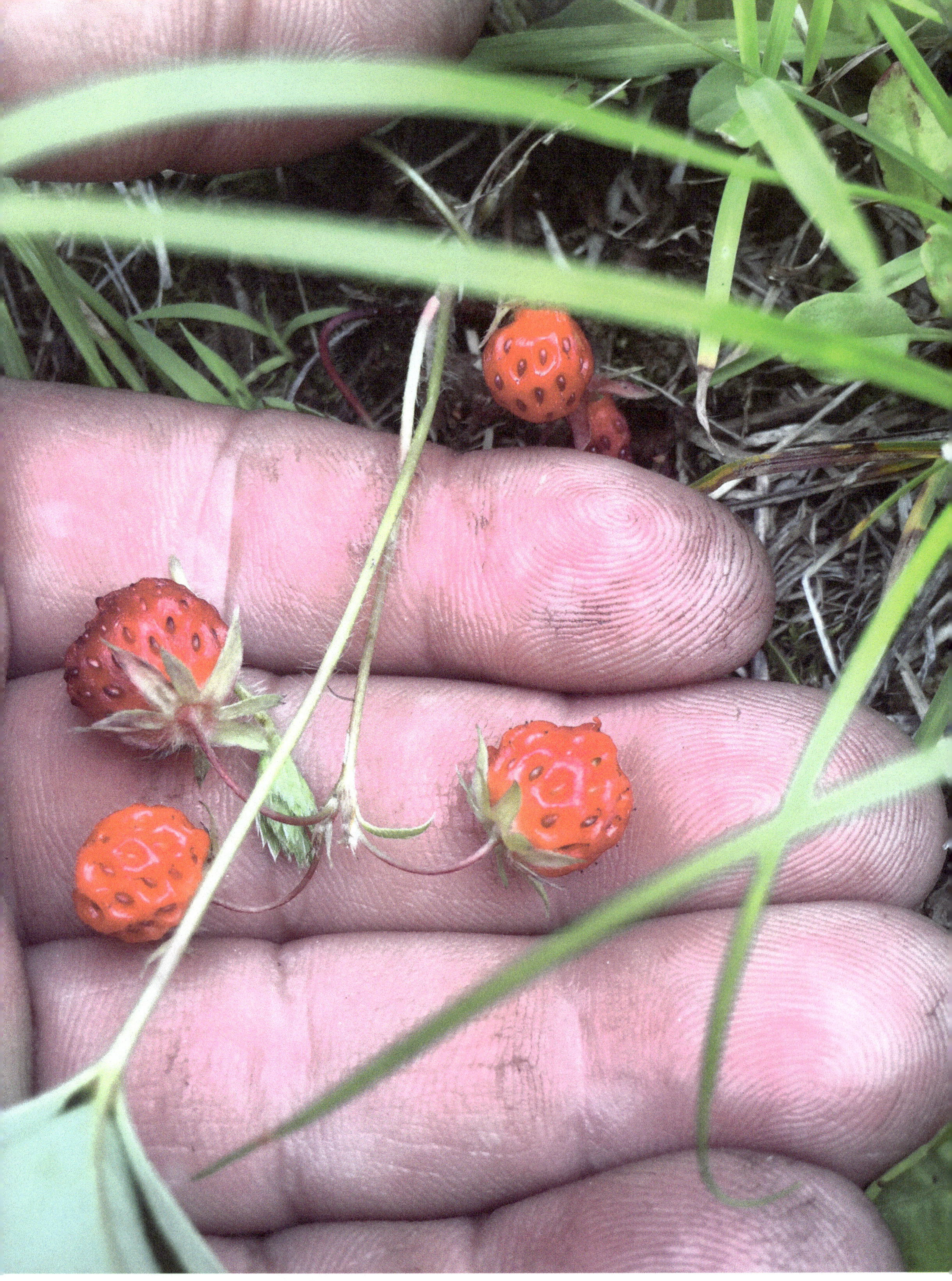

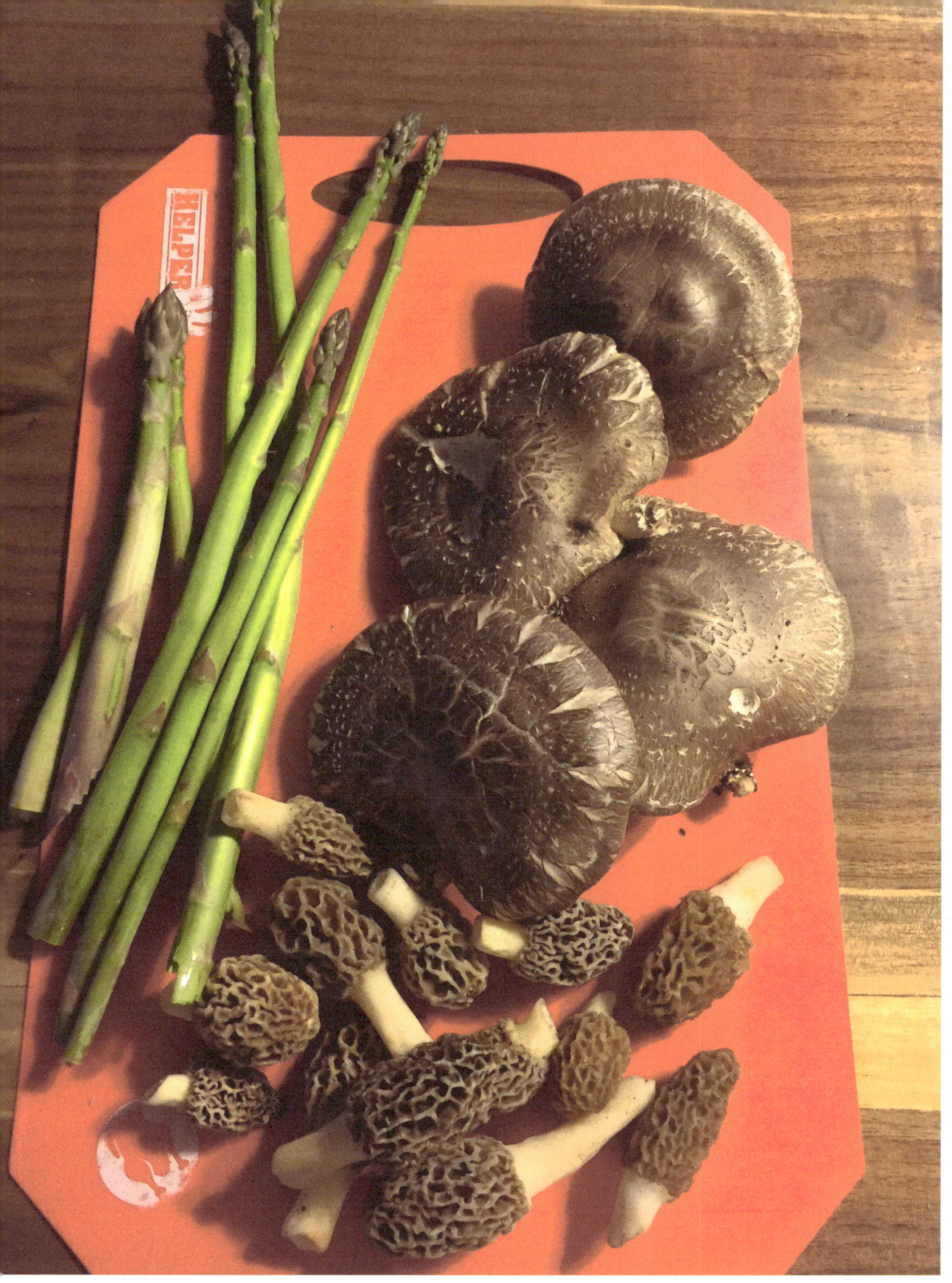
HELPER

I normally head out to begin foraging in the spring. I like to go out as soon as the weather breaks and the snow melts, with the ground beginning to thaw. On the sunny slopes on the south side of the pasture near me, I like to look for dandelions. They're one of the easiest plants to find, with their low-lying, bright yellow flowers giving them away. I grab my basket and pick the tender greens that emerge in the pastures among the clover. I cut the dandelion just below ground level, piercing it through the root.

For folks who tend their lawn with such care, dandelions are looked at as the enemy. Although people seek them out and attack them, they're of great value to nature and the ecosystem. They're rich in iron and very healthy to eat. They're also one of the first flowers of the season that bees focus on when gathering pollen.

I sauté them with some garlic, extra virgin olive oil, black pepper, and a little sea salt. They're also wonderful in salads. They tend to taste a little bitter, but you could always fix that with a bit of honey. While I'm not a winemaker, I do know people that make dandelion wine from the yellow blossoms.

Mustard greens also come up in the spring. They're one of the early plants to make an appearance in the season. These greens grow on the edges of fields and meadows, and they're easy to distinguish because of their tall height. They have a very peppery taste and are good steamed with olive oil and garlic. Mix them with a salad, or you can make a beautiful and tasty omelet with them using fresh eggs, parsley, and then adding the mustard greens.

As spring continues to progress, I enjoy picking fiddleheads, the small fronds that appear at the base of an ostrich fern. The fiddlehead resembles the curled ornamentation (called a scroll) on the end of a stringed instrument, such as a violin. It's also called a crozier, after the curved staff used by bishops, which has its origins in the shepherd's crook.

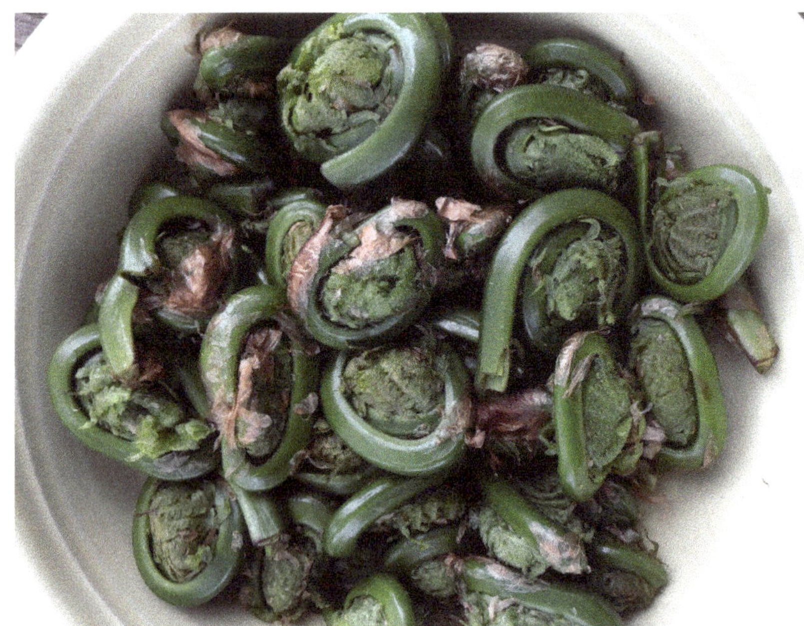

*Just picked fiddleheads.*

The ostrich fern grows along swamp edges and river streams. Fronds grow down at the crown of the fern in the early spring, generally in May. As you go down, you pick them while they're curled up, and then gather them in a basket. To prepare them, partly boil them and blanche them until they're fork-tender. Then place them in a bowl and add olive oil, balsamic vinegar, salt, pepper, and a little cumin. Chill them in the refrigerator.

They have a taste similar to asparagus. They're one of my favorites, and my family enjoys them every spring. Fiddleheads are also nutritious. They have antioxidant properties, are a source of omega-3 and omega-6 fatty acids, and are high in iron and fiber.

A good time to mark their territory is during the summer. When fully grown, the ostrich fern is easy to spot. It's one of the tallest ferns that grow in the woodlands. When you identify them, you can mark the area with a small piece of red flagging. When spring rolls back around, you know exactly where to locate them.

My father taught me to look for a particular plant when I was a child. He showed me how to pick it and where to find it. I think it's the most delicious plant you can pick in the woods. It's called burdock, or Italian carduni. It's a very big plant in the artichoke family. It has large, elephant-sized ears. It grows along sunny banks in the pastures, and you usually find it around farms. It grows a tall stem during the summer months and has circular, burrow-like seedpods that cling to your clothing. When we were kids, we used to pick them and throw them at each other. It was a fun game since they stuck to your clothes. It wasn't so much fun if they got in your hair, since they aren't easy to get out.

Burdock is very nutritional. It's rich in iron, as well as vitamin A, vitamin D, and vitamin C. This plant is harvested at the base of the root. You can also harvest the entire root, which is a very long taproot. Peel it and boil it, similar to a potato. All it needs is some salt and pepper, or another seasoning, to enjoy it.

I prefer to pick the stems. They look very much like celery when I'm done preparing them. I remove the leaves and cut them up into four-inch pieces. I blanch them in hot water until tender and then drain them. I put together an egg mixture with fresh parsley, fresh garlic, salt, and pepper. I dip the burdock stems in the egg mixture, coat them in breadcrumbs, and fry them in olive oil. They're a real treat for one and all. I've made them every year for the last 25 to 30 years.

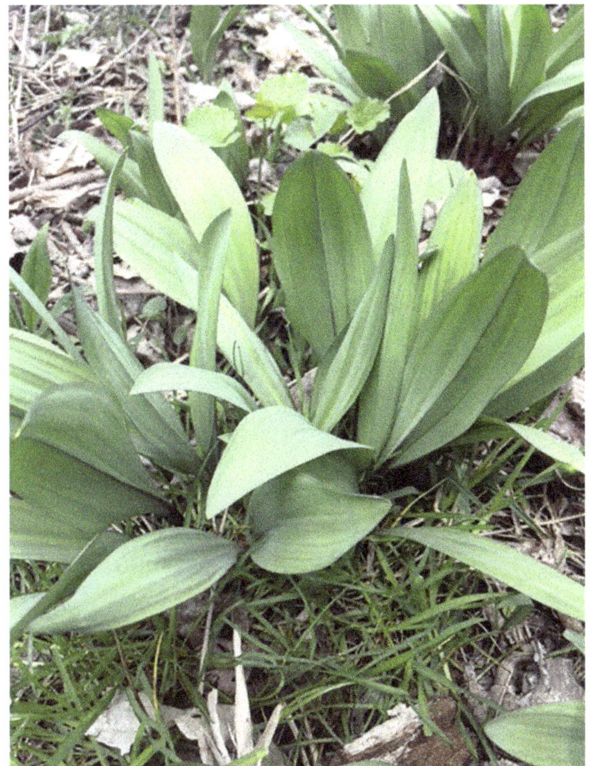

*Wild ramps.*

As summer approaches, I enjoy searching for and harvesting a few more plants. One is asparagus, another perennial plant. Many people don't know that asparagus grows wild, and it's delicious and sweet. I find a great deal of asparagus growing along the Hudson River. I pick them from certain areas and pockets every year. A feature of asparagus is that it produce seeds. Wind and animals spread them to different areas, where they will grow into new plants.

The asparagus is a wonderful plant in the fern family that you can enjoy in an omelet or steam, bake, or broil. They're easiest to identify in the summer. Once they come out of their fronds, they become tall, ferny-looking plants, with a lacy quality. When you do identify their location, mark those areas so you can come back the following spring to pick their tender shoots.

Ramps are another spring/summer plant I look for when foraging. They're a scallion-like leek with a sweet, oniony taste. They grow in abundance along the edges of swamps. You can harvest ramps with a small spade. Shake the dirt off and give them a quick rinse. You can store them in the fridge for a few days. Prepare them by sautéing, stewing, or even canning them for a longer shelf life. One option is preparing them as an omelet with fresh eggs, parsley, and black pepper. To prepare as a side dish, steam them with olive oil, garlic, salt, and pepper.

I do a great deal of trout fishing and use ramps by cutting them up with fresh parsley, adding some black olives, and stuffing them into the fish. Drizzle the brook trout with olive oil, sprinkle with paprika, and bake in the oven. Your taste buds will dance with the flavor.

In the early summer months, I forage for wild scallions. You'll find these plants in meadows and grassy areas. They're in the allium family, and you recognize them by their hollow, tubular stems and onion-like aroma. These wild scallions are even more flavorful than the ones you can buy from a nursery.

To harvest, snip them at ground level. To eat them, cut them into quarter-size pieces and allow them to dry on a piece of burlap or a few paper towels. Another option is to mix them with cream cheese for a delicious spread. Store them in a mason jar for future use.

I use the scallions in cooking. You'll find a great dish to add to your dinner table in the recipe section. I mix them with cilantro and mango. I add fresh wildflower honey to this scallion-mango-cilantro salsa and serve it over pan-seared salmon or trout.

## *General Foraging Guidelines*

There are definitely some important rules to abide by when foraging:

- Get to know your area. Learn the weeds, flowers, herbs, leaves, bushes, and trees in your locality. Educate yourself as much as possible about the environment where you live.
- It's important to know how to recognize the plants and fungi of your neighborhood correctly and know their uses. Look at everything as part of one big system. What plants do you notice usually growing with others? What tree is native to the area, or was it imported from somewhere else? Does a plant add to the nutrients in the ground or absorb what's there? Having this type of all-inclusive knowledge will help you understand how each tree, bush, etc. adds to the ecosystem of the area.
- Know any poisonous plants in the area. A great rule of thumb is that if you can't identify a plant, don't eat it! Better safe than sorry.
- Edible plants can be tricky. Be 100 percent certain you know what you're thinking about eating. There are edible and non-edible plants that can look eerily similar. Don't be fooled into getting sick.
- Practice good conservation. You should learn the endangered flora and fauna of your area. First, if they're illegal to pick, you shouldn't pluck them out of the ground anyway. If you're considering taking something that isn't endangered but is rare, don't take it all. In both cases, feel free to spread its seeds around for more to grow.
- Never take more of an edible plant than you need. Again, you don't want to deplete something from an area, and you want to be able to go back and find it in the future. This is especially true of any plant you take from the root. That usually means the plant will die. These plants should be plentiful in the area so they can continue to propagate even after you take what you want. If you aren't sure how much of the plant is around the area, it's probably best not to take any.
- Be aware of what happens in the zone you're searching in regards to insecticides, pollution, chemicals, industrial waste, etc. When those things go on the plant, they're going to end up in you to some degree. Washing plants only does so much. Many varieties of edible plants absorb those nasty things in the air and water.
- Consider the chemical angle with the soil where the plants are growing. You might be in a pristine area, but if you happen to find wild edibles growing in soil brought in from somewhere else, you have no way of knowing what that dirt contains regarding contamination.
- Avoid trying to collect plants from reserves and protected areas established by the government or other organizations. They're set up to protect what's in them. Often, a hefty fine is the penalty if caught.
- When you have the opportunity, throw seeds around from the native plants as a way of encouraging new growth. A true forager knows to give back to the earth whenever he or she can. You can even adopt a little section of wilderness and put it under your protection to help see that the native plants continue to thrive.

- Don't litter. Bring everything out that you take with you. Feel free to pick up after someone who isn't as conscientious as you.

Be careful when preparing your edibles:

- Thoroughly wash the sections of the plant you want to eat or use for cooking.
- When you're starting out, eat one plant at a time. Ideally, you should do no more than one new plant a day. You want to see what your body likes. If you eat more than one new thing at a time, you might have a reaction to one of them, but you won't know which one.
- A good idea is to rub the plant on your skin first. If your skin is fine, rub some of the plant on your lips. If that goes well, then eat a tiny piece of it. If there's no reaction from consuming it, then you should be good to go!

## *Harvesting Edible Plants*

Like any domesticated vegetable, grain, or fruit, you should only pick edible wild plants when they're at their peak flavor. It will take practice, but you'll learn that most wild edibles have their best times to be picked. It's something you can learn from reading about the plant you're interested in or through trial and error. A great deal depends on what part of the plant you're interested in utilizing and how you want to use it. You also want to be aware of when the vitamins, nutrients, and minerals are at an optimal level when you harvest the plant. Here are some general tips:

- Start to harvest a plant only when there's enough foliage so that the plant can continue to grow.
- It's best to pick your plants in the early morning before the dew evaporates as the day becomes hotter.
- When you harvest an edible plant before it flowers, its leaf production will continue to flourish.
- There's a small window of time after an edible plant's buds appear but before they open when they have the best flavor and concentration of its oils.
- Know the few poisonous species in your area. When you know the bad plants by sight, you'll feel more comfortable searching for the edible wilds in your area.
- This might sound too scientific, but learn plants by their Latin names instead of their common or local names. This way you can be very specific about a plant and identify it through your plant book. The Latin terminology can also help you identify certain poisonous plants, as they often have the same Latin words in their title. The Latin names for plants don't change, while the local names can over time.
- Don't limit yourself to identifying edible plants by eyesight along. Use your different senses. You can determine a great deal about a plant by how it smells and its texture. The one sense you don't want to use unless you're very sure about the plant is taste. Even a small bit of certain plants can make you extremely sick or worse.
- Learn where different plants grow. A plant that grows in the hills and the woods isn't going to thrive in a wetland. This knowledge will help you identify a potential area for the plant you're looking for in the wild. You won't be wasting your time looking somewhere that it just won't grow.
- It also pays to learn what plants commonly grow with others. When you know plants and their companions, it makes the detective work of finding what you want a little easier.

- Understand how the look of edible plants changes throughout the seasons. In this way, you know when they're at their peak, or if they're past their prime. It also enables you to find a plant when it's first growing so you know when it will be in season. For perennials, you can mark the location and come back to them next year too.
- Even if something is an edible plant, that doesn't necessarily mean you can eat the entire plant. Certain plants have good things you can eat off it while other parts of it are downright dangerous. Again, study your resources when selecting what parts of a plant you want to harvest.

## *Supporting Foraging*

- Be sure not to take more than you need. If you take every type of an edible plant, it's going to take a while for it to grow in the area again. Don't over harvest. No wild edible is unlimited. Even if there seems to be a plentiful supply of a certain species, try to limit yourself to a harvest of 10 percent or less of the available plants. Again, only take what you will use.
- Be careful of foraging for rare edibles. There might seem to be enough in the area where you're looking, but that might be it for the entire range.
- If you only want to use certain parts of the plant, only collect them. If you need leaves, pluck them off. There's no need to uproot the entire plant. A general recommendation is not to take more than 25 percent of a plant if you aren't harvesting the entire thing.
- There's nothing that says you can't grow wild edibles in your garden at home. Many edible plants are great at being transported and thriving where you plant them. As you would for any other vegetable or fruit you cultivate, make sure the conditions you prepare are conducive for the plant you want to raise. This is also a way to help increase the population of the scarce plants in your area. With renewed awareness of foraging wild edible and medicinal plants, growing them in your garden will help preserve their numbers.

## *Safety*

- Keep away from toxic areas, whether due to too many pesticides or industrial pollution. We still have too many areas like this. Stay away from busy roads for your foraging adventures, as the plants absorb the toxic properties from vehicle exhaust.
- As you look for wild water plants, know the condition of the water where they grow. Eating a plant from contaminated water is as bad as drinking a glass of the stuff. Many toxins can get into plants through its water source that can't be taken out by washing or cooking.
- If a plant doesn't look healthy, it probably isn't. Pick the robust plants, and you'll save yourself from the disease, insects, pollution, or toxins that affected a sickly plant.
- Pay attention to where you forage. If you're on private land, ask for permission. While not exactly a safety issue, you need to observe the laws of public lands and be respectful of private property.

## *Get Better at Foraging*

- Like most skills, the more you forage, the better you'll get at it. Every time you go out, concentrate on finding a new edible plant as you're looking around. As you find something new, learn all you can about its nutritional and medicinal properties. The more you know, the better your search efforts will be.
- As a forager, you're one of the safeguards to be a guardian of our planet. Be on the lookout for plants that are vanishing or in danger and do what you can to reverse the situation. We want the earth to continue providing sustainable foraging for many, many years to come.

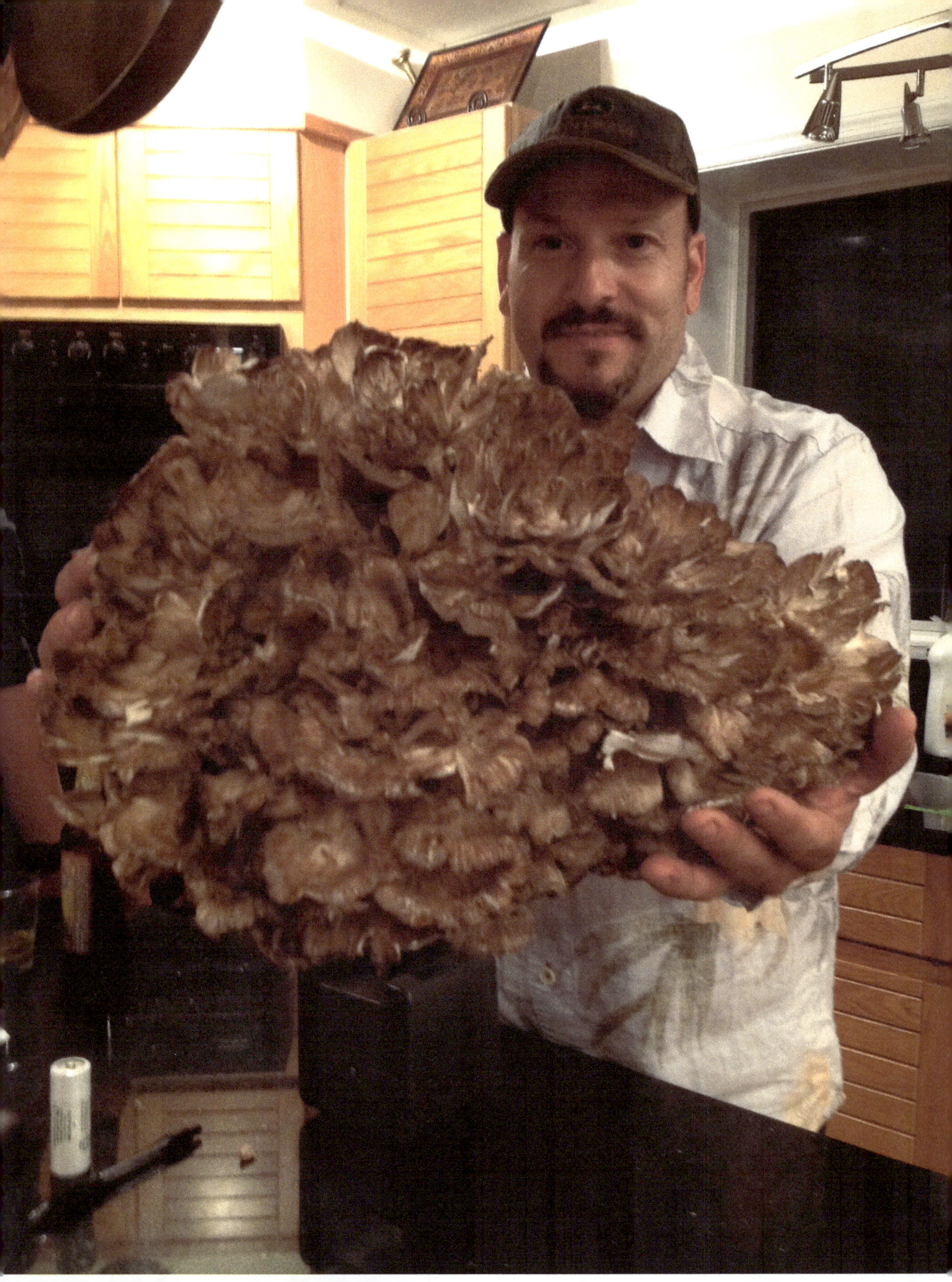

# Mushrooms

*"Mushrooms are miniature pharmaceutical factories, and of the thousands of mushroom species in nature, our ancestors and modern scientists have identified several dozens that have a unique combination of talents that improve our health."*

**— Paul Stamets**

## *Chanterelle*

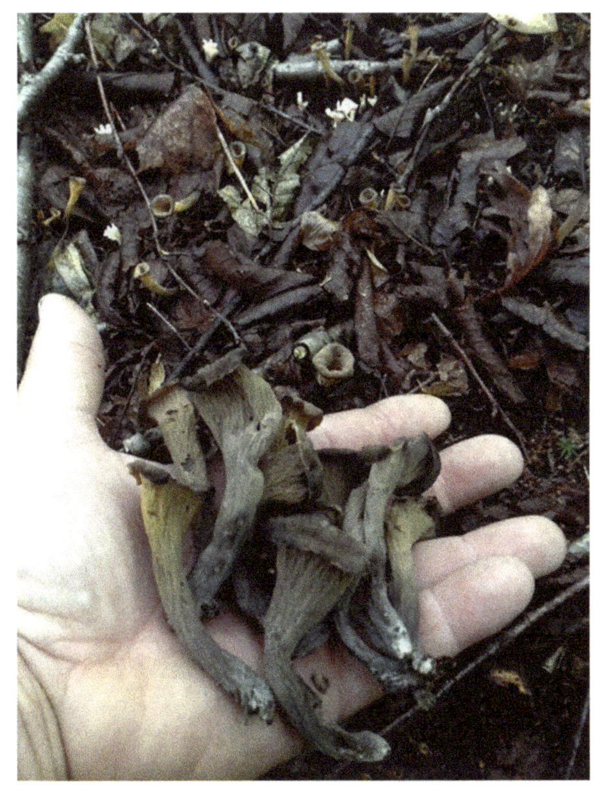

Much of the wild plants I talked about in the last chapter are found in pastures or near wetlands. There's also a great deal of tasty vegetation in the hilly areas. I head into this type of terrain around mid-June looking for a particular fungus. (While "fungus" might not sound appetizing, this scientific designation contains plenty of great eating selections.) The fungus I look for is chanterelle. They grow abundantly amongst the birch and hemlock canopy. These are highly prized by my palette and my family. I've been picking them for several years in abundance, and I usually mark my territory at a little log where I know they grow, as they emerge year after year.

It's a good idea to carry a field guide with you when foraging, especially with fungus. Chanterelles come in several different colors. Black chanterelles, or black trumpets as they're also known, grow in clusters. You'll find them below birch trees, especially the black birch. They're the most flavorful of mushrooms. The small black trumpets that emerge from the soil grow level with the leaves that form the ground cover. This means they're camouflaged and hard to distinguish at first. However, once you see them, they seem to jump at you.

You harvest the chanterelles by snipping them at the base. You might want to bring a big basket with you because you can pick them in abundance. It's not unusual to walk out of the woods with several pounds of black trumpets. Once you get home, lay them out on a small table next to a small fan or near a

*Left: Getting ready to clean foraged hen of the woods and put in jars for winter.*

*Above: Just harvested black trumpet.*

breezy window so they'll dry out within a few days. Store them in a mason jar with a folded paper towel that acts as a dehumidifier for any extra moisture that might remain in them. I use them in a lot of my recipes, including one I'll share that includes shrimp and scallops.

I pick other chanterelles that grow amongst hardwood maples and under a mixed canopy of birch. Their cone and vase-shaped appearance plus their bright yellow color give them away on the forest floor. I also pick these from the base but do not dry them. I cut them up into small pieces and use them fresh, or I freeze them. They pair well with poultry. I cook them with rosemary, black pepper, butter, olive oil, and fresh shallots.

I also blanch them with water mixed with white vinegar, which is a preservative. I place them in a jar with fresh oregano, garlic, mint, and olive oil. Doing this extends their shelf life, and I can continue to enjoy them when they're out of season.

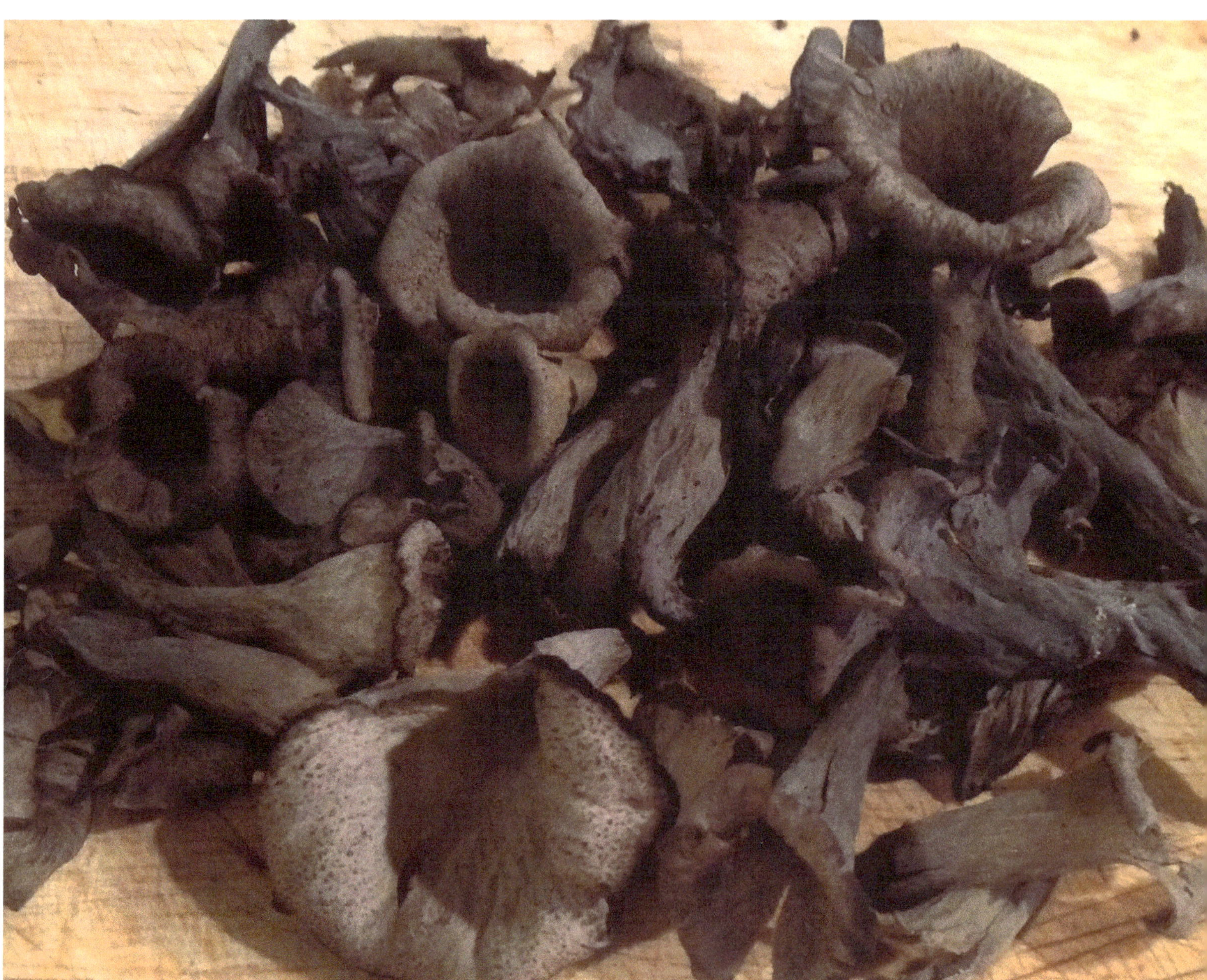

*Black chanterelles, or black trumpets as they're also known, grow in clusters.*

## *Morels*

Morels are another one of my favorite mushrooms from early in the season. They're highly prized and greatly enjoyed by my family and me. I usually pick them in abundance if Mother Nature cooperates and the weather is ideal. They're commonly an earlier producing mushroom that comes up in late spring and early summer. I can find them from May right up until the end of July. These might be the most popular mushrooms people forage for across the United States. This mushroom has a small, cylindrical, conical shape, and if you stand one upright, it looks somewhat like a piece of coral you'd find in the ocean.

Morels only grow in certain areas. You'll find them where the wood has burned, as with forest fires. They emerge after the ash has disintegrated into the soil. What's one of the best indications that you're in an area with morels? When you walk into a mature woodland of hardwood trees, look for some dying or decaying trees, like elms that have succumbed to Dutch elm disease. Look for skeletal trees. Elms tend to lose and shed their bark while they're still standing, and it's very easy to determine in the spring if a large tree that's standing upright is dead. I get excited when I see the unfortunate circumstances of a dead tree, because I know that I could reap the bounty and the beauty from below.

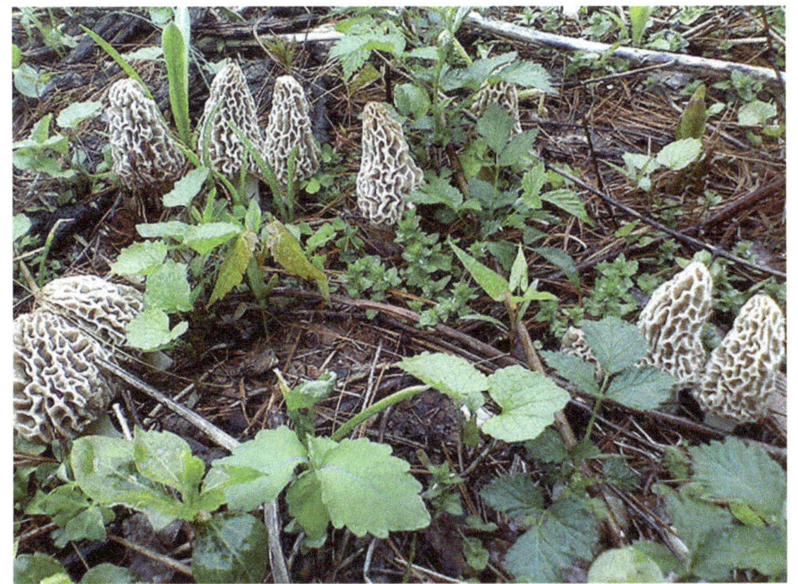

As I approach a dying or dead elm tree in the spring, I walk carefully, not wanting to disturb or to crush any of the morels that may be lurking below. When I notice a few of the morels poking through some of the leaf matter, I reach down and start to harvest them. Once I have them all, I make sure I check off the area in my mushroom logbook. This way I know where to come back the following spring because morels will continue to grow until the tree completely disintegrates.

I've also found morels under dead or dying ash trees. Remember, they do camouflage themselves on the forest floor, so you need to tread carefully through the ground cover to find them. Overall, I have my best luck locating them under ash and elm trees.

*Top: Just harvested basket of blonde morels.*

*Bottom: Nice find of blonde morels under a stand of dead elms.*

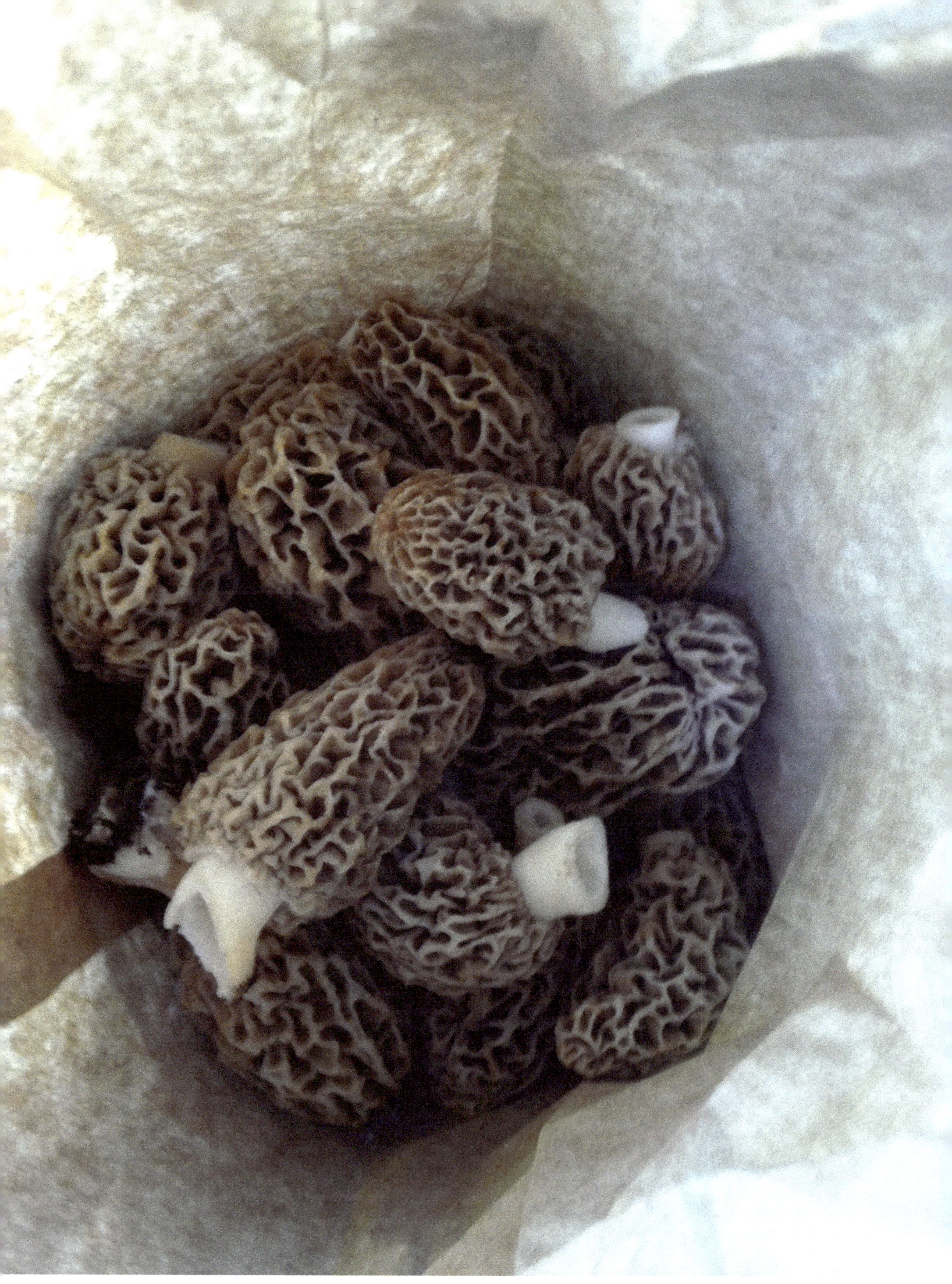

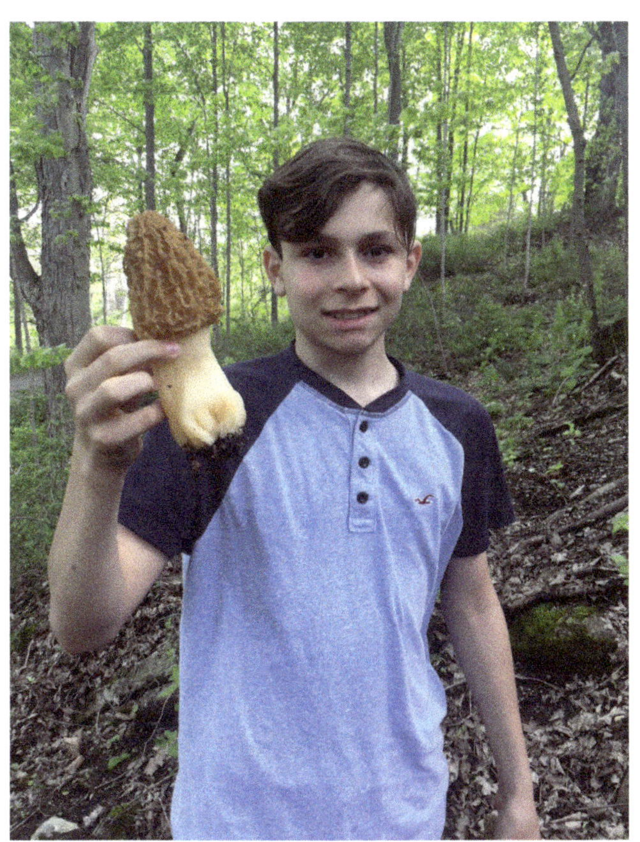

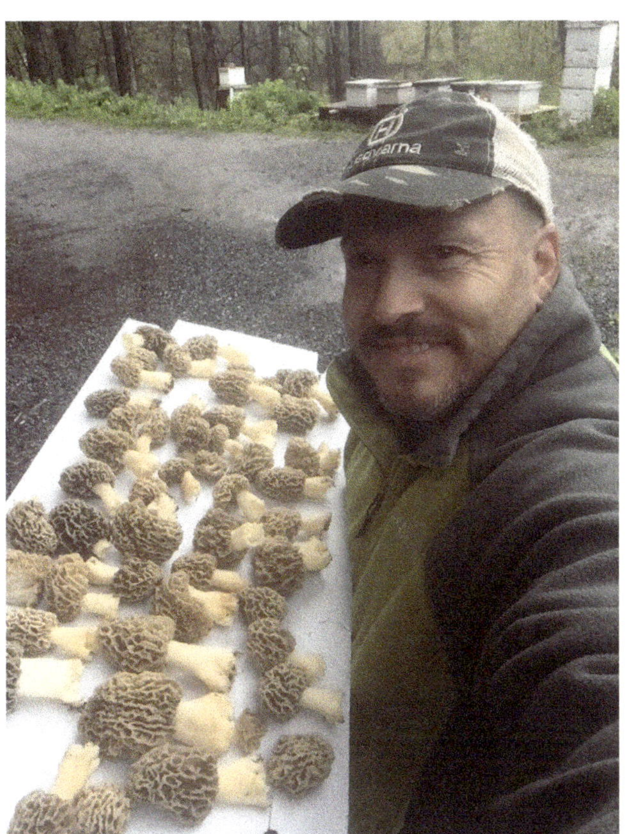

*Left: Fresh picked morels.*

*Above: Julian with giant blonde morel and a nice spring harvest.*

*Page 136 and 137: Father and son giant blonde morels.*

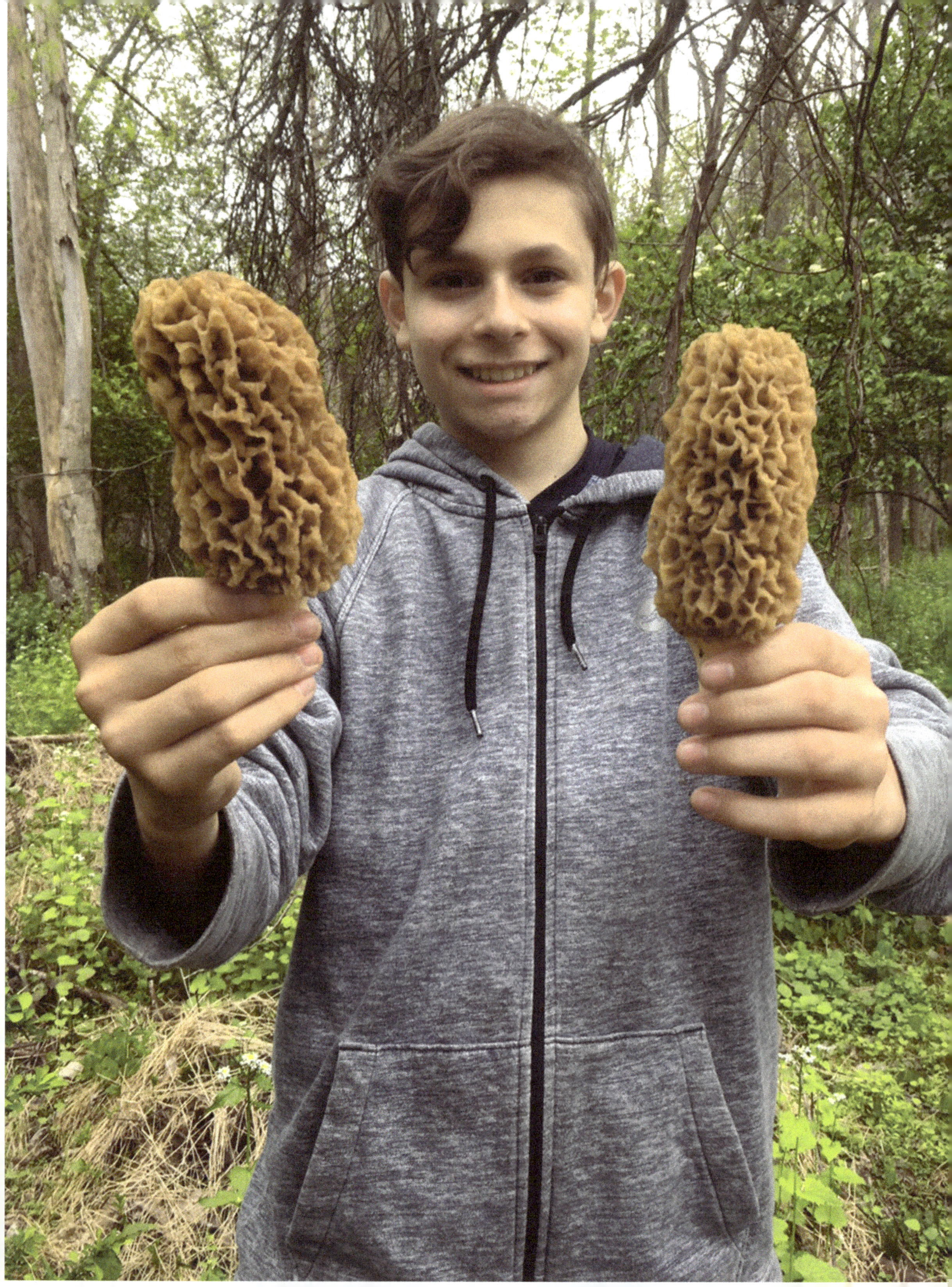

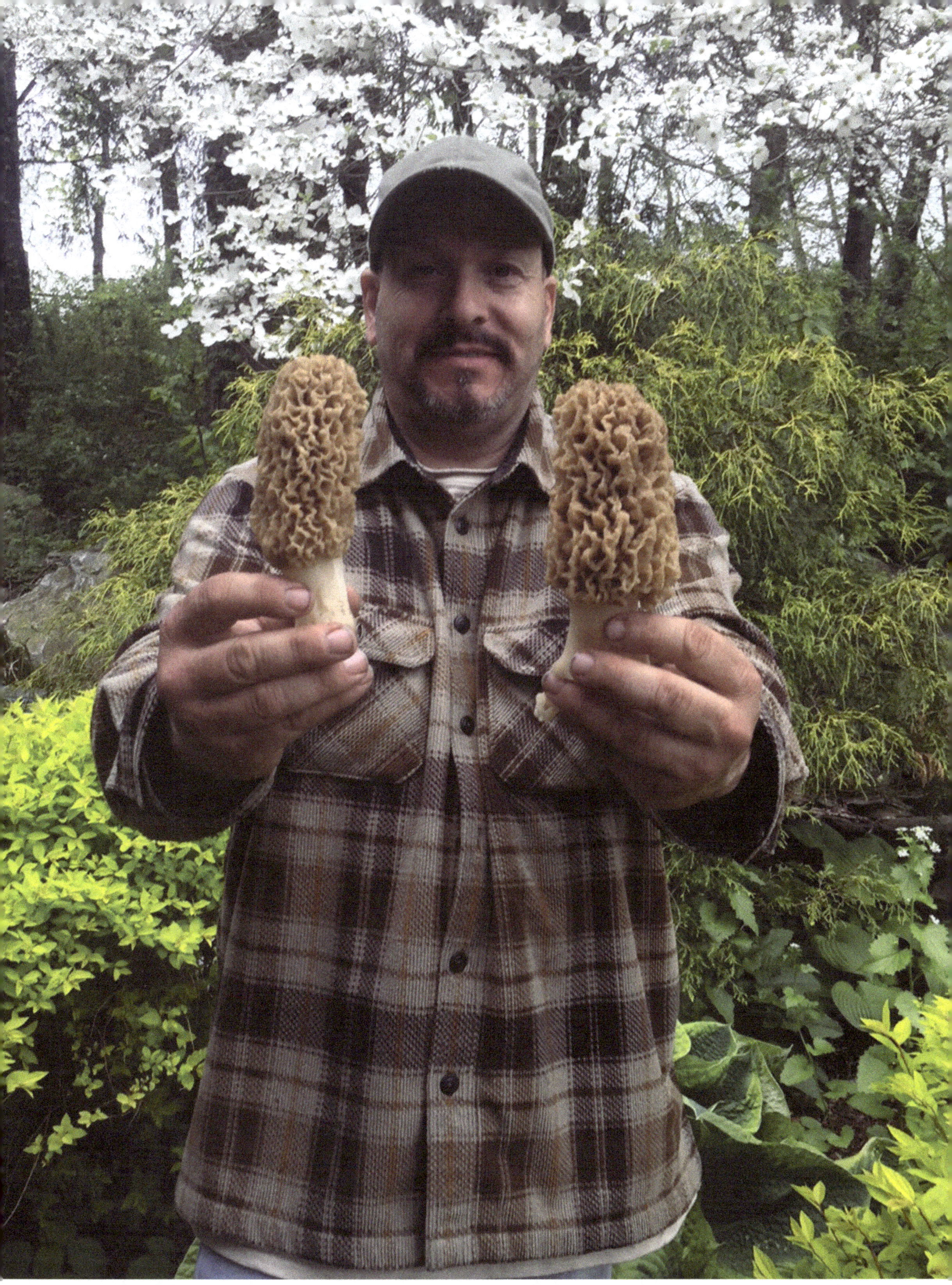

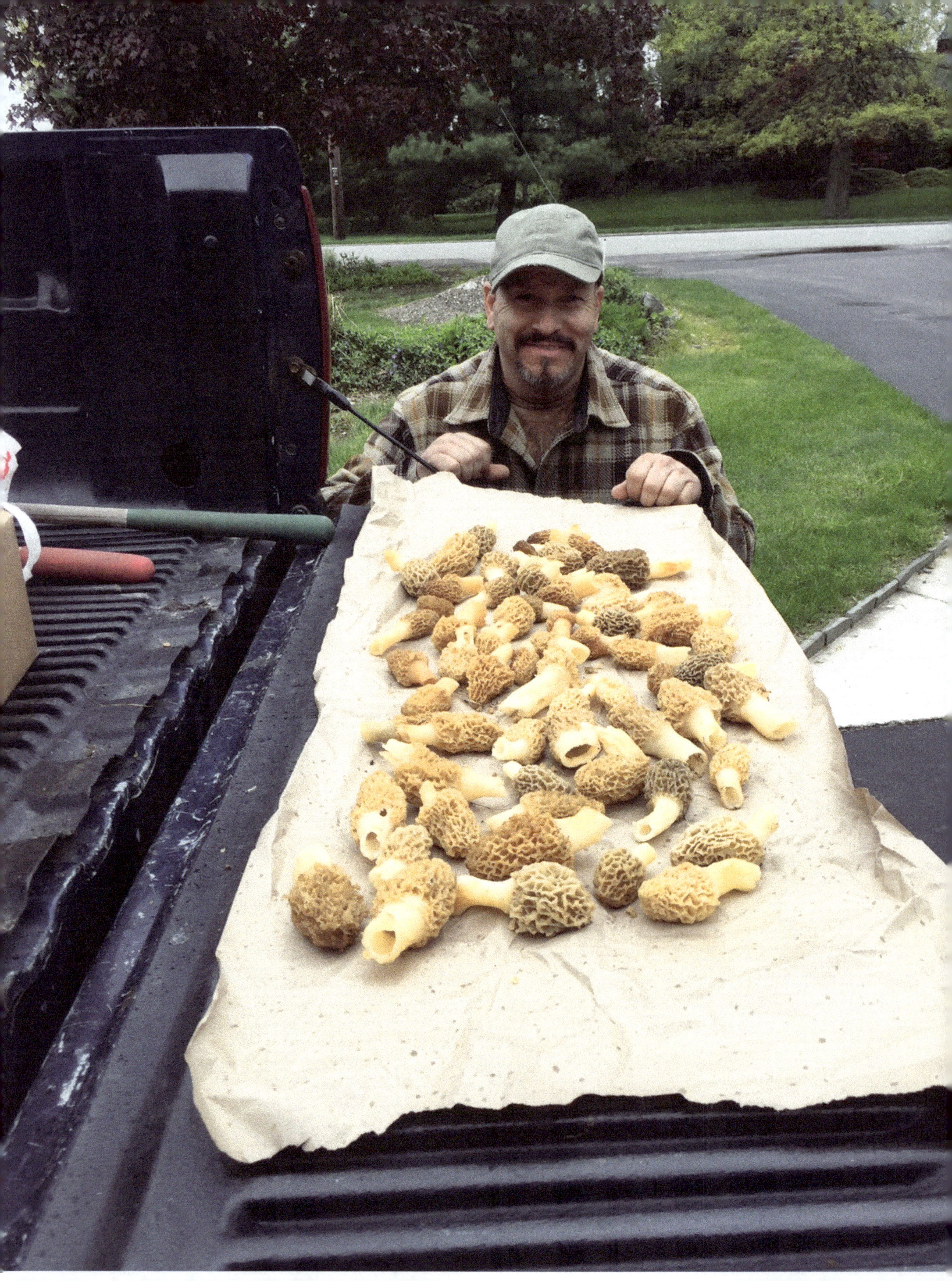

## *Phoenix Oyster*

As the season progresses, we get into July and August. During this time of year, I look for another mushroom, called the Phoenix Oyster, which grows about midway up dying maples. It can also be found on black birch and poplar trees. Like the morels, I pinpoint the locations where I find these mushrooms because they'll continue to emerge every year until the tree has completely deteriorated.

The oyster mushroom is cream colored, stacked against each other, and delicious to eat. It's also a good mushroom to jar or freeze. I enjoy cooking oyster mushrooms several different ways. I like to slice them up and cook them with Marsala wine, butter, olive oil, salt, and pepper and serve them with chicken. Basically, I'm making a chicken marsala with them. Another way that I prepare them is to blanch them in hot water and take them out when they're fork-tender. I then mix them with some virgin olive oil, balsamic vinegar, oregano, fresh mint, and garlic. I toss them in a salad and enjoy them with some fresh greens.

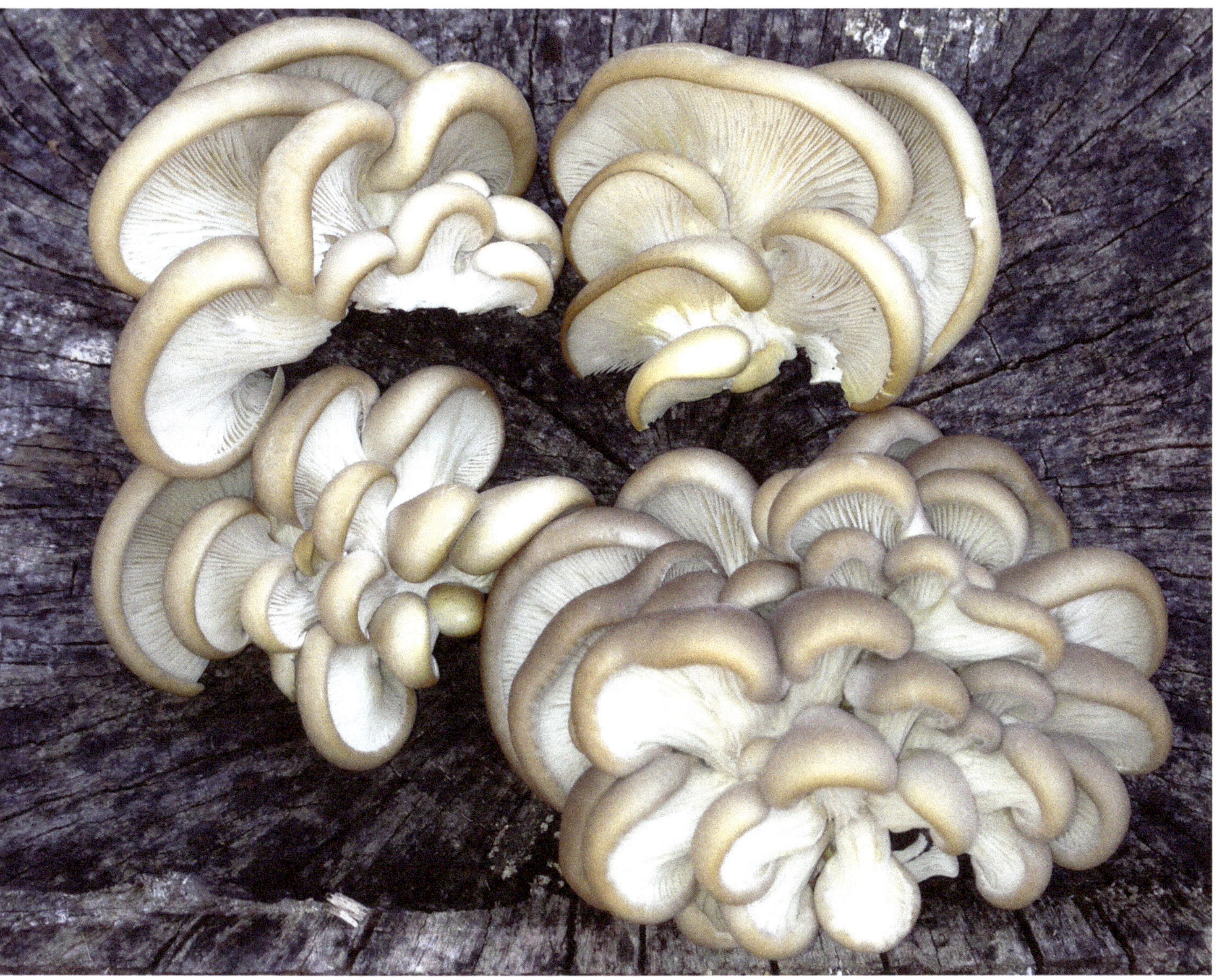

*Page 138: A good spring morning — over 50 morels.*

*Above: Just harvested Phoenix Oysters.*

## *Chicken Mushroom (Sulphur Shelf)*

I pick another mushroom this time of year known as the Sulphur shelf or the chicken mushroom. Many chefs and foragers prize this mushroom. You can distinguish it easily by its bright yellowish-orange appearance. It grows on hardwood trees, particularly oak. Its appearance is like the oyster mushroom, but much brighter orange in color. You pick the chicken mushroom when it's tender and young. Sautéed or stewed, it can be prepared similarly to the oyster mushroom. Gather these when they're young, because once they become mature, they tends to get a little woody and not very flavorful.

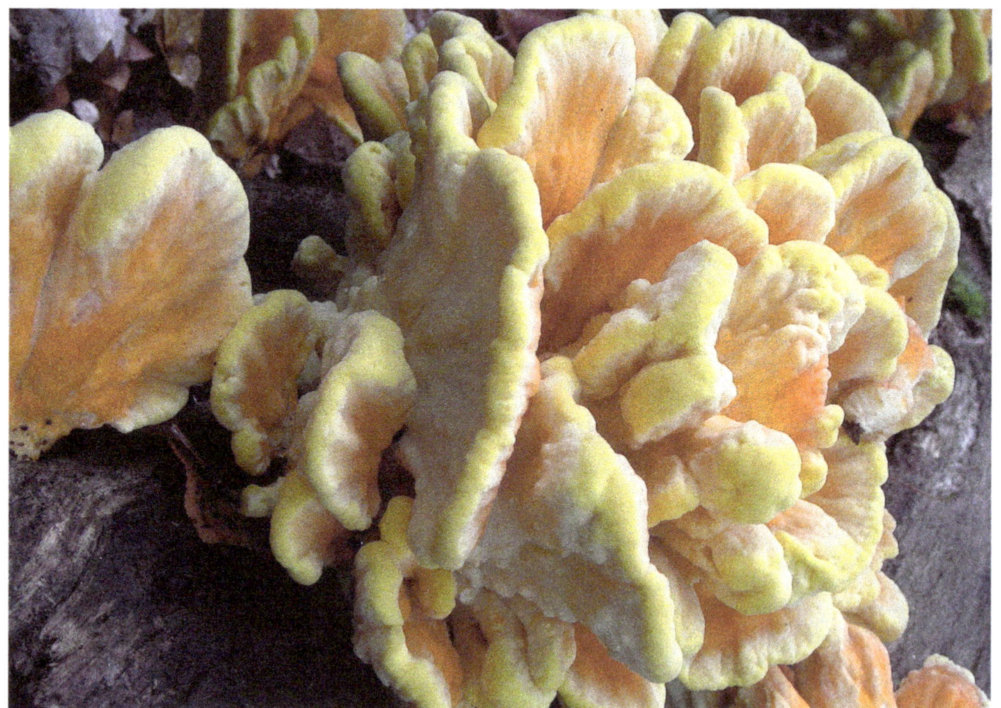

## *Maitake Mushroom (Hen of the Woods)*

One of my favorite mushrooms comes out in the autumn, depending on the weather and the rainfall. It is the maitake mushroom, which also goes by the name of hen of the woods. My father showed me how to find these mushrooms when I was just a little boy. We would go into the woods looking for them. A few times he had to use his jacket to carry this mushroom because it was so heavy and the bags we brought wouldn't hold it!

This mushroom grows throughout the United States, as well as China and Japan. When people from those lands find them, they do a dance around them with excitement. Well, to tell you the truth, I do as well! It's a very versatile mushroom that freezes well, can be dried, and made into a tincture or powder. This mushroom has many beneficial vitamins and minerals that are extremely healthy for you. To me, they're worth their weight in gold.

The hen of the woods is found mostly on mature, downed oak trees, particularly black oaks and white oaks, although other downed trees can host them. The way I find these mushrooms is to look for bigger, mature canopies of oak trees. Usually, they're on very large oak trees.

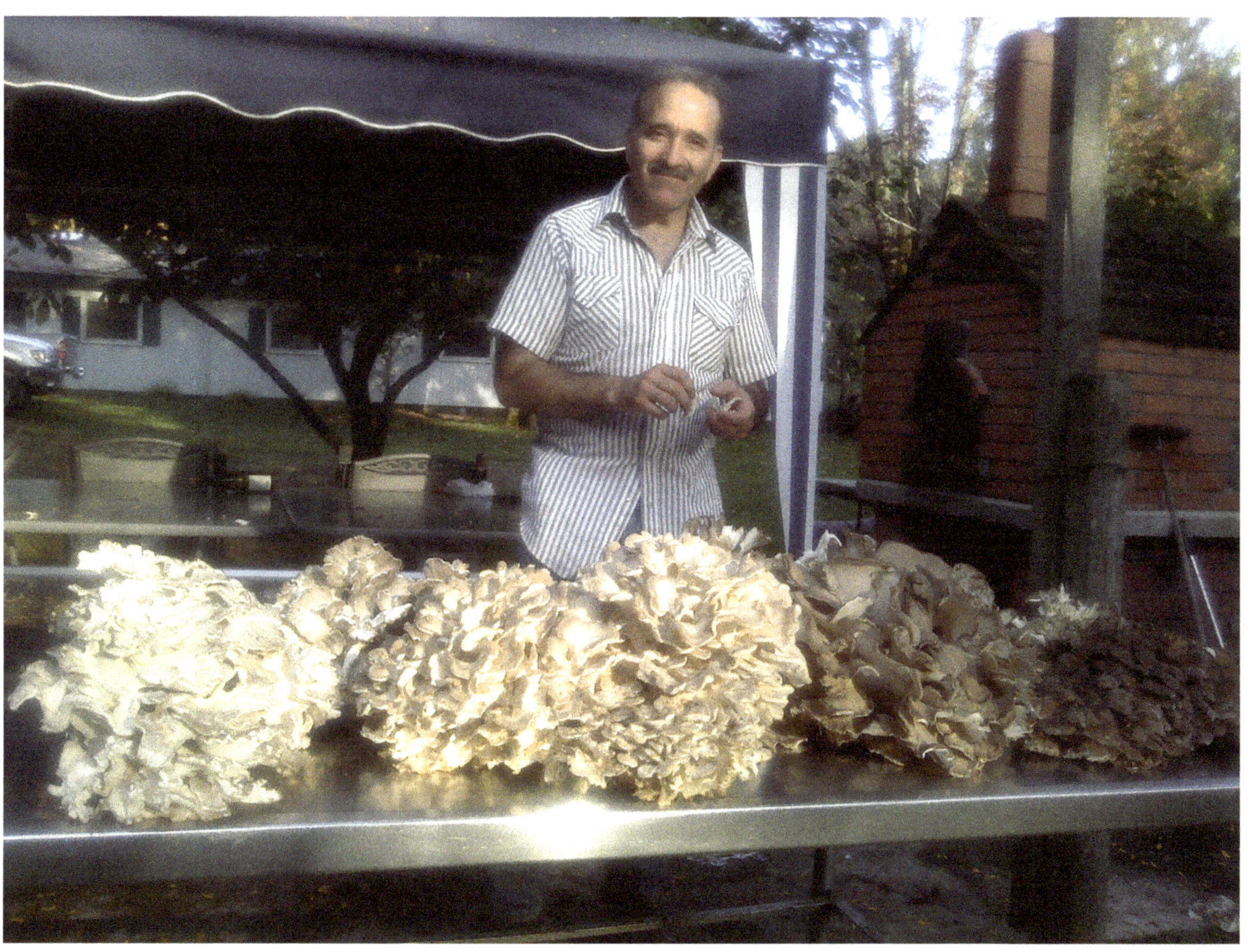

*My brother John with 100 pounds of hen of the woods to be processed.*

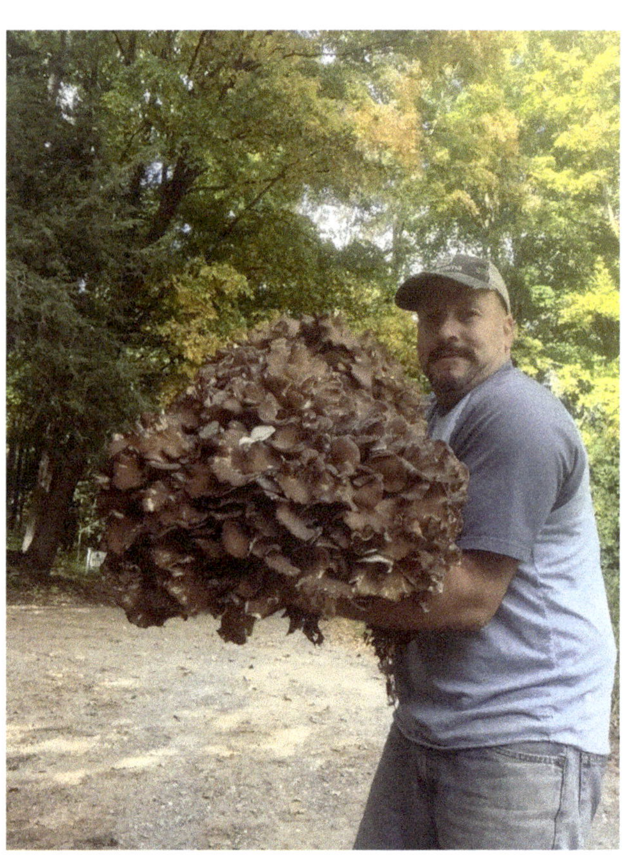

When I find one, I map it and mark it in my logbook. You harvest the mushroom by cutting it from the base, leaving some of it there to regenerate some spawn and spores for the next year.

The spawn produces different colors. Sometimes they're blonde, while others are brown. There's no look-alike for this mushroom, so it's very easy to distinguish its appearance.

When the time is right, which is usually in October, they seem to be fruiting nicely. I first go to the trees I've marked in the past. I check each and every one of them. Sometimes, I find new ones along the way.

I blanch them in water and white vinegar. I then pack them into a jar and add a dressing. The dressing is a combination of fresh garlic, mint, oregano, olive oil, a little piece of cayenne pepper, and apple cider vinegar. I pack the mushrooms into the dressing and put them into jars. I boil the jars for 15 minutes. In this way, I have mushrooms I can use throughout the winter. It's delicious and it keeps for almost two years.

*Above: My largest hen of the woods to date, at 65 pounds.*

*Page 143: Just harvested hen of the woods.*

*Page 144: Jarred hen of the woods.*

*Page 145 and 146: King stropharia giant wine caps. This mushroom is found in Europe and North America.*

*Page 147: Beautiful bicolor bolete mushrooms found in July under some black birch trees.*

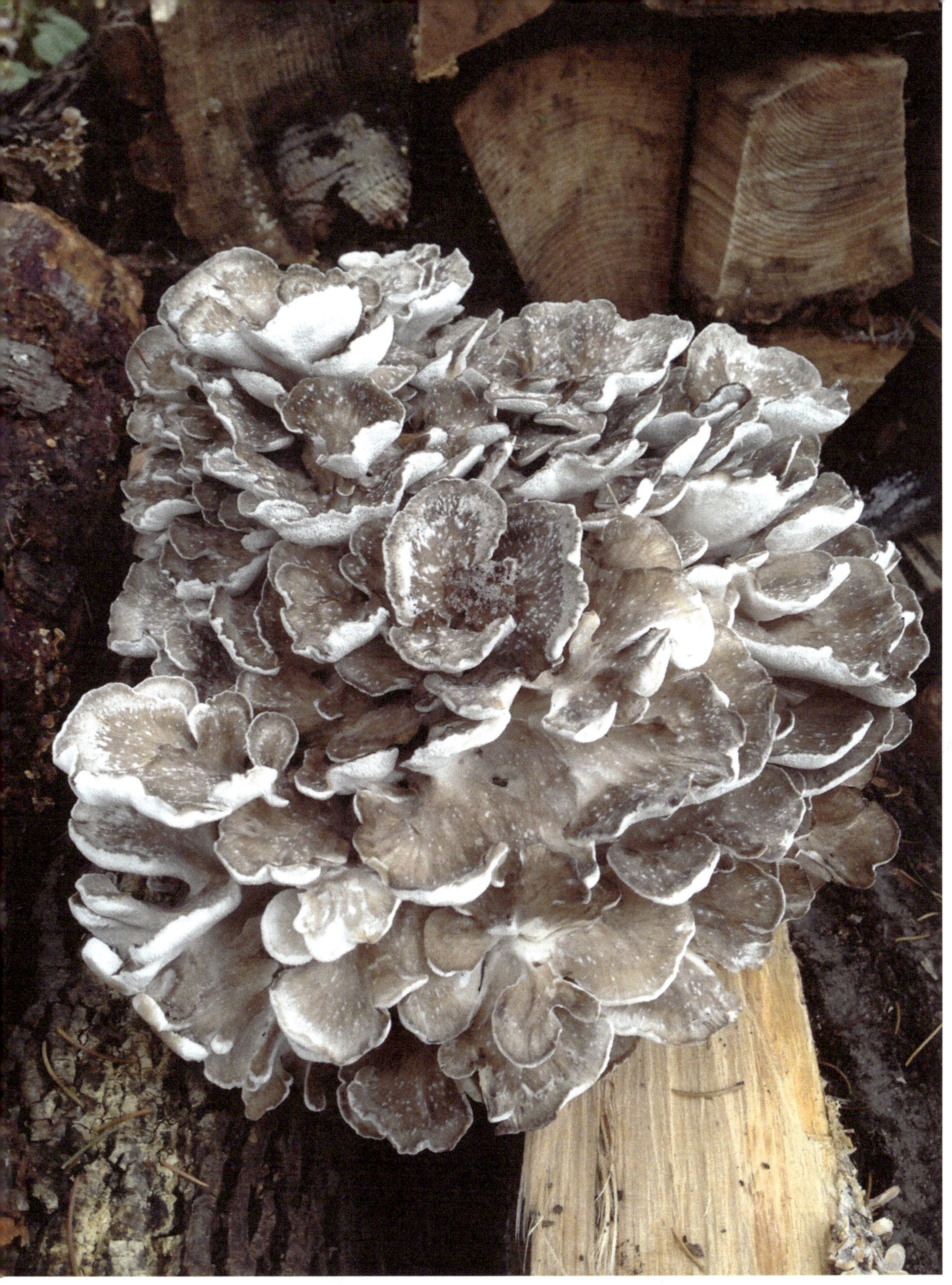

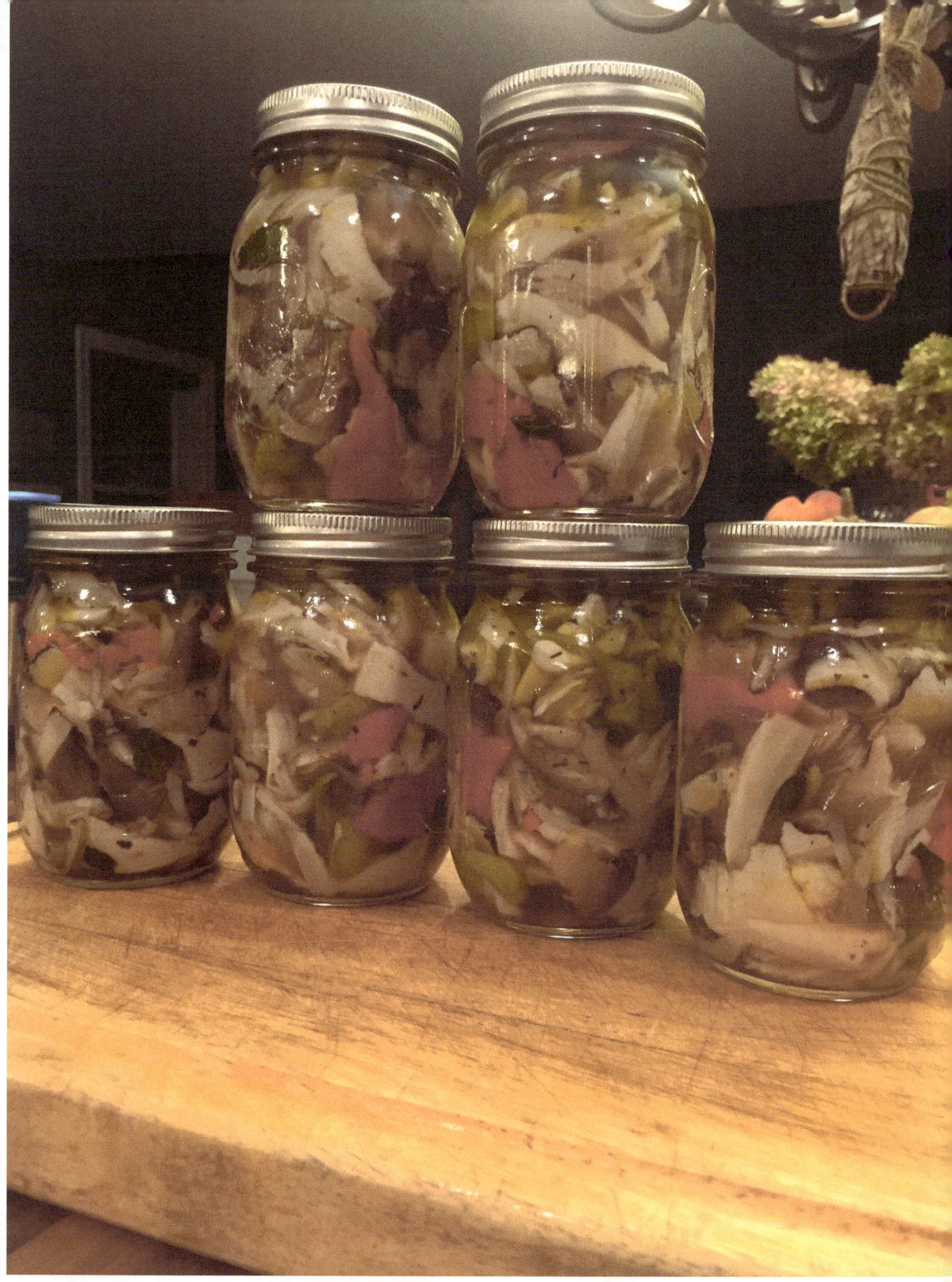

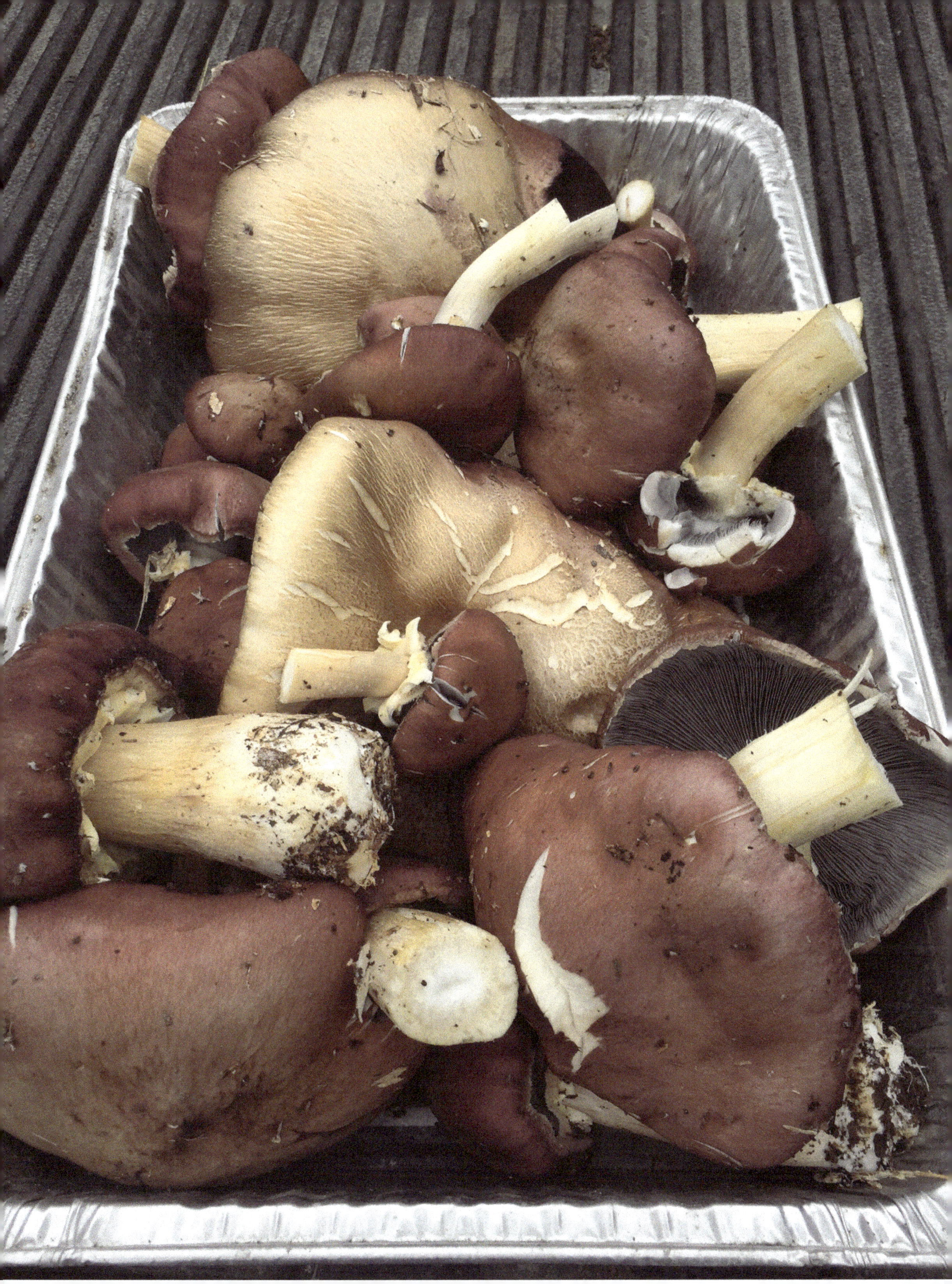

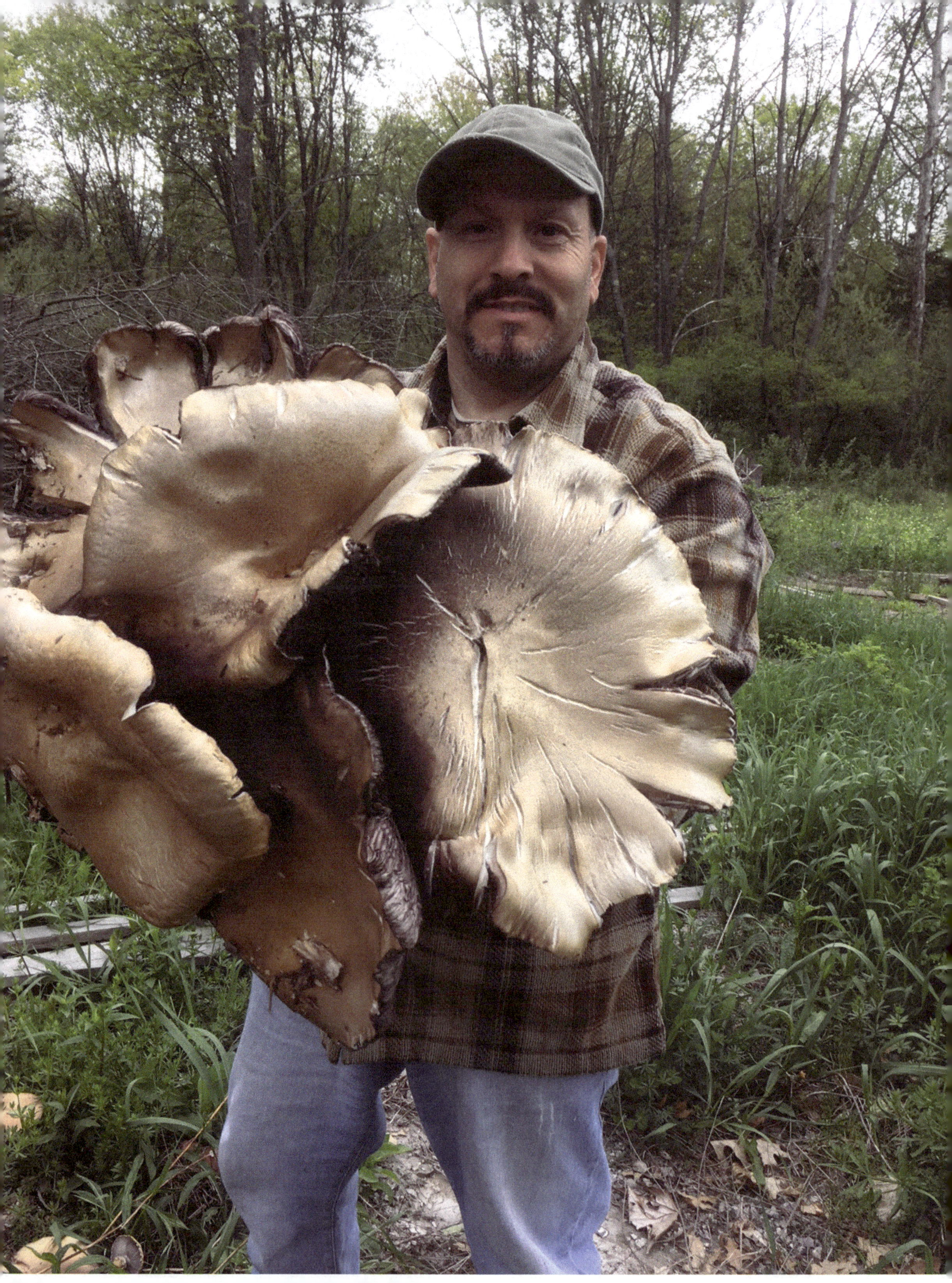

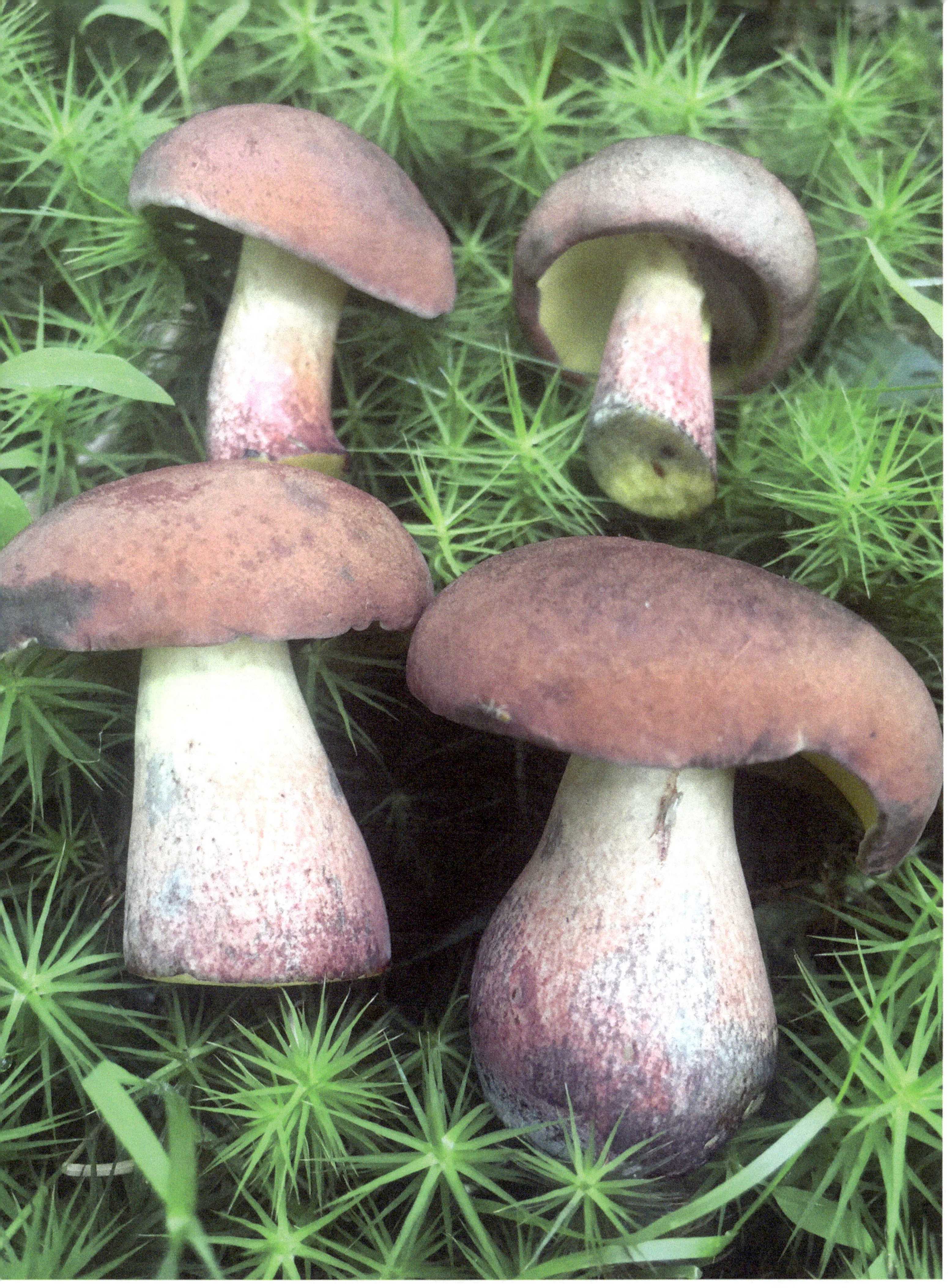

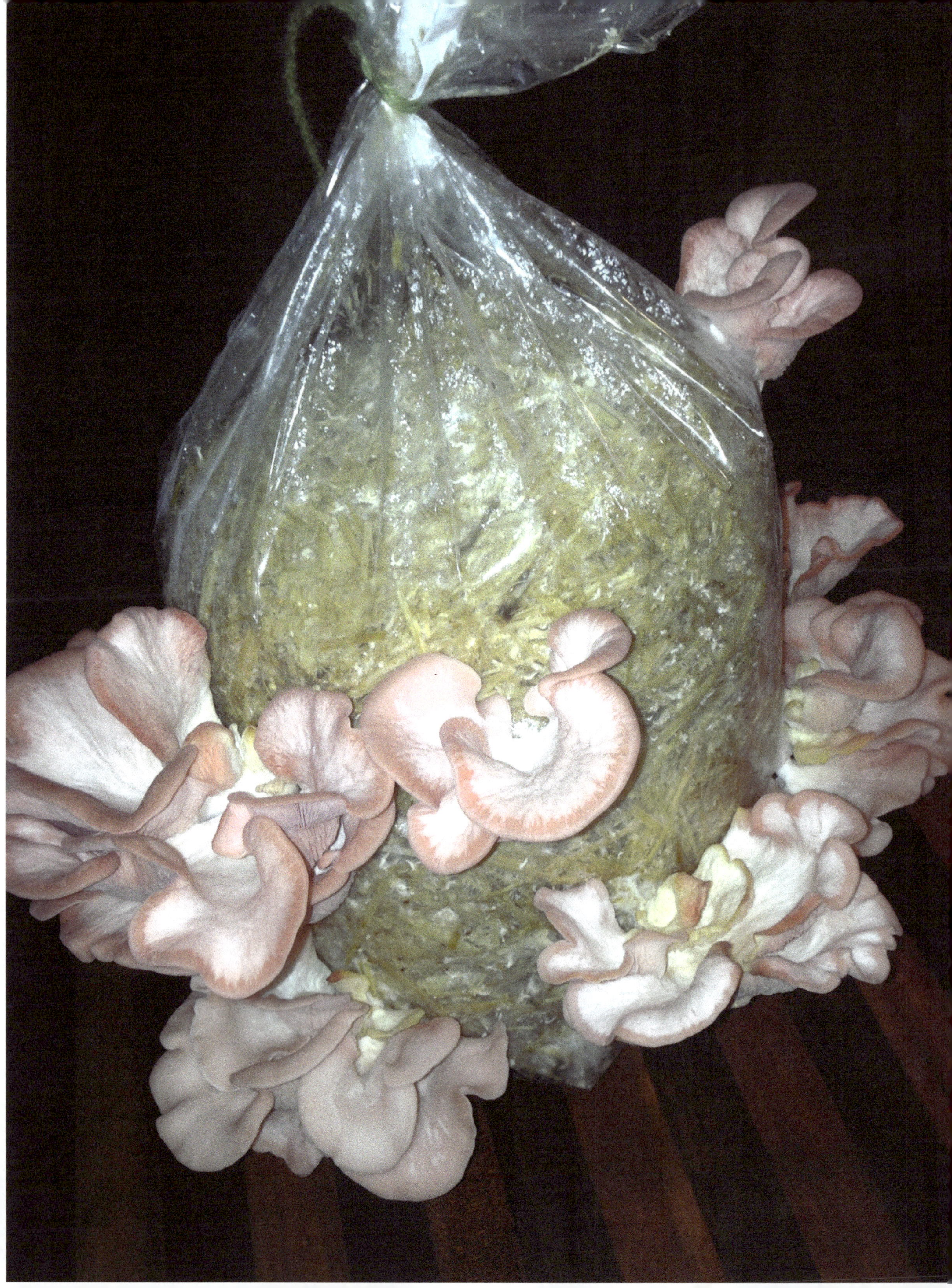

## *Growing Mushrooms*

While I love mushroom foraging, I also like to grow some of my own. The ones I've grown with great success and little effort are oyster mushrooms. You can purchase the spawn from different suppliers. They sell a large variety of different mushroom spawn, but the one that I like to use is Fungi Perfecti. You can also order some sterile plastic bags, and go to the local Agway or garden supply store to buy a bale of straw. You take the straw and boil it in small amounts to pasteurize it. Next, place the pasteurized straw into the plastic bags, add some spawn, close the bag with a tie, and let it rest for a week until the mycelium starts to grow among the straw.

You know the mycelium is starting to grow when it covers the straw and turns it white. You then prick the bag with a small paring knife and place it in diffused, indirect sunlight on a windowsill. Soon, it will start to fruit beautiful oyster mushrooms. I've grown a few different varieties such as pink ones and brown ones. They're very tasty, and they mature fairly quickly. You can enjoy them fresh, but they also freeze well, and you can put them in a jar in a similar way to what I did with the hen of the woods.

One of my favorite and most rewarding mushrooms to grow is shiitake. There's a little bit of work involved with the shiitakes, but you'll be greatly rewarded in your efforts. To get started, you have to go into the woods, select a few young oak trees, and cut them into four-foot lengths. They shouldn't be more than five inches across in circumference. I lay them to rest on the forest floor for about two weeks, as they contain antifungal agencies when they are live, green wood. After the two-week resting period, the antifungals leave the log, and they're ready for inoculation.

Inoculation might seem like a strange term to use with mushrooms, but that's exactly what you do. Drill a nine-sixteenth-inch hole, one inch deep, into the log every 10 inches. Make four different lines of holes going down the log. Now you have four different fruiting sites. I then purchase the shiitake mushroom spawn from Fungi Perfecti. It comes in two different ways. You can get it as a grain spawn, which is very soft and can be injected into the inoculation sites. However, the one I found that works the best is the wooden dowel inoculation plug. It's very easy to use and fun for growing your own mushrooms.

It's a small oak dowel that's been inoculated with the shiitake spawn. Once you receive it, you can store it in the refrigerator until you're ready to use it. Bang the spawn plugs into the holes you drilled. Knock them in with a hammer. Next, melt some cheese wax, which you can also obtain from the mushroom spawn distributor. Heat it up and brush it on each inoculation area. This holds in the moisture and pasteurizes the inoculation spot, killing off any foreign fungus. You'll ensure the growth of beautiful fruiting shiitakes in the months to come.

Once you fill in the inoculation sites in the oak logs, pick a spot for them. I like to choose an area that has a few evergreen trees, like hemlocks or spruce. Hemlocks have boughs that cast some shade onto the forest floor in the winter months. It seems to be a prime location where my shiitakes have always done well. If you don't have any evergreens or spruce trees in your area, store them underneath any hardwood tree, such as maple, oak, or ash.

I've discovered that it's best to lay them flat on the ground. The moisture stays constant in the logs until they're ready to fruit. Depending on the variety of shiitake and how long the spawn run takes, it generally means you must let your logs rest for about six months before the mushrooms begin to fruit. Seeing the butt ends of the logs starting to turn white when the mycelium is starting to run is a good indication that your logs are ready.

*Pink oyster mushroom fruiting on a straw.*

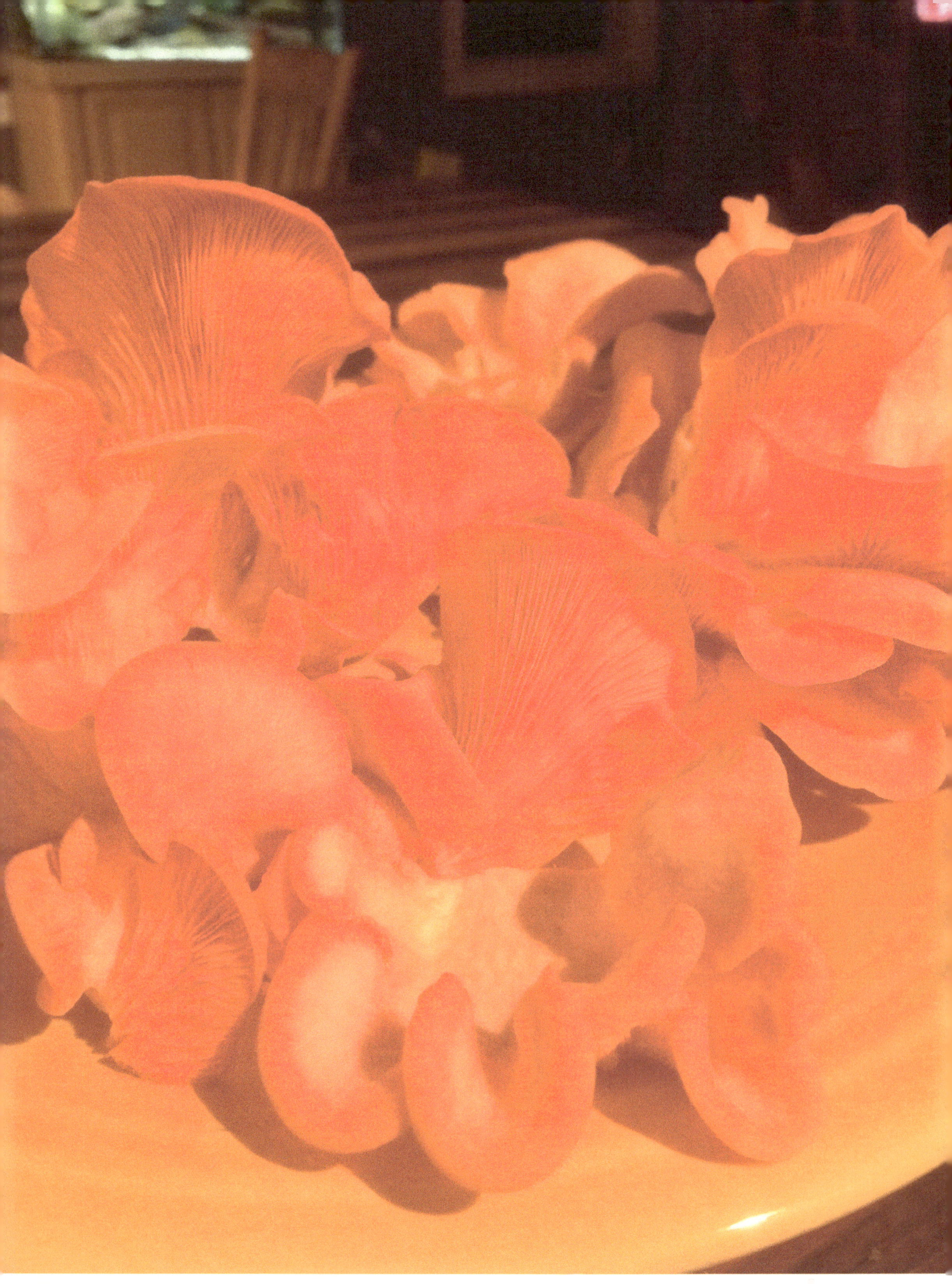

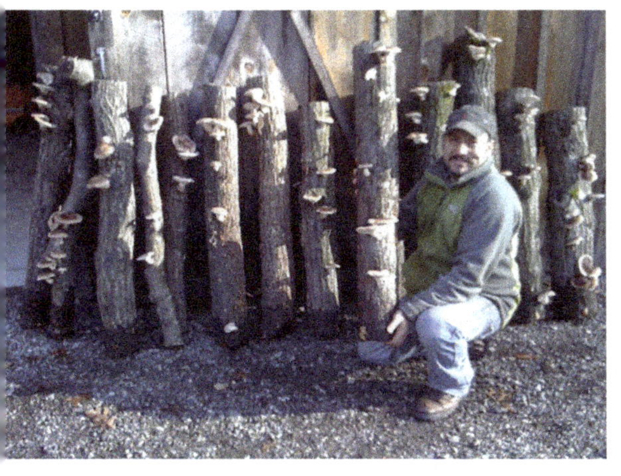

When you see the mycelium starting to come out of the end of the logs, it's time to remove them from the forest floor and allow the fruiting process to begin. Stand the logs upright. Lean them on a tree or the side of a barn so that they're out of direct sunlight and in the shade. As soon as the mushrooms start to fruit, they won't have to compete with the forest floor or the ground. You'll soon have nice, uniform shiitakes that will fruit. Once you harvest the shiitakes, you can eat them fresh, sauté them, put them in salads, or dry them for further use.

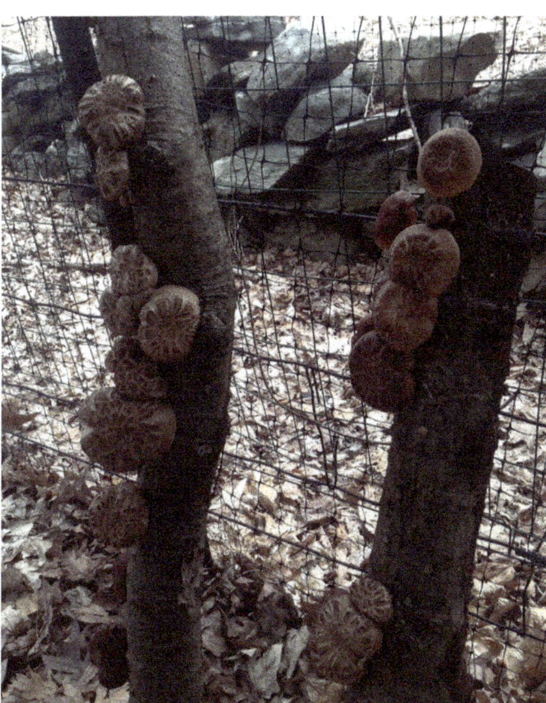

Clearly, all wild mushrooms aren't edible. Many species are truly desirable and quite delicious. However, some will give you gastronomical problems, or will also cause you to break out in a rash. In fact, some of them are quite deadly. One of the ways you can distinguish mushrooms is by making a spore print for identification.

When you harvest any mushroom, place one of them on a white index card with the gill side down. Put a small container over it to retain the humidity. Overnight, they'll leave an imprint of a spore print. Some of them could be yellow, salmon pink, or brown. Others could be purple to black. A few will leave a green spore print. This is a good indication to distinguish which mushrooms are edible.

How does this work? Well, immature gills sometimes are an off-white, while matured gills of many different mushrooms are the same color as the spore print. It's not always the best way to identify them, but it's the only way to distinguish them other than checking out the photos of the mushrooms in a field guide. Many good guides are available on websites or in book form. The bottom line is that if you come across a mushroom you aren't familiar with, check it out before you consume it.

The few I've talked about are commonly found. These are the oyster mushroom, hen of the woods, chicken mushroom, chanterelles, and morels. These are the highly-prized mushrooms that I hunt for, and they all make for great eating.

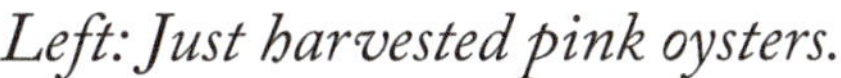

*Left: Just harvested pink oysters.*

*Above, Clockwise: Several logs that have just fruited some beautiful shiitakes, shiitakes fruiting on an oak log.*

*Page 152 and 153: Shiitake mushroom plug spawns and oyster mushrooms fruiting on inoculated straw.*

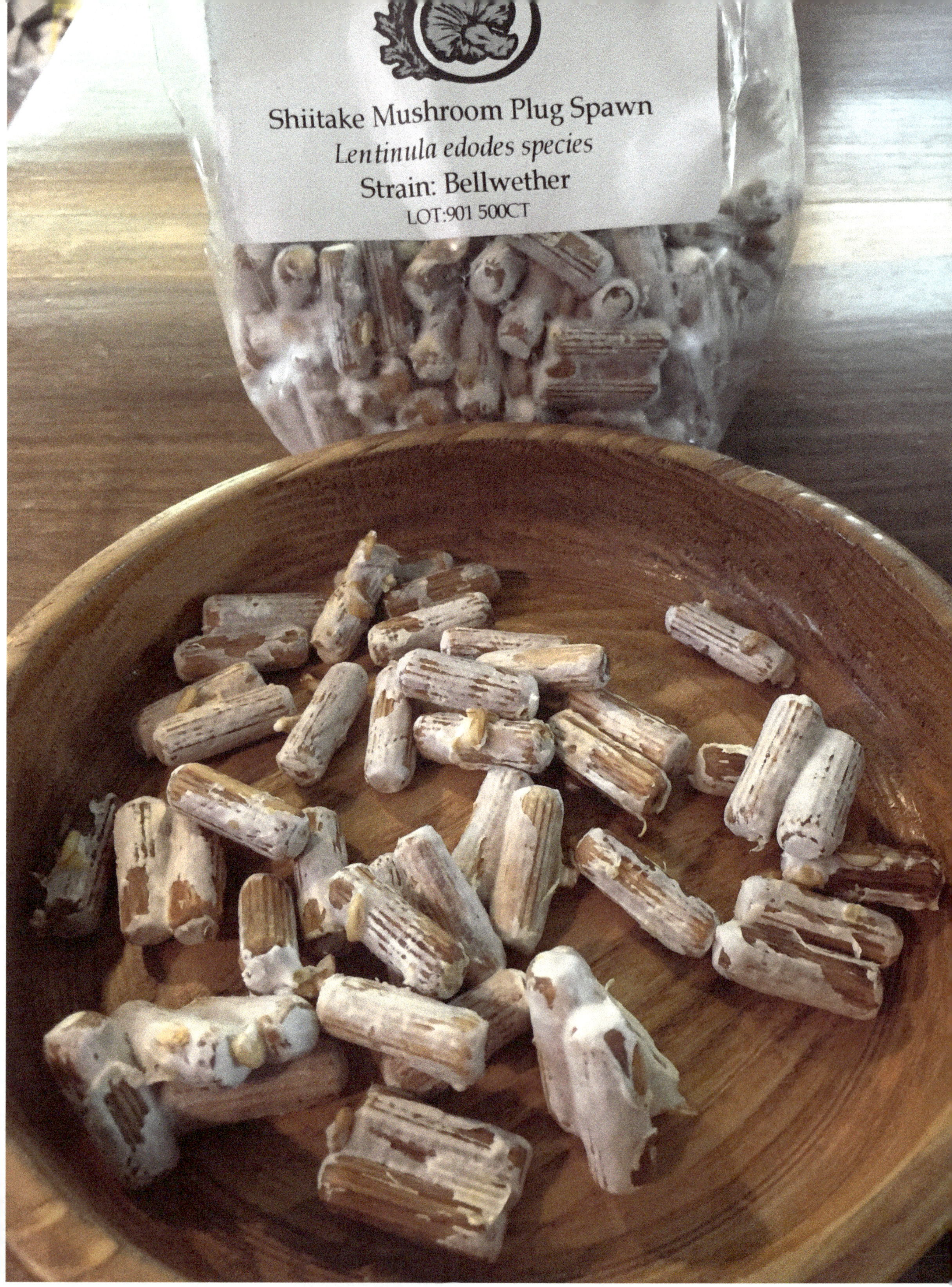
Shiitake Mushroom Plug Spawn
Lentinula edodes species
Strain: Bellwether
LOT:901 500CT

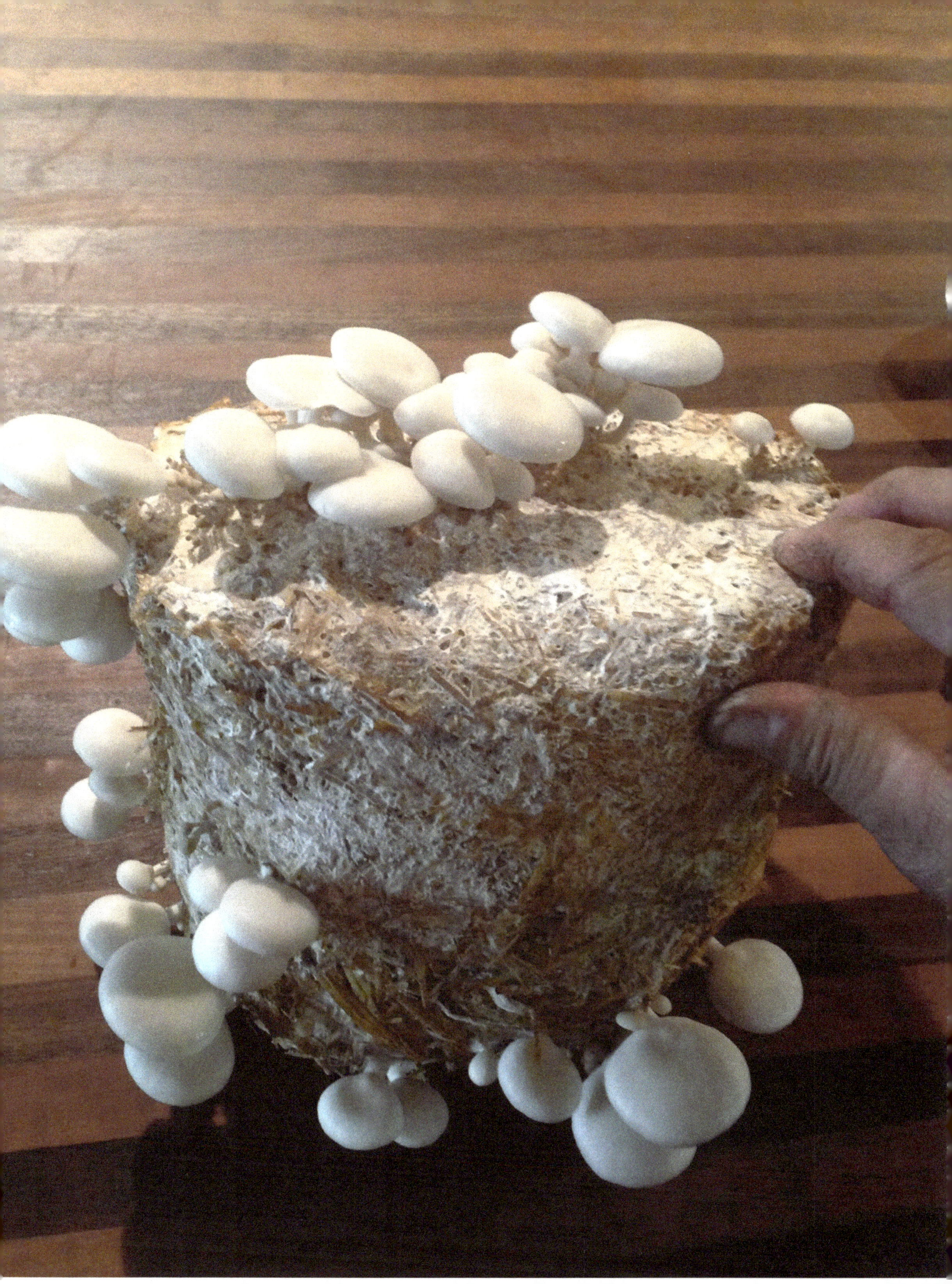

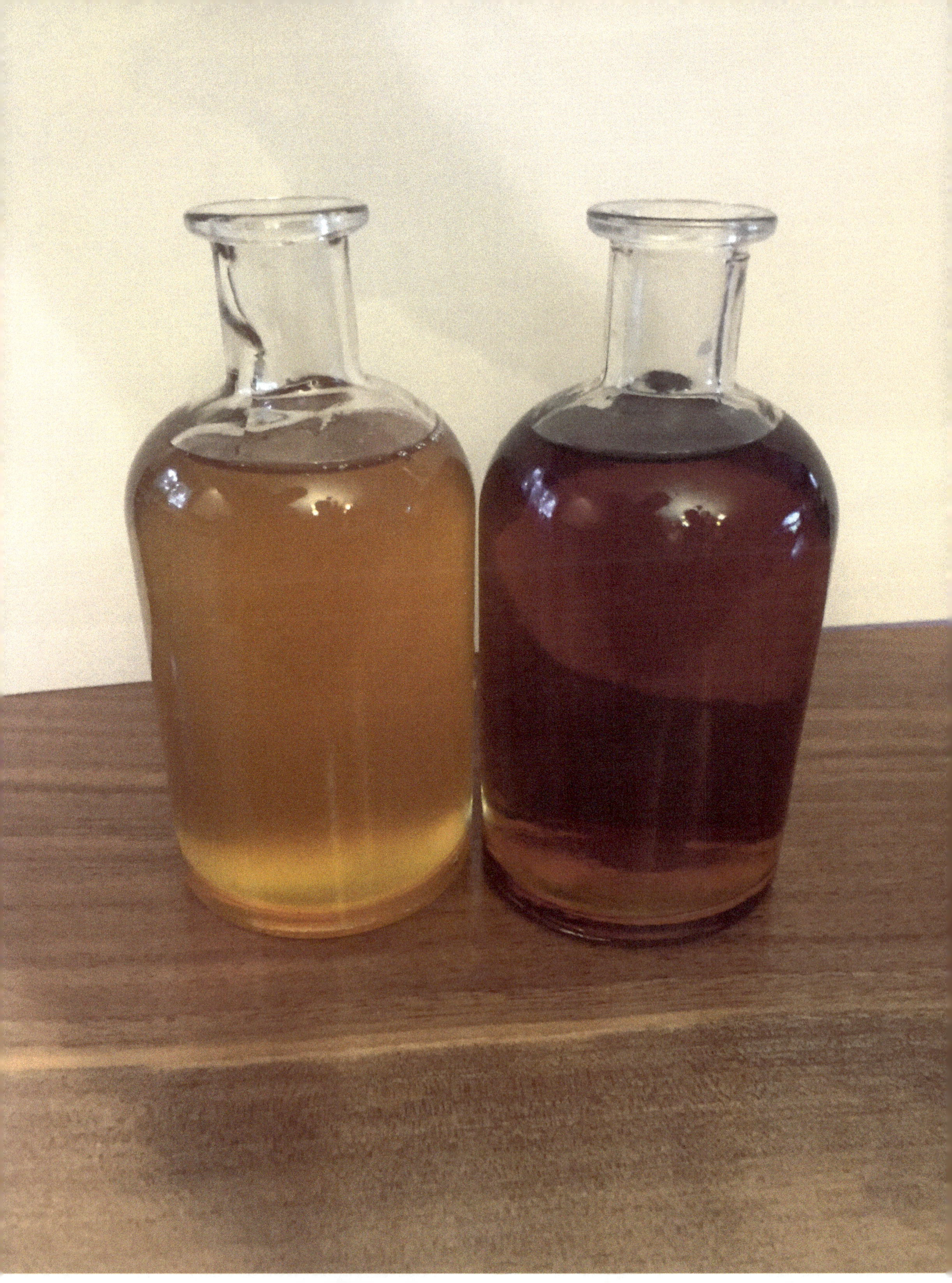

# Maple Syrup

*"Blood is thicker then water, but maple syrup is thicker then blood so technically pancakes are more important than family."*

**Author Unknown**

A very enjoyable process I love doing in the winter is gathering maple sap for syrup. This is best done in the mid-February through March time frame here in the Northeast. If you have sugar maple trees in the area, this is a lot of fun to do. All you need to do is tap a hole about a quarter of an inch into a tree. The tap is called a spile, and you tap it into the tree about two feet above the ground. Attach a small piece of tubing to it and direct it into a catch, which would be a bucket or any container to hold the sap.

If you're in an area with many trees, you can do this on a large scale. You can connect tubes from tree to tree and bring the sap into one mainline. That mainline goes into a large collection vat. Within a few days, you can start to boil the sap in the vat.

On a smaller scale, you can make the syrup on a burner in your kitchen or outside on a propane burner. Another option is to make an arch out of concrete cinder blocks with a wood fire and a large pot. This method works very well. Whatever way works for you, the idea is to pour the sap into a pan or pot and let it boil down for several hours or until all the water moisture has evaporated from the sap. Then, it slowly thickens into syrup.

The first tapping of the spring produces a light-colored syrup. The lighter syrup is the early sap that flows. As the season progresses and the snow starts to melt, the trees begin to come out of dormancy. The last bit of sap that you take out of the tree will boil down to a darker color. In case you ever wondered what it meant when you buy syrup in the store, this is how they determine the different grades of syrup.

You can store maple syrup in bottles for up to a year. You do need to know it's a time-consuming process. It takes 30 gallons of sap, boiled down and evaporated, to make one gallon of syrup. That might seem daunting, but it's very delicious and enjoyable to make.

I like mixing the fresh maple syrup with honey. I then add a few cloves and a cinnamon stick. To make the best dressing ever, mix this with a little bit of balsamic vinegar, black peppercorns, and some good olive oil. It's very tasty. Or you can use it straight up, without the vinegar, on your pancakes, hot oatmeal, French toast, or in a hot cup of tea.

*The syrup to the left is early sap flow and is grade A, light. To the right is late sap flow, which will be grade B, dark amber.*

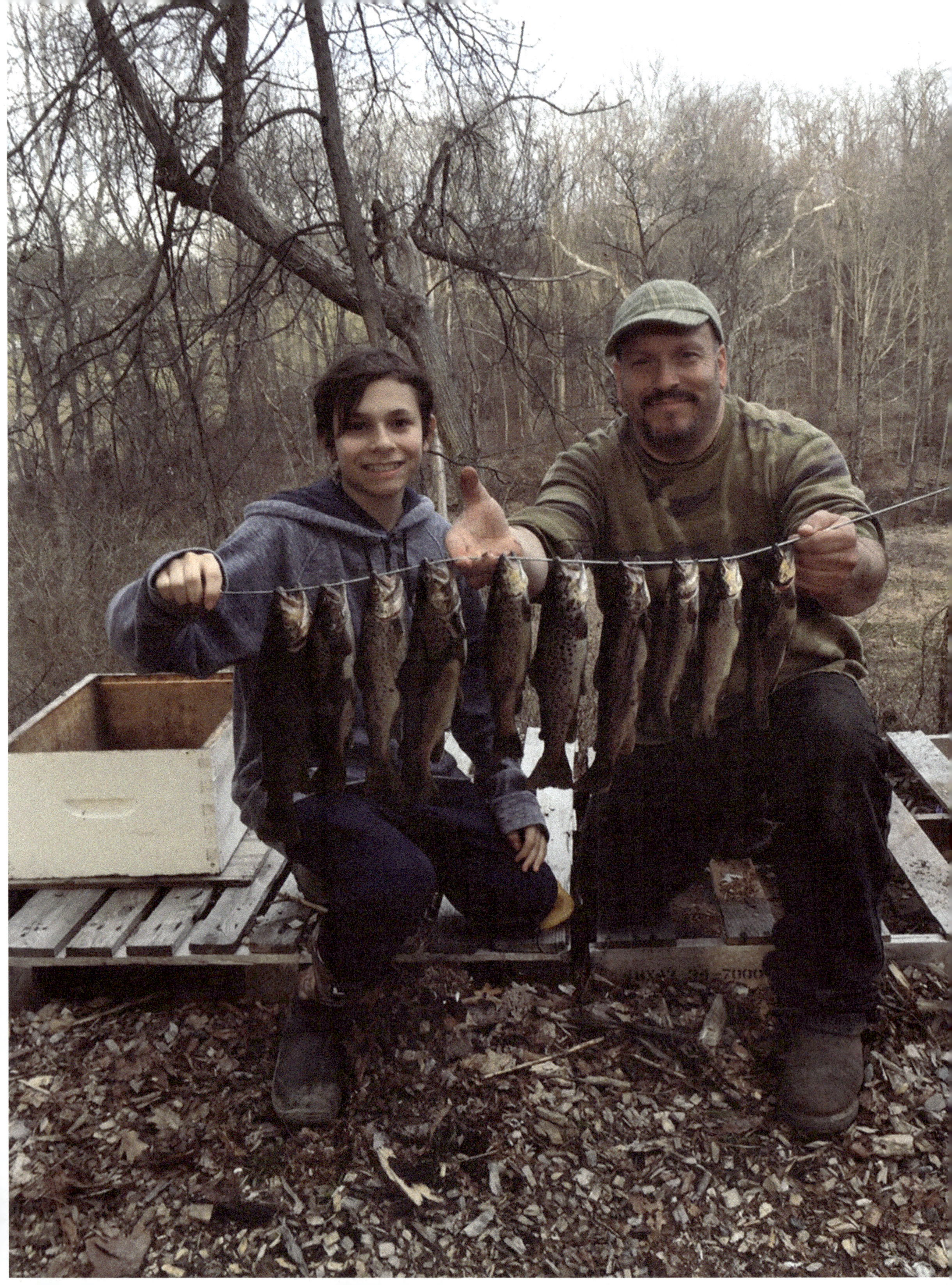

# Fishing

*"Give a man a fish, and you feed him for a day; teach a man to fish, and you feed him for a lifetime."*

**— Russian Proverb**

Nature's bounty isn't limited to forests and fields. Our waterways hold an abundance of food that is delicious and nutritious.

Fishing is a wonderful sport. It's very relaxing. I think it's a good idea to raise kids with fishing, as there needs to be more tackle boxes instead of Xboxes these days. Fishing brings children closer to nature and keeps them out of trouble. My son enjoys fishing with me, as well as my daughter. They both have their own poles. During our free time, when we're not doing sports, working in the garden, or tending our bees, we enjoy fishing. It's our favorite thing to do, and we also like to reap the benefits. We'll keep a trout, fillet him, put him in the smoker, and enjoy him with our family. There's nothing better than having wild, organic, fresh fish to eat over the spring and summer.

## *Trout*

Fishing usually starts for me in the month of April. In my area, April 1 is the beginning of trout season. Trout is one of the most finicky fish to catch. You really have to know what you're doing to snag trout in the streams, especially the native trout that have spawned in the stream from adult trout in the water beds.

You can fish for trout in a stream several different ways. You can use spinners, live bait, or flies that simulate live flies. These are tied by hand and made to look like insects. Fly fishing is also very challenging, but you need to have plenty of space to cast a fly rod. Out West, where the streams run through meadows and valleys, there's not so much interference from trees and overhanging limbs. It's a great place to fly fish for trout. Here in New York, the low-lying streams and creeks that run through the heavy brush and timber forests make fly fishing very challenging. As soon as you whip out that fly rod, you can get tangled very easily.

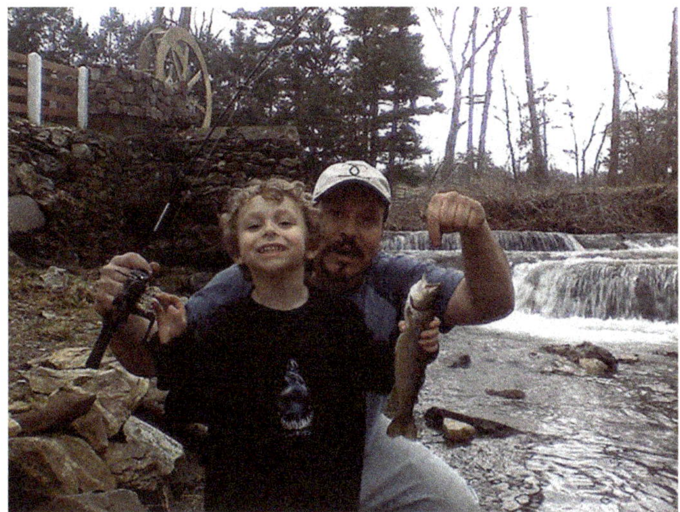

Over the years, and with lots of practice, I've learned to cast differently with the fly rod in congested areas. I stretch out as much line as possible and let it float

*Left: Me and Julian with some nice brown trout caught in the stream in the Hudson Valley.*

*Above: Julian's first trout caught on the first day of the season at age 5.*

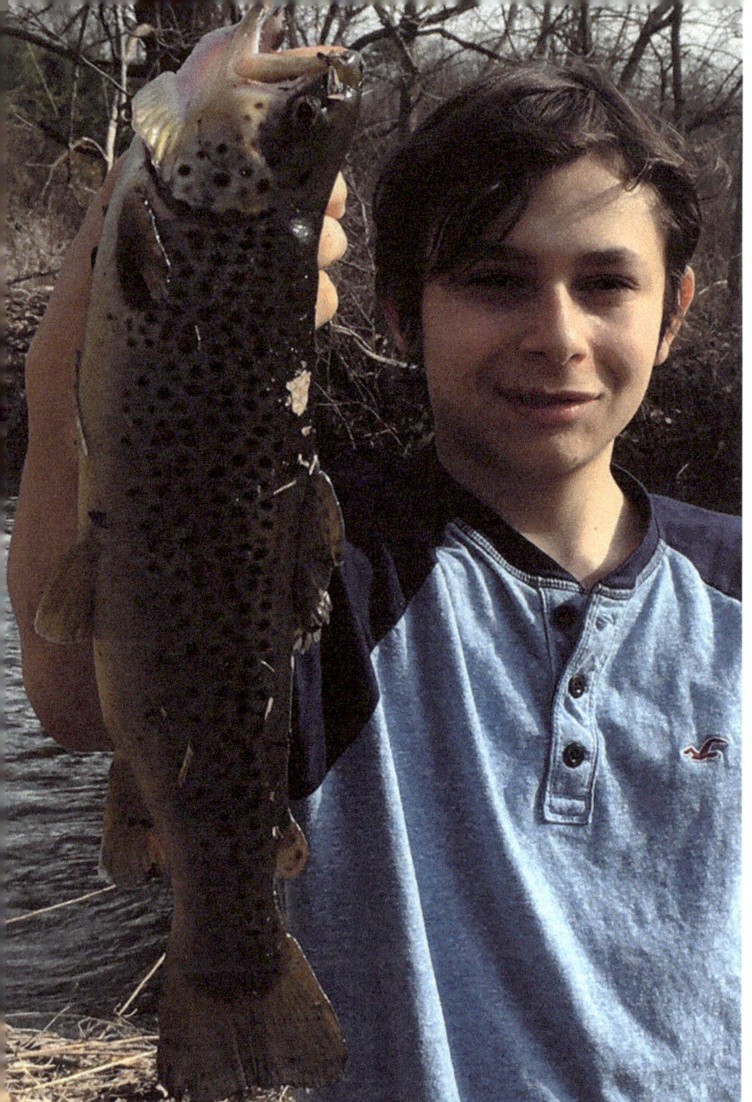

downstream. Then, I lift my rod slowly, taking out the slack of the fly line, and snap the tip forward instead of retracting back and forth as you do with a typical fly rod cast.

There are other alternatives to getting that nymph in the right pocket behind the stone where the trout are laying. It's called a roll cast. The roll cast is very efficient in heavy, congested woodlands where the trout are lurking. I've had much success with this style of fishing with my fly rod on the creeks and rivers around my area in Dutchess County.

One of my favorite ways to fish for stream trout is by using a spinner. A spinner is a little, fixed lure that has a blade that propels as you pull it through the water. The color of my choice is black with a gold spoon. The gold spoon has always proven to have great success against the native trout that live in the rivers and streams in my area.

I've been doing this for quite some time, so I've learned how to simulate live bait in the creek or the streams. When you're fishing with a spinner, the biggest no-no is to cast downstream and retrieve your spinner upstream. That's very unnatural for the fish, as trout face upstream with the current coming over their face. With any natural food that's floating down the river,

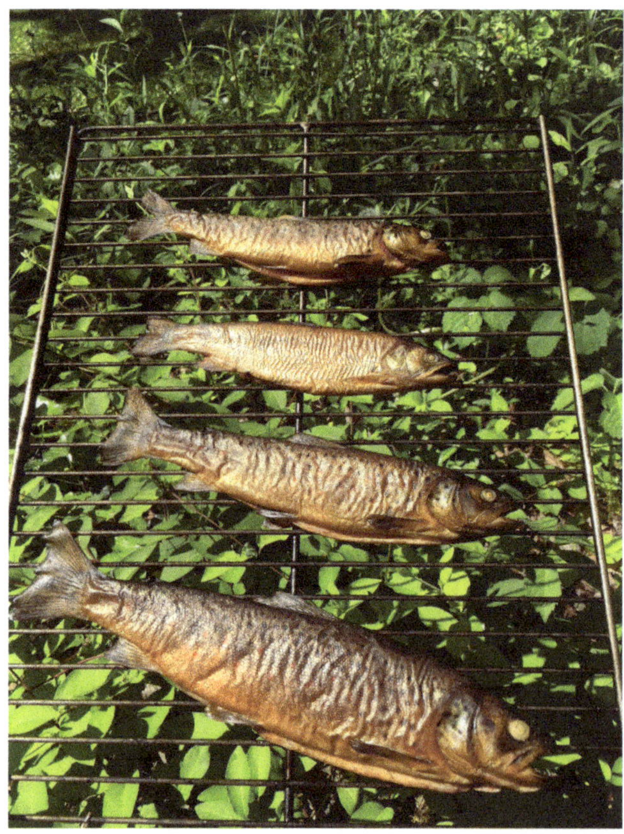

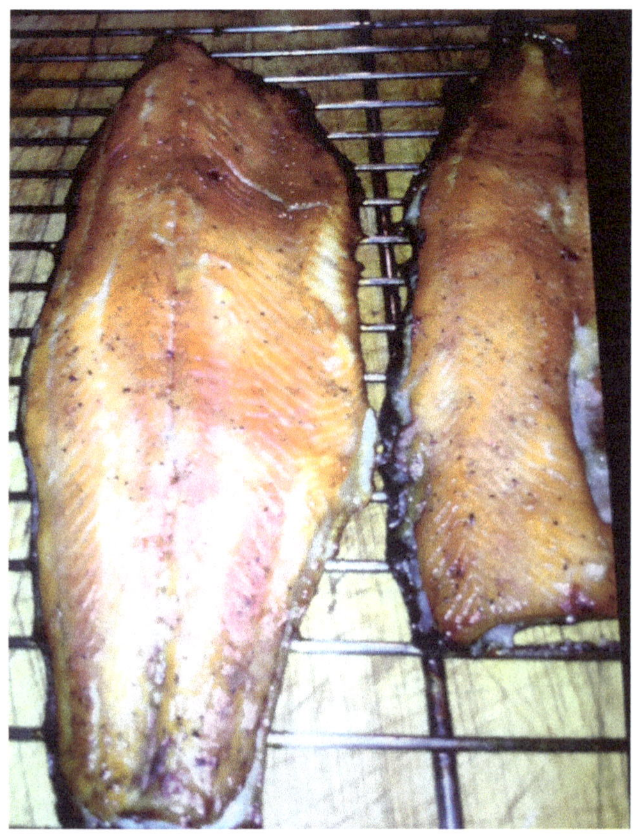

a trout can inspect it several times as it passes by the fish. The trout will then spin around and snatch up that bait.

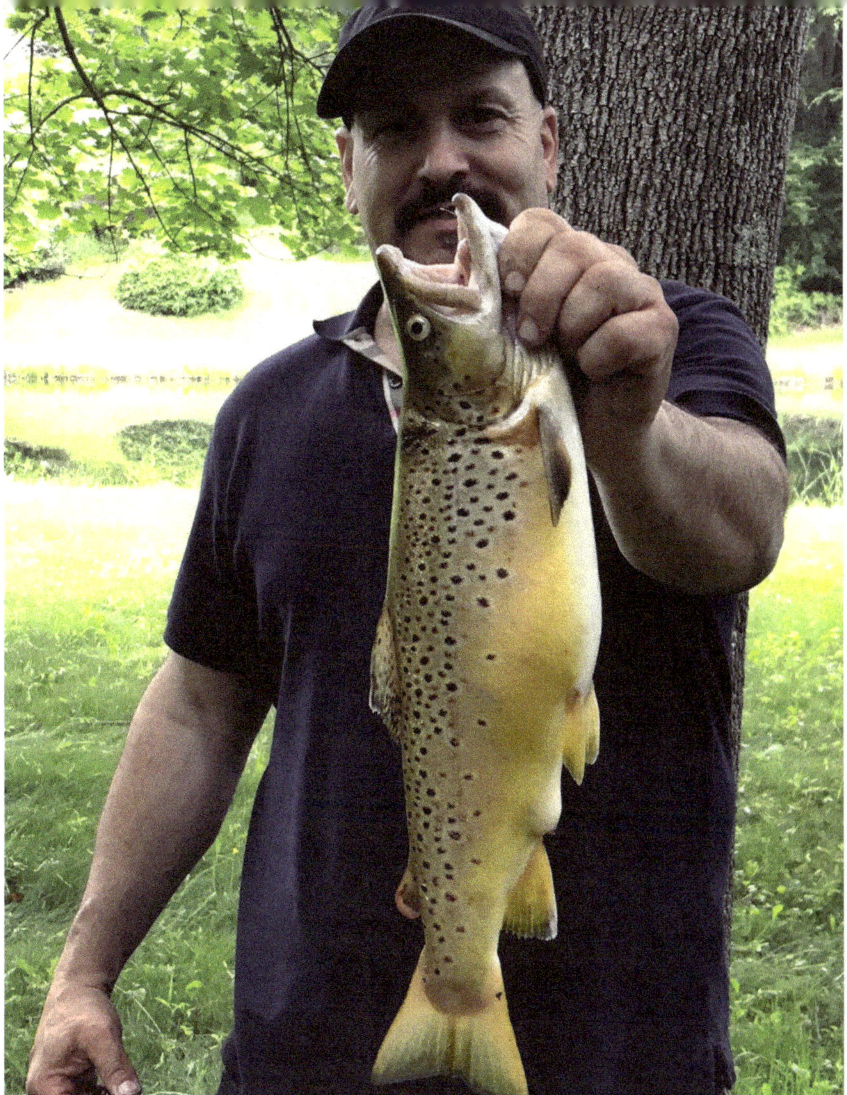

If you try to cast downstream and bring the lure across the surface of the stream, passing by the trout's tail first and over his head, you will never catch a trout. It's very unnatural for any sort of grub, insect, or worm to be floating upstream past their tail. It will only spook the fish, making him not bite the bait at all.

When it comes to reservoir fishing, which is usually in the month of May, I tend to jump on my rowboat and hit some of the local reservoirs. One of my favorites to fish is the Croton Falls Reservoir. This reservoir holds trophy brown trout weighing up to 15 or 20 pounds.

I have three different ways that I fish for trout from a rowboat. One is that I'll cast a spoon. The spoon I usually use is called a crocodile. It's a gold spoon, and it also comes in silver. Silver seems to have a nice flash in the depth of the reservoir. I usually cast out and let the spoon sink. I count to 30 before I close the bail of the reel and start to retrieve my spoon.

During retrieval, I twitch my rod every two seconds, giving it a jerk to simulate the natural baitfish in the reservoir, which is called a sawbelly. These sawbellies swim in very large schools, and the trout will come up and take one of the injured sawbellies or one of the weaker ones. Twitching the lure simulates an injured sawbelly. I get a good bite usually within 15 to 20 casts and land a beautiful trout out of the reservoir.

Another way I fish for trout in the reservoir is to go to the edge of it and row out into 20 to 30 feet of water. I check with a depth finder, which is a battery-operated tool you place in the water to read its depth. In the early spring, during May, I like to fish in 25 to 30 feet of water.

These fish are coming out of the deeper water from their long winter rest and start to feed heavily on baitfish. Once again, the baitfish consist of shiners and native sawbellies. I bring some sawbellies that I purchase from the bait store, and I'll hook them just in front of the dorsal fin on a number-10 treble hook with no split shot. This is called live lining. I then cast out my 30-foot mark and place my rod along the side of my boat.

I like to use two poles when I fish with live bait. This gives me a better chance of scoring a nice trout in the reservoir. Once I make my cast, I place my pole down, and I hook my line into a mechanism called

*Page 158 top: Julian with a nice brown trout.*

*Page 158 bottom: Trout in and out of hickory smoker.*

*Above: Native brown trout caught using light tackle in a brook.*

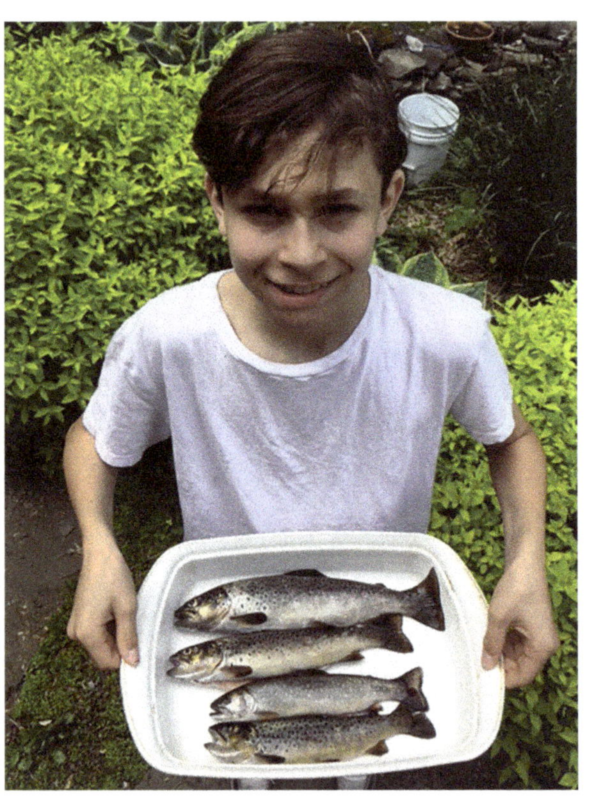

a strike guard. In this fashion, my reel is wide open, and my line is clipped into a little ball bearing, which enables me to grasp it with very little effort. As soon as I get a bite, the trout will release the line from the ball bearing. When the bail is open, the fish can take line freely.

When the strike guard has been triggered off, it makes a click. That tells me a fish has taken my bait. Once I can see the line peeling off my reel, I lift it up and remove the strike guard, as it's just clipped onto my pole. I place the guard down on my lap, alongside my boat seat. When I notice that the fish has stopped taking line, I slowly close my reel. I reel up the slack, and then I set the hook.

Once I set the hook, I feel the fish tugging. As this happens, my drag — which is the mechanism in the reel — will start to go, and the fish will start to take line with the drag. The drag prevents the line from snapping. It's very important to set your drag before you go out into the reservoir to fish.

I work the fish and get him closer to the boat. I always bring a net. After I get the fish to the boat, I always land it from the tail, getting the net around the tail and scooping up the trout. I size him up when he's in the boat. If it's something I don't want to keep, I carefully release the fish back into the reservoir, unharmed and uninjured, for another time.

If he's a keeper, I run my stringer through his bottom gill, tie him off, and place him back in the water contained on my stringer. That way, he'll keep fresh and stay alive until I get him home to dress him out, fillet him, place him in a brine, and get him ready for the smoker or the barbecue. I could also prepare him with some white wine, shallots, garlic, olive oil, wrap him in foil, and bake him in the oven.

## *Largemouth bass and crappie*

As the season progresses and June turns into July, the water warms up, and the trout move into deeper water. That's when I pursue the largemouth bass and crappie. The largemouth bass is fun to catch. They tend to frequent the shallow waters and the edges at this time. I usually fish for them in the lakes and ponds, but also from my rowboat.

The bass will congregate in the sandy flats along the edges as they begin to spawn. During the spawning ritual for bass, they become very aggressive, and they'll bite just about anything. My go-to lure for the bass is a Rapala. It's a wooden float lure called a stick bait. It has a plastic lip at the tip of it. When you cast it out, and you go to pull it, it dives under the water. They come in several different colors. Black and orange is a flashy mix. Green and silver is also one of my favorites. I think the green makes it look like a frog jumping through the water.

*Above: Trout caught in the morning and smoked in the afternoon.*

*Page 161: John Alfano with sons Jaden and Matthew and a largemouth bass.*

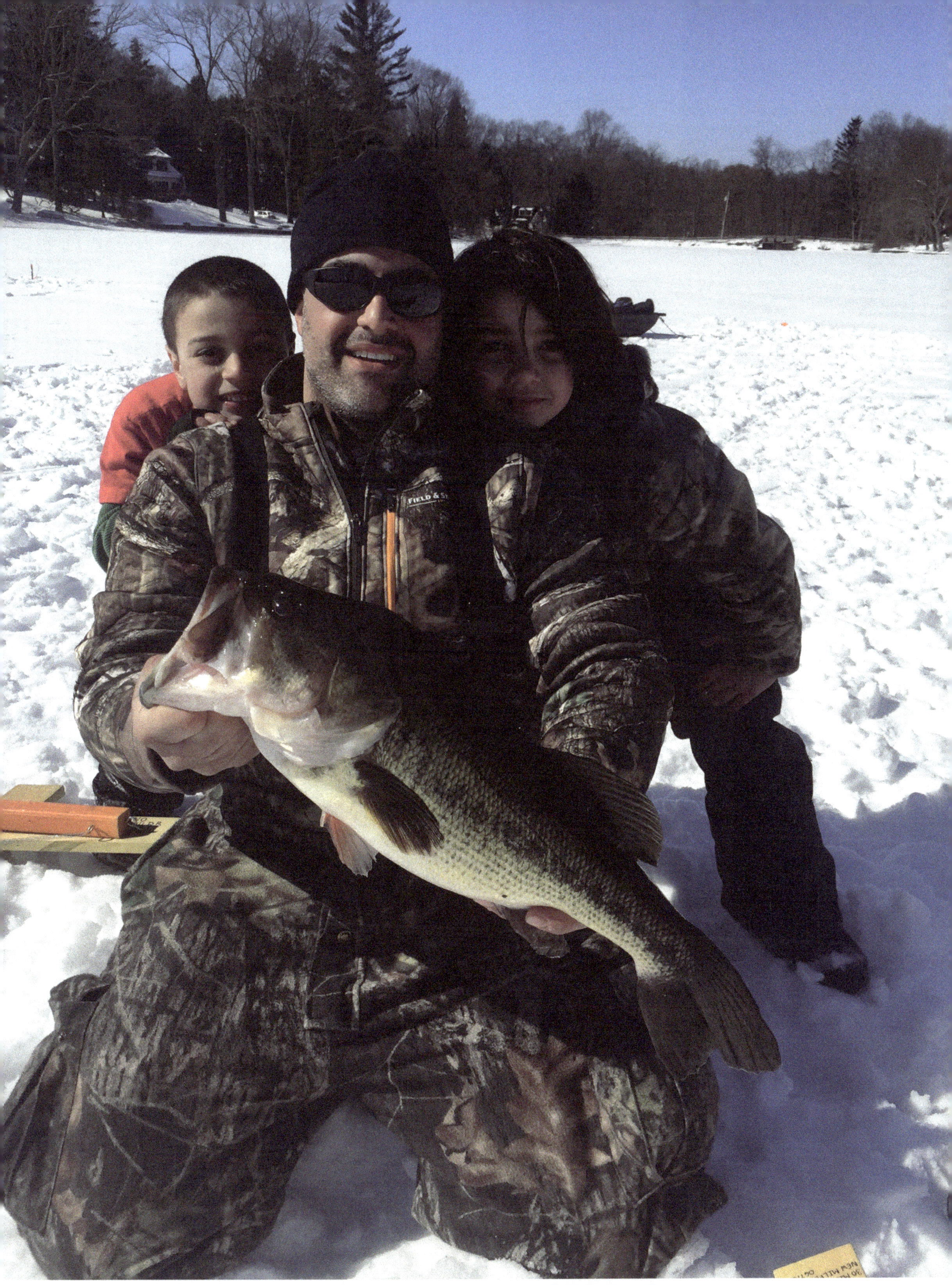

The bass will come out of the shallows and crash the lure. Bass are fun to catch, as they usually leap out of the water two or three times. Bass aren't generally one of my favorite fish for the table, but they sure are fun to go after. Anybody can catch them during the month of June while they're spawning, because they're very aggressive in protecting their nests. I always tend to put the bass back to catch another day.

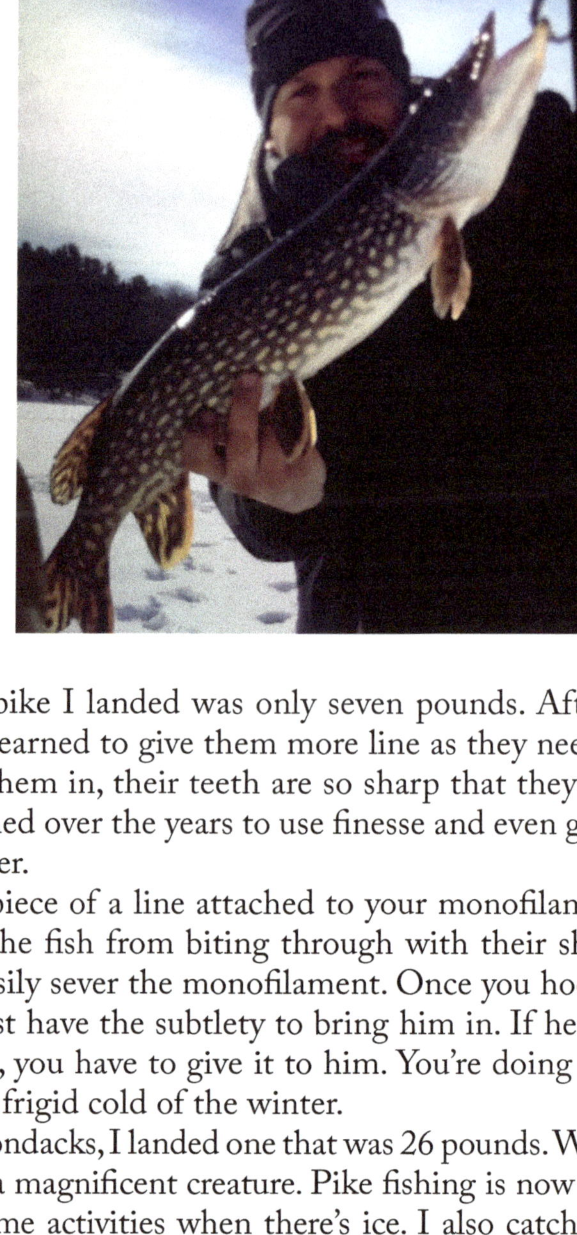

## *Northern Pike*

Northern pike is a game fish I really enjoy catching. I go for the pike as the season gets on, the weather starts to become cold, and we have some ice. I enjoy catching northern pike in several different places. Bantam Lake in Connecticut is one of them.

John Alfano, my good buddy, fishing partner, and lifelong friend, asked me to go fishing with him there about six years ago. After he had taken me on this fishing trip, I was able to get a northern pike at the end of my line. We were using large shiners for bait — bigger bait than I've used for anything. Once I landed my first pike, I was hooked. It was the most challenging fish to get through the hole in the ice, because of the long length of the fish and some of them having such a big girth.

Ever since then, John and I have traveled to different destinations to catch the elusive northern pike. The first pike I landed was only seven pounds. After I became better and had more experience catching them, I learned to give them more line as they needed it. If you try to horse them in, their teeth are so sharp that they can sever the line. I've learned over the years to use finesse and even go as far as using a steel leader.

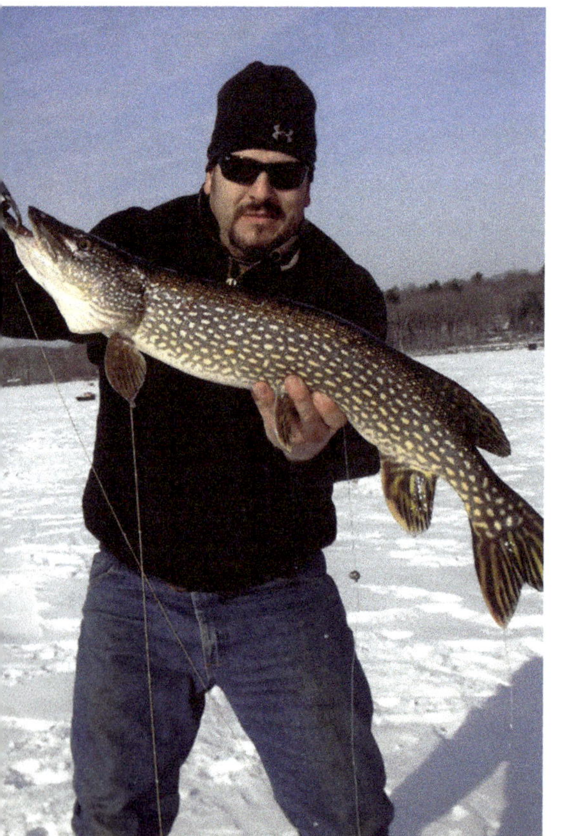

A leader is a small piece of a line attached to your monofilament line that will prevent the fish from biting through with their sharp teeth, as they would easily sever the monofilament. Once you hook a northern pike, you must have the subtlety to bring him in. If he decides to take more line, you have to give it to him. You're doing this with your hands in the frigid cold of the winter.

Recently in the Adirondacks, I landed one that was 26 pounds. What a beautiful fish! It was a magnificent creature. Pike fishing is now one of my favorite wintertime activities when there's ice. I also catch the occasional largemouth bass, trout, and panfish through the ice.

*Top: My first pike.*

*Left: Northern pike caught through the ice with live bait.*

*Page 163: This is the largest northern pike I've ever landed to this day, at 26 pounds, 46 inches long.*

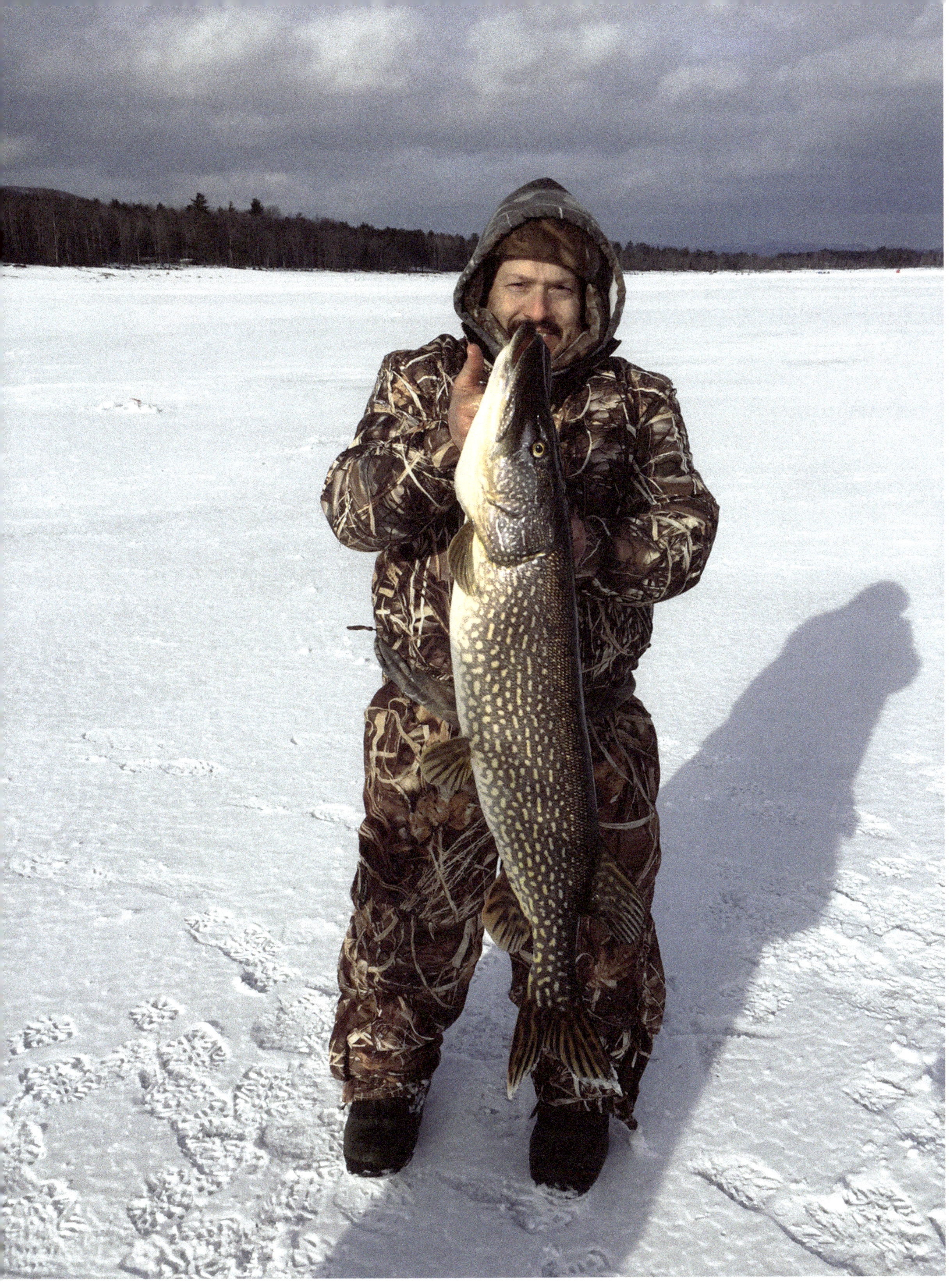

## *Perch*

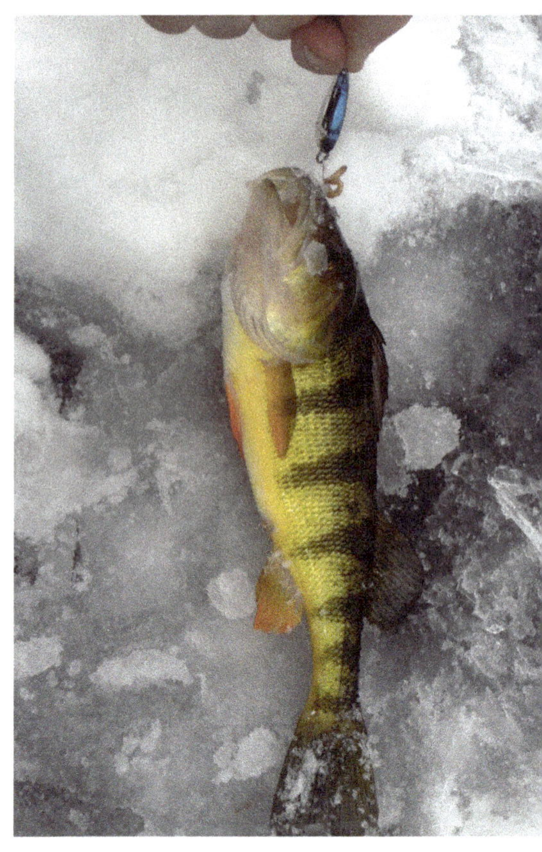

Perch is another go-to fish that I enjoy catching, and they're very delicious to eat. You catch perch in a different fashion, using a jigging pole with a small jig tipped with a grub. Perch is one of my favorite fish to eat that I catch through the ice — it's called the "poor man's lobster." You can fillet perch, boil them in salted water with a bay leaf, chill the fillets, and dip them in cocktail sauce. It's like eating a delightful shrimp or a piece of lobster. You can dip them in butter as well. Pan-fried perch is also a tasty dish.

## *King Salmon*

Another favorite to catch is king salmon. They reside in the Great Lakes, especially Lake Ontario. As a ritual, the salmon tend to spawn later in the season, around September into October. They leave Lake Ontario and swim upstream. As they make their journey upstream, fighting the current and rocks, they get to their spawning grounds. This is called the salmon run and attracts many fishermen there to harvest the salmon.

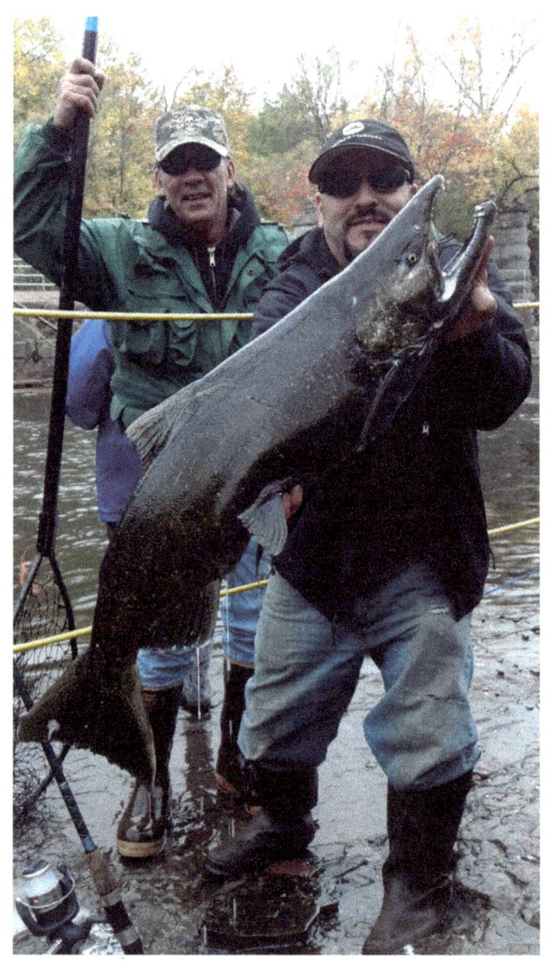

The salmon spawn and fight their way to reach females, to get to the gravelly banks and beds where they'll deposit their eggs. Once they lay their eggs, they perish. It's a great way to harvest some beautiful salmon in the river, and there's nothing more fun and exciting than getting a salmon at the end of your line that weighs between 25 and 30 pounds. One will take your bait up and down the river. It's very exhilarating, challenging, and incredibly rewarding if you land the fish.

One of my favorite places to visit every fall to catch salmon is Point Breeze, up towards the Canadian border and not far from the Niagara River. Its Oak Orchard Creek is one of the rivers I like to fish, and I enjoy fishing the Salmon River. It also holds brown trout that come up to spawn, and steelhead, which is a type of rainbow trout. However, the king salmon is the biggest and the most fun to catch.

I head upstream. Polarized glasses enable me to look into the water. This way I can spot and stalk some of the fish. I use my salmon rod with 17-pound test monofilament once I notice some of the fish hanging out in the pools. At the end of the monofilament, I have a swivel with six-pound test line. It's much thinner and makes the bait more appealing to the fish as it flows through the water.

I use a salmon egg sack, very fine material tied to a small ball that consists of six or seven fresh salmon eggs. The spawn sacks can be made or bought locally at a bait shop. All the bait shops will sell spawn sacks during the salmon run, because they're the preferred bait to use. You can also catch the salmon on a fly rod, but that's very challenging.

I like to cast upstream and let the spawn sacks bounce along the bottom, appealing to the salmon. As they pass by, the salmon suck them up. When you feel the bumping of the tip of your rod, you lift the rod and set the hook. The salmon are aggressive, so many times you'll have a miss. They'll pick it up and sometimes spit it out. Once you get your hook set into the jaw of a salmon, you have to really hold on and make sure that you set your drag.

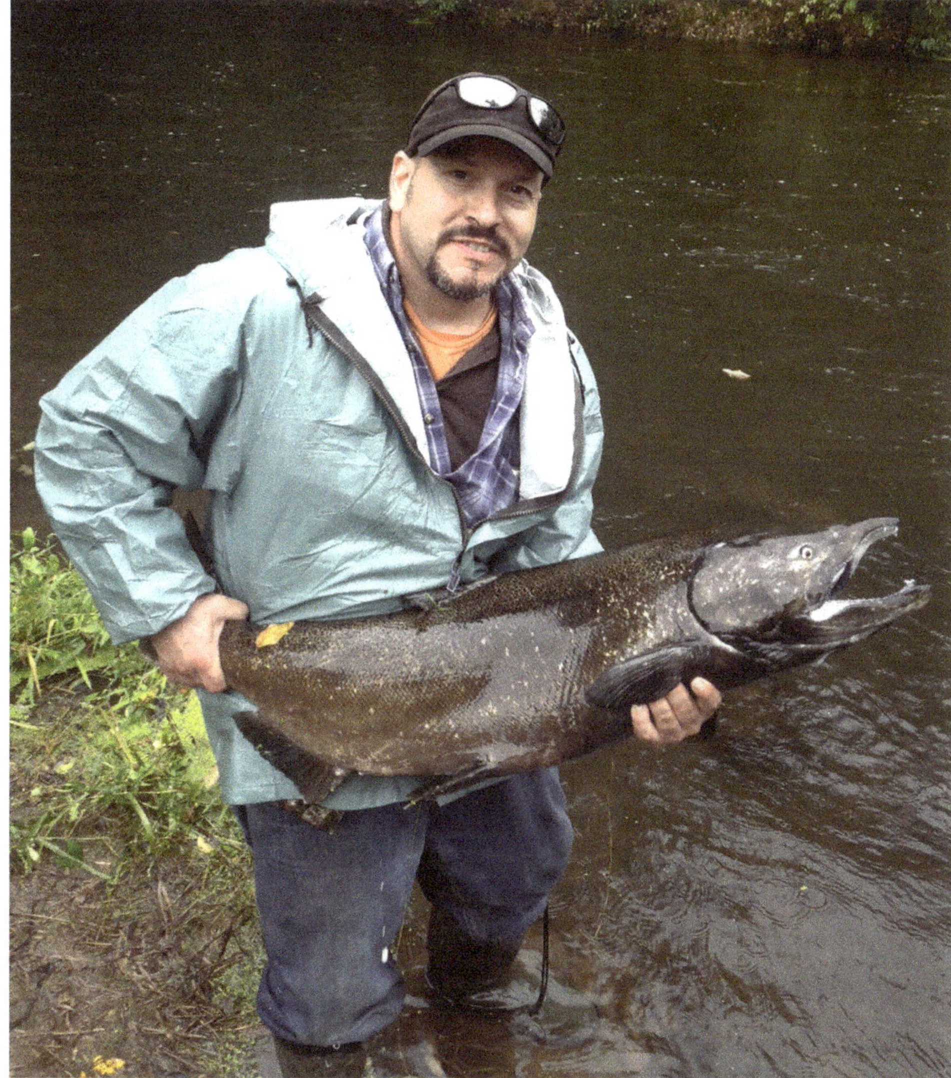

When you hook a fish, let it go without muscling him in because he could easily break the six-pound test leader. As the salmon runs up and down the pool, knowing that it's hooked, gently and gingerly try to get him into the net. It's very rewarding and pleasing to catch that salmon in the net.

When I catch any female salmon, I usually return them to the water safely so they can continue to do their spawning ritual. I generally keep the males, as they're plentiful in the streams, spawning with all the females. If I catch a salmon, I like to keep it in the cold river on a stringer. That keeps the fish safe, cold, and fresh until I'm ready to prepare him for the smoker.

When I get the salmon home, I fillet it, removing the carcass and the bones. I brine the salmon in maple syrup, kosher salt, and black peppercorns for two days with a little bit of Worcestershire sauce. I smoke the salmon either over hickory or alder for four to six hours. It's truly delicious. I can also bake the salmon, pan-sear it, or broil it. When I smoke it, it lasts for quite a while in airtight packages. Then, I can freeze it and use it throughout the season, or give it away to friends and family.

*Page 164 top: Perch caught through the ice on a jig.*

*Page 164 bottom: 38-lb. male king salmon caught drifting a spawn sac in the Salmon River, Upstate NY. My fishing partner John Phillips helped land it with a net.*

*Above: Male king salmon caught in September during the salmon run in Oak Orchard Creek in Point Breeze, NY.*

# *Recipes*

In this section, I share with you some of the bounty and the recipes that have been passed down from my family for you to enjoy.

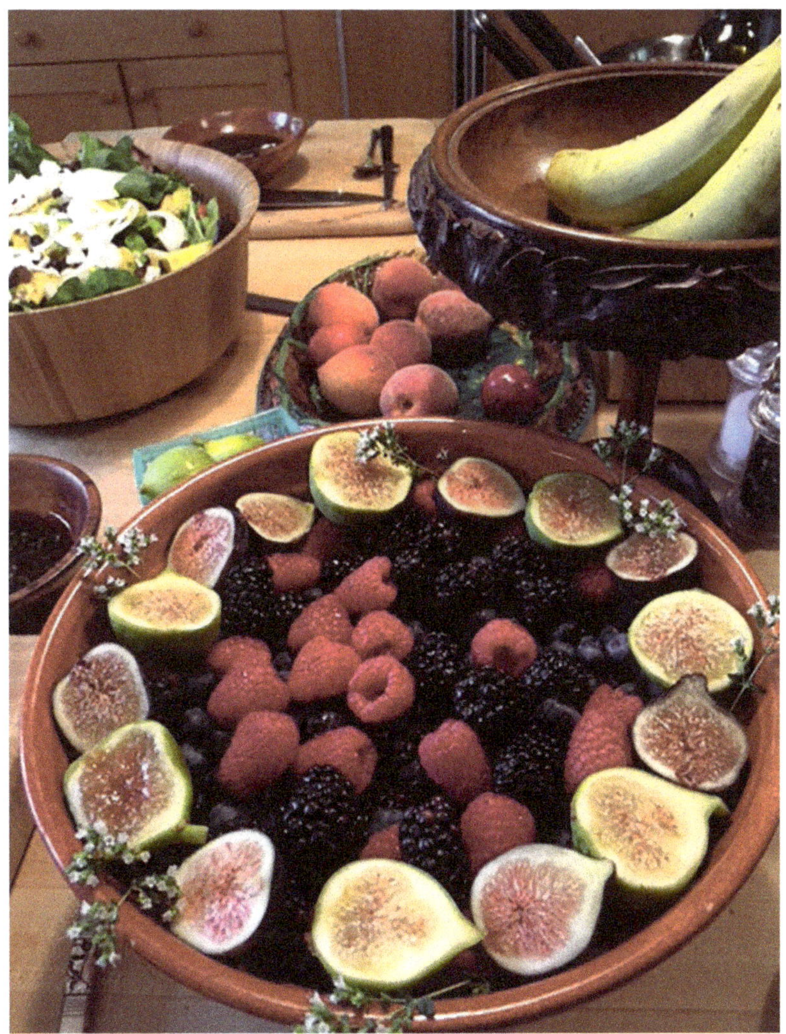

*When the berries are in abundance and figs are ripe, we enjoy them with goat cheese drizzled with honey.*

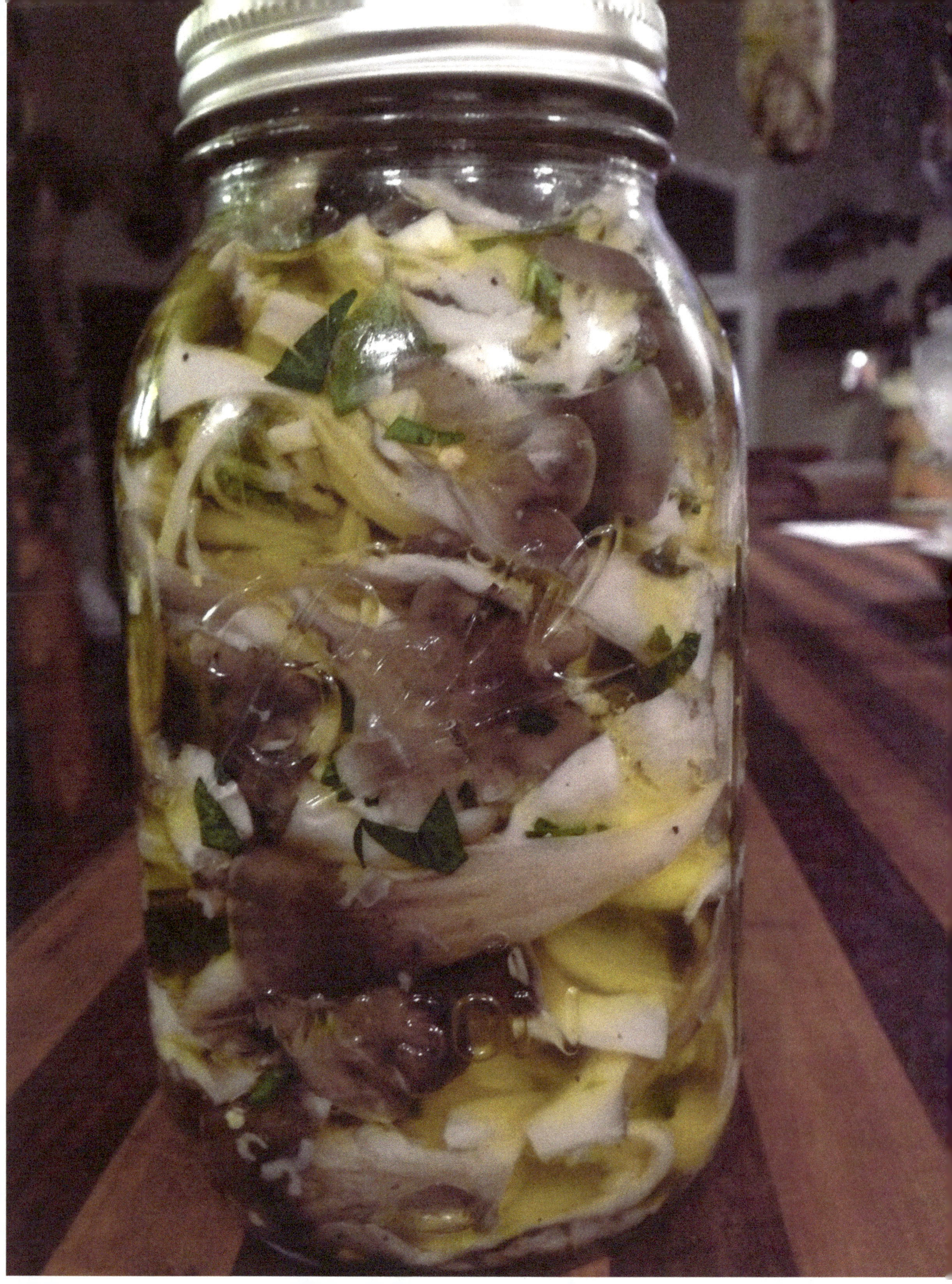

*Hen-of-the-woods mushrooms can be harvested in abundance. If you follow these steps, you can enjoy them long into the cold winter months when they're not available to pick fresh.*

## *Hen of the Woods*

5 pounds hen-of-the-woods mushrooms
1 gallon water
4 cups white vinegar
4 cups olive oil
2 tablespoons salt
1 cup apple cider vinegar
1 teaspoon oregano
1 teaspoon marjoram
1/2 cup fresh chopped mint
1/2 teaspoon black pepper
6 cloves garlic, chopped
1/2 teaspoon cayenne pepper

1. Bring water and vinegar to a boil in a large pot.
2. Add mushrooms and boil for 10 minutes.
3. Remove mushrooms and place in a colander to drain.
4. In a separate bowl, combine the olive oil, salt, apple cider vinegar, oregano, marjoram, mint, black pepper, garlic, and cayenne pepper.
5. Mix well.
6. Add blanched mushrooms and stir together.
7. Place mixture in jars and top off with the remaining oil mixture.
8. Cap the jars and boil them for ten minutes to pasteurize.
9. They will keep for 2 years.

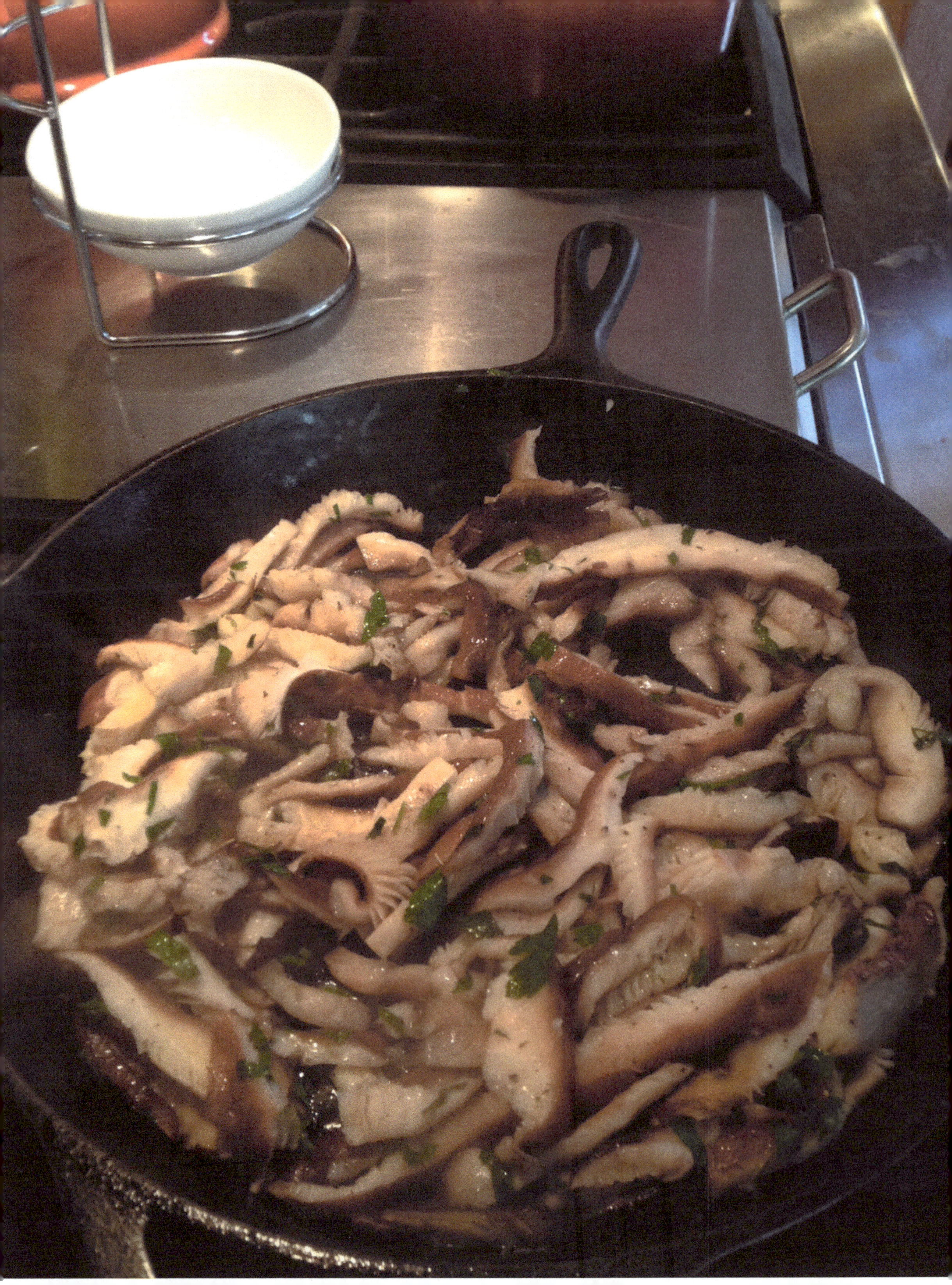

## *Sautéed Shiitakes*

10 to 15 shiitakes, chopped
2 cloves minced garalic
1 cup extra virgin olive oil
3 sprigs parsley
1/2 cup white wine

1. Mix all ingredients into sauté pan until golden brown.

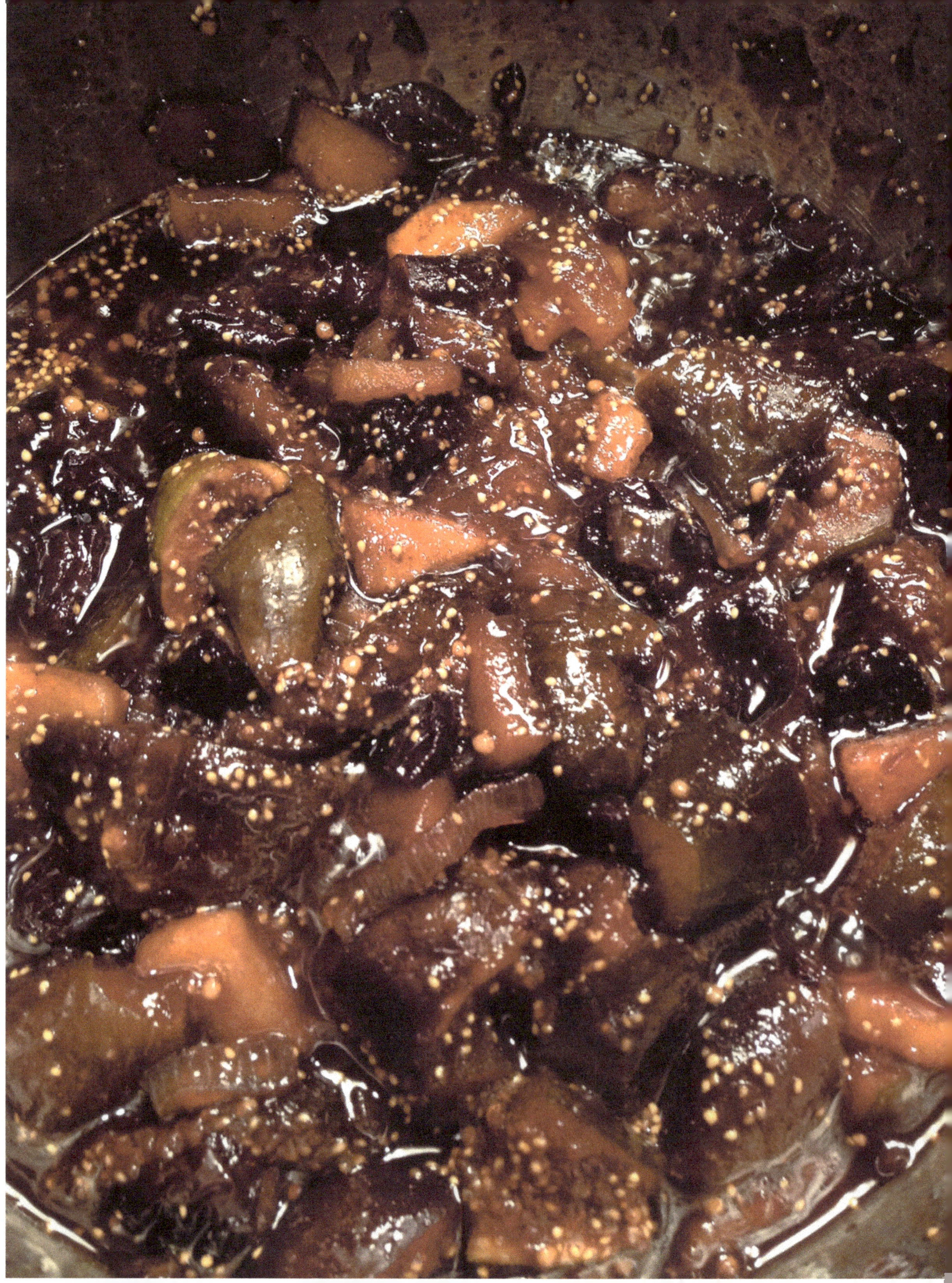

## *Fig Chutney*

2 pounds fresh semi-ripe figs, chopped
2 shallots, sliced
1 cup dark honey
1 teaspoon ground clove
1/2 teaspoon nutmeg
1/4 teaspoon salt
1/2 cup brown sugar
4 tablespoons butter

1. Place butter in sauce pot and add shallots until transparent.
2. Add diced figs, honey, brown sugar, and spices.
3. Cook down on medium heat until thick and bubbly.
4. The mixture can be ladled into jelly jars, capped and then boiled for 10 minutes.
5. They will seal and can be enjoyed for up to a year.

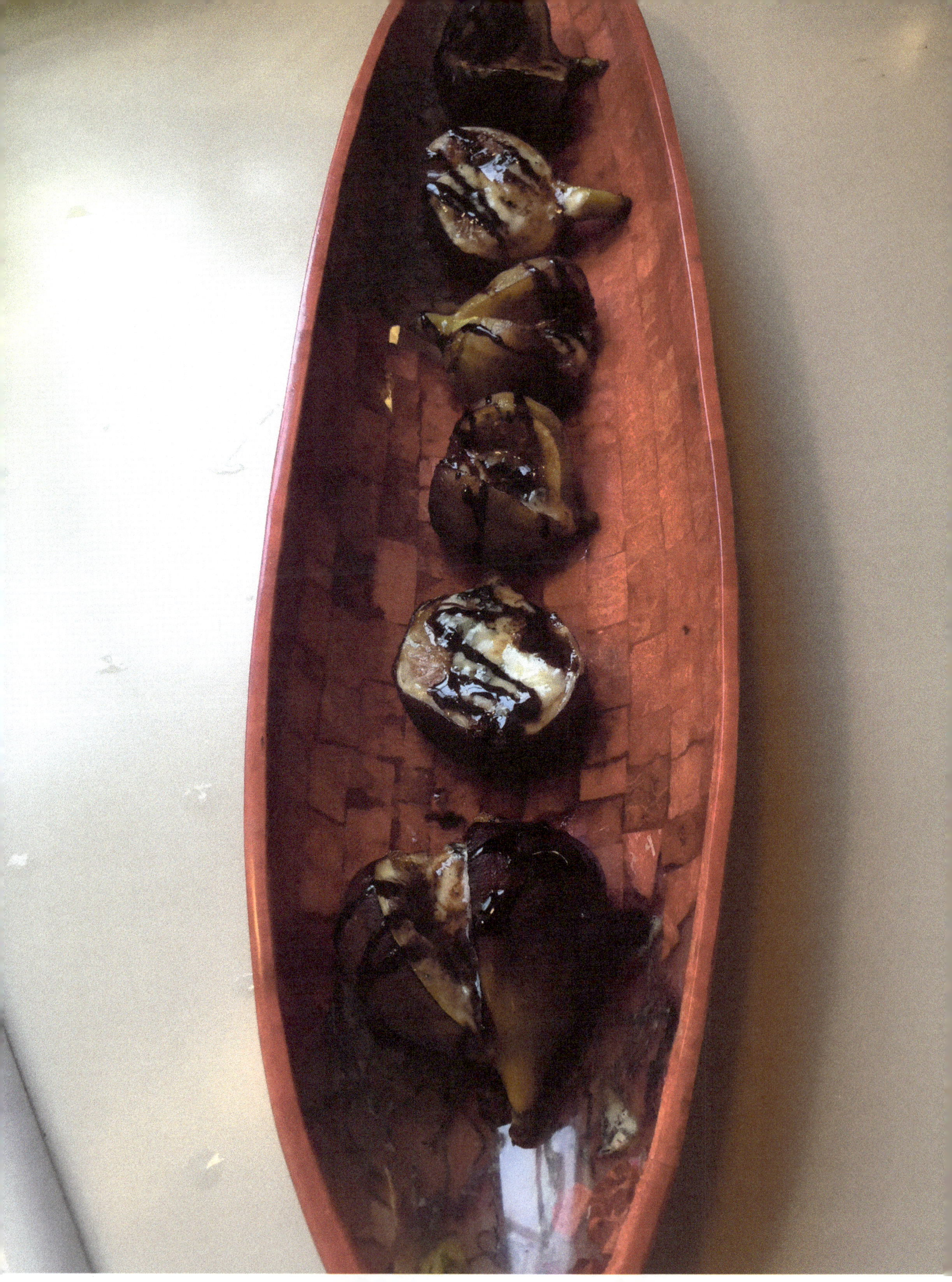

## *Stuffed Turkish Figs with Gorgonzola*

Figs
Gorganzola
Olive oil
Honey
Reduced balsamic glaze

1. Slice figs.
2. Place one piece of gorgonzola in each fig.
3. Drizzle with olive oil, reduced balsamic glaze, and honey.
4. Bake for 15 minutes at 350 degrees.

# *Sautéed Oyster Mushrooms*

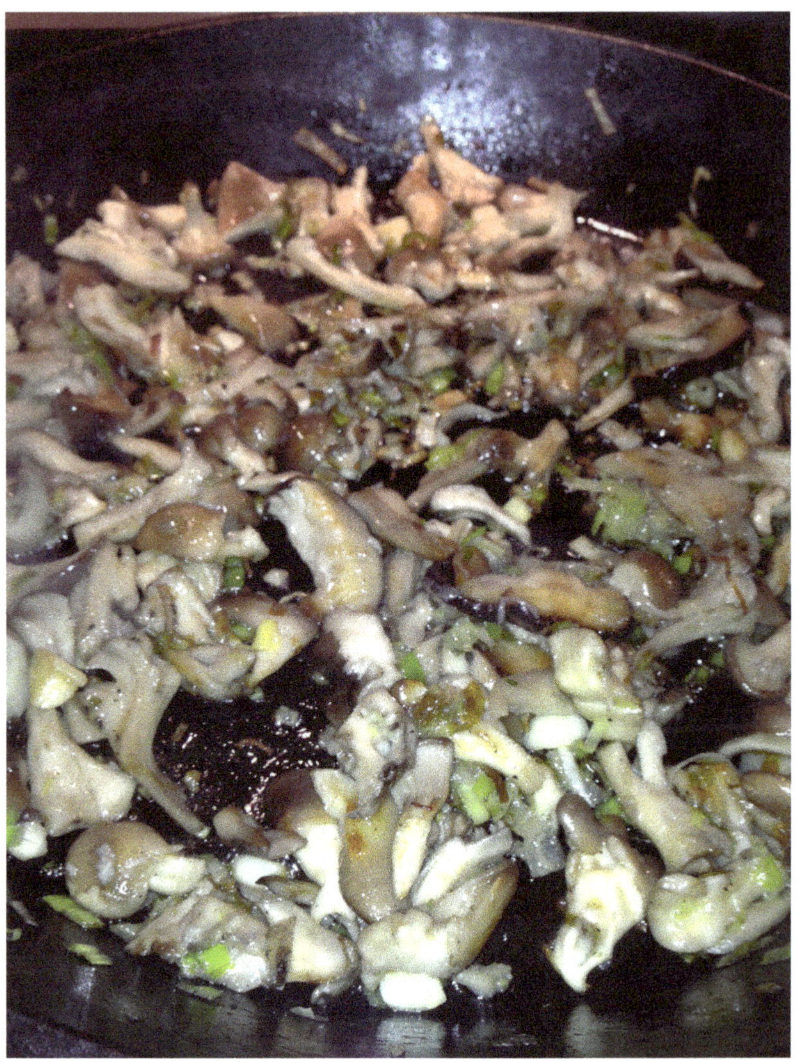

2 tablespoons butter
1/2 cup olive oil
2 cloves garlic
4 sprigs chopped parsley
Dash salt and pepper
2 cups sliced oyster mushrooms
1 cup white wine

1. In a large skillet, combine the butter, olive oil, garlic, salt, and pepper.
2. Cook over medium heat until garlic is sautéed.
3. Add sliced oyster mushrooms along with one cup of white wine.
4. Cook until golden brown.

## *Chicken Madilana*

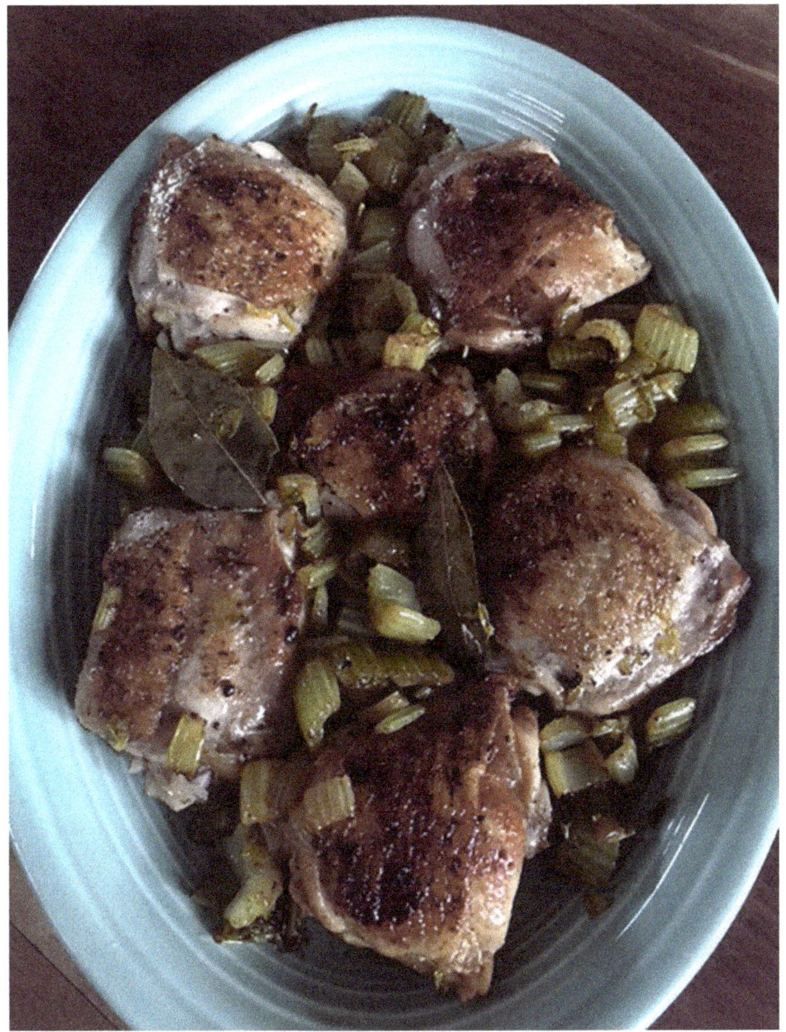

6 to 8 chicken thighs
1/2 teaspoon salt
1/2 teaspoon pepper
2 cloves garlic, crushed
1/2 teaspoon onion powder
3 cups chopped celery
2 bay leaves
Sprig of rosemary
1/2 cup chardonnay

1. Dust chicken thighs with salt, pepper, garlic powder, and onion powder.
2. Brown chicken.
3. Combine celery, garlic, bay leaves, rosemary, and chardonnay and add to chicken.
4. Cover and let cook for 25 minutes until celery starts to turn brown.
5. Serve over brown rice.

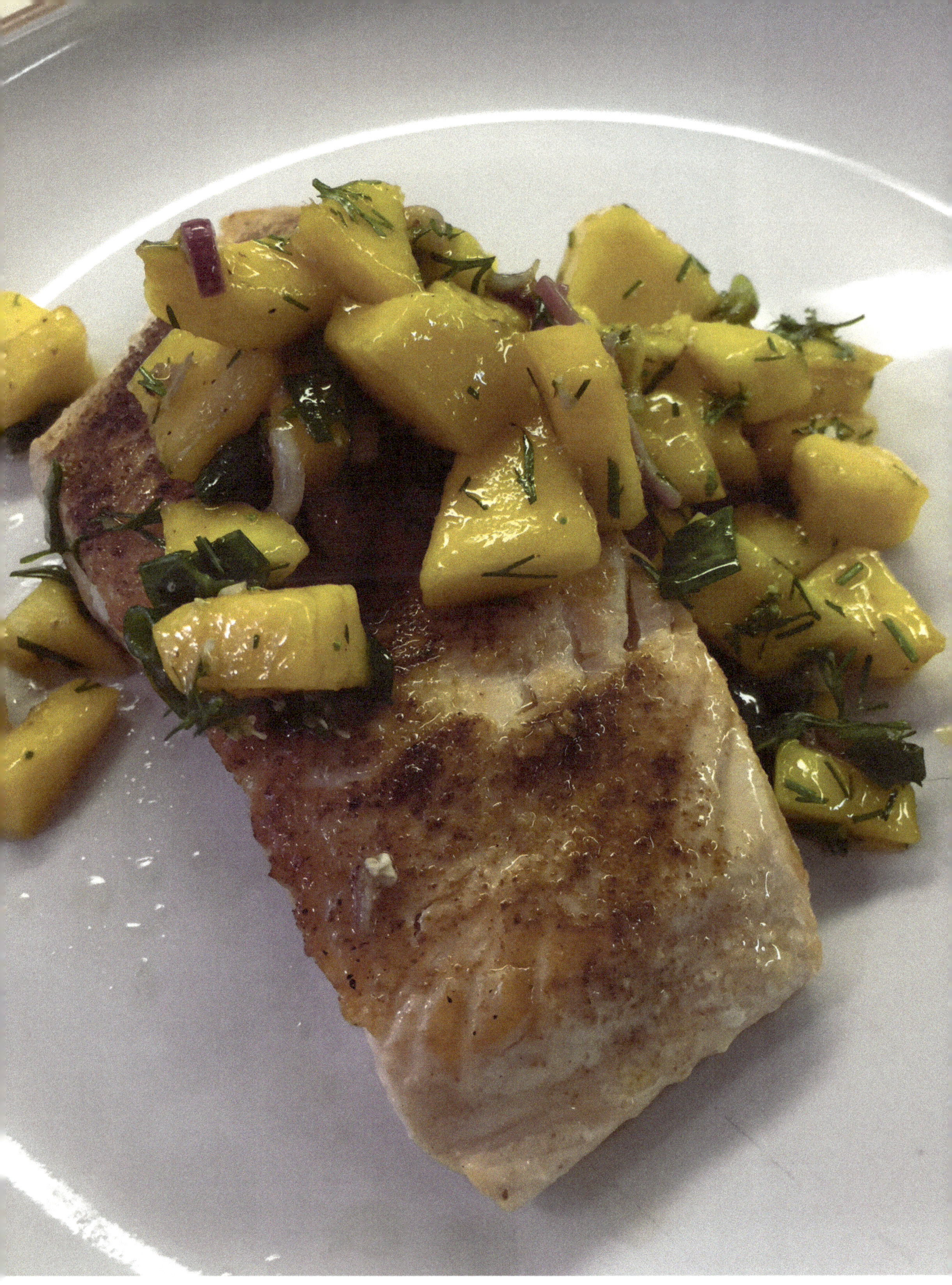

## *Grilled Wild Salmon with Mango Cilantro Salsa*

2 pounds salmon fillets
2 tablespoons olive oil
Old Bay Seasoning
1 mango, cubed
6 sprigs fresh cilantro
2 green scallions, chopped
2 tablespoons wildflower honey
1 tablespoon apple cider
Dash salt and pepper

1. Coat salmon fillets with olive oil.
2. Sprinkle with Old Bay Seasoning.
3. Place salmon on grill until golden brown.
4. Set aside.
5. In a small bowl, mix all of the other ingredients.
6. Serve salmon with salsa over the fish or on the side.

## *Smoked Salmon or Trout*

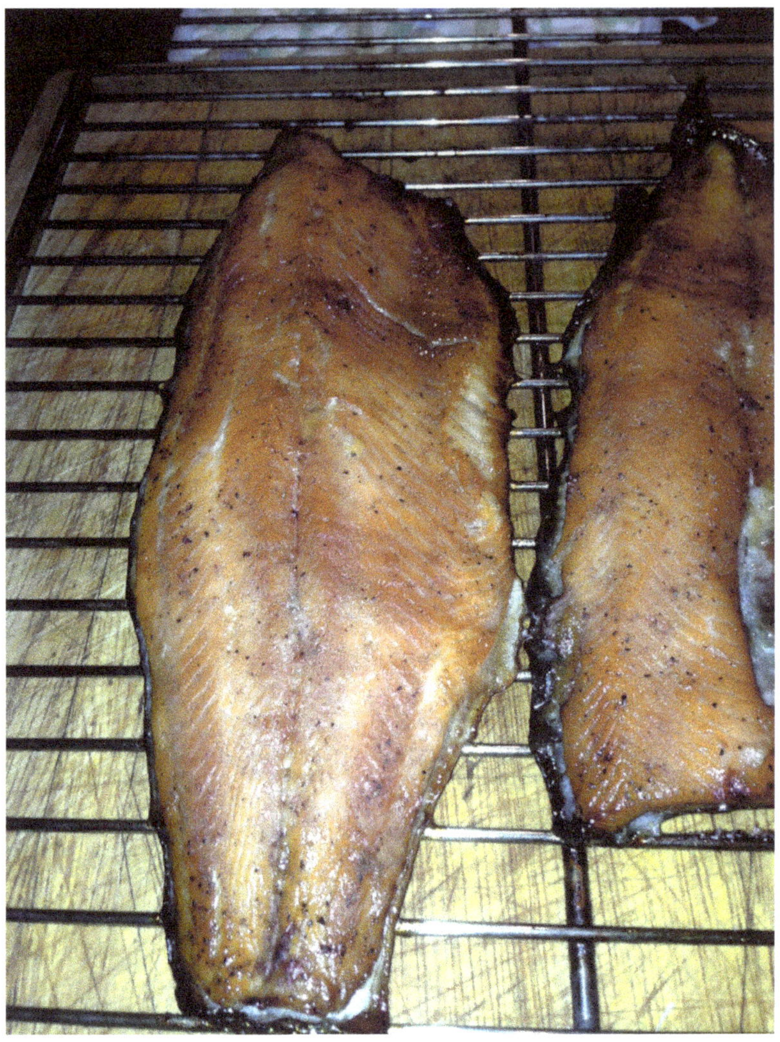

3 pounds salmon, fillet or butterflied
2 cups water
1/2 cup sea salt
1 teaspoon ginger powder
1/2 teaspoon garlic powder
1 teaspoon black pepper
1/2 cup soy sauce
1/2 cup honey

1. Mix all ingredients well and marinate salmon.
2. Place in refrigerator overnight.
3. Place salmon in smoker the following morning at 225 degrees using alder or mesquite chips.
4. Let smoke for 3 hours.
5. Cool and enjoy with horseradish sauce.

## *Apple Wood Smoked Blue Fish*

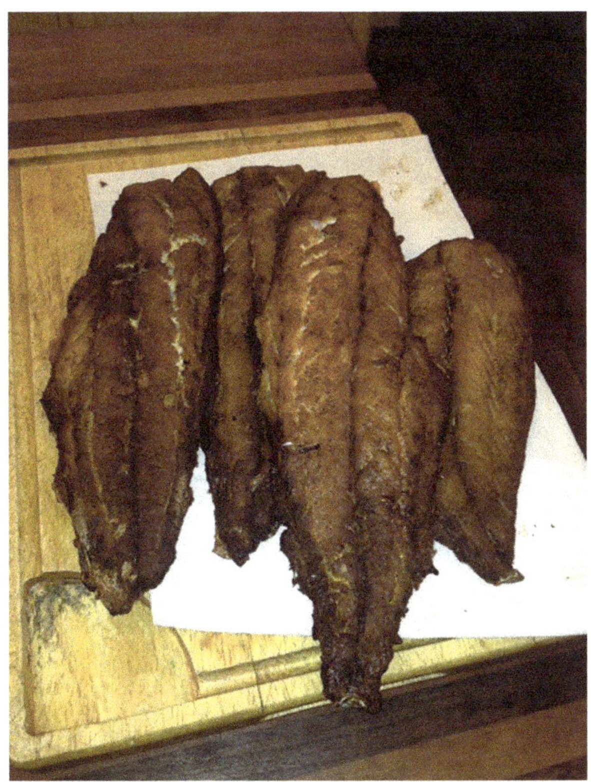

Blue fish fillets
4 cups water
1/2 cup sea salt
1/2 cup honey
1 tablespoon black pepper
1 cup apple cider

1. Place the blue fish in a mixture of all the other ingredients overnight in the refrigerator.
2. Place the fillets in a smoker with apple chips for 4 hours on low heat.

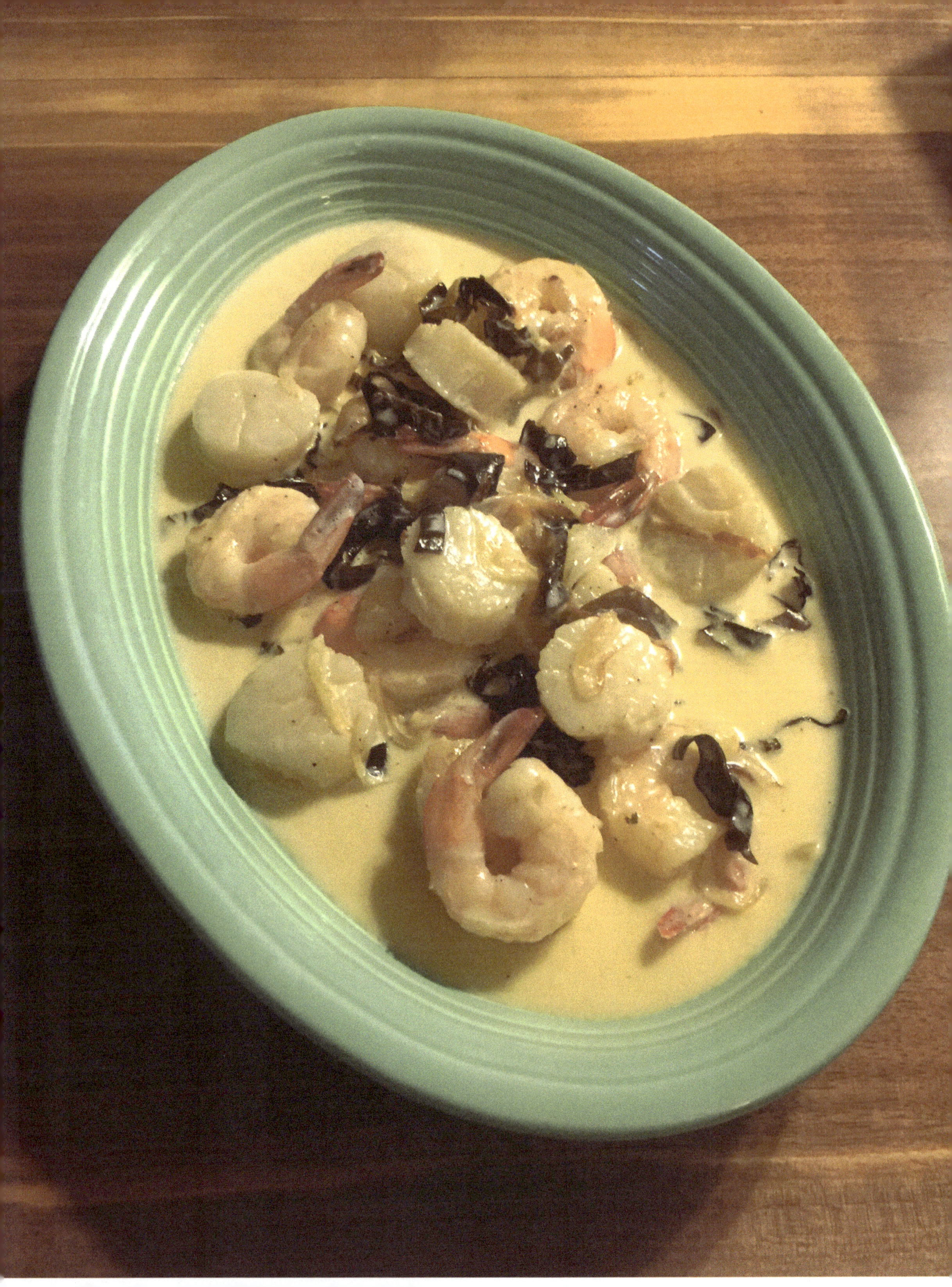

## *Black Trumpets, Scallops, and Shrimp*

2 cups black trumpets
1 cup chopped shallots
2 cups heavy cream
2 tablespoons butter
Fresh parsley
Salt and pepper
1 pound deveined and peeled shrimp
1 pound sea scallops

1. Sauté shallots in butter.
2. Add salt, pepper, shrimp, and scallops.
3. Sauté everything together for 10 minutes until the shrimp starts to brown.
4. Add black trumpets and cream.
5. Bring to a slightly bubbly mixture on medium heat.
6. Serve with risotto or brown rice.

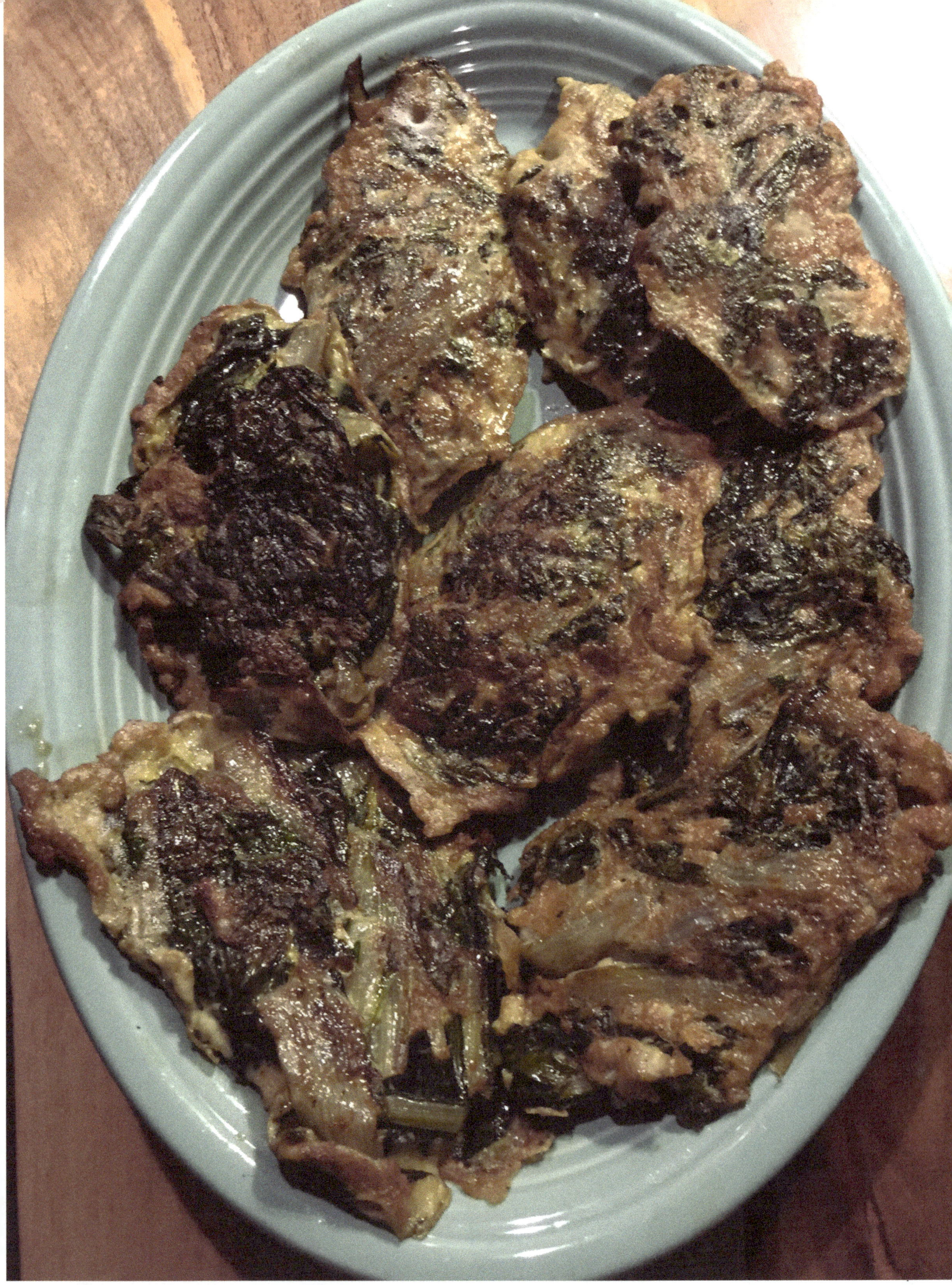

## *Mama Lucy's Swiss Chard Patties*

4 pounds Swiss chard
1/2 cup olive oil
5 eggs
1/2 teaspoon salt
1/2 teaspoon pepper
2 cloves garlic, minced

1. Sauté Swiss chard, olive oil, garlic until tender and garlic starts to brown.
2. Remove from stove.
3. In separate bowl, beat five eggs, salt, pepper, and garlic.
4. Combine Swiss chard with egg mixture.
5. Drop into oiled pan with tongs until golden brown.

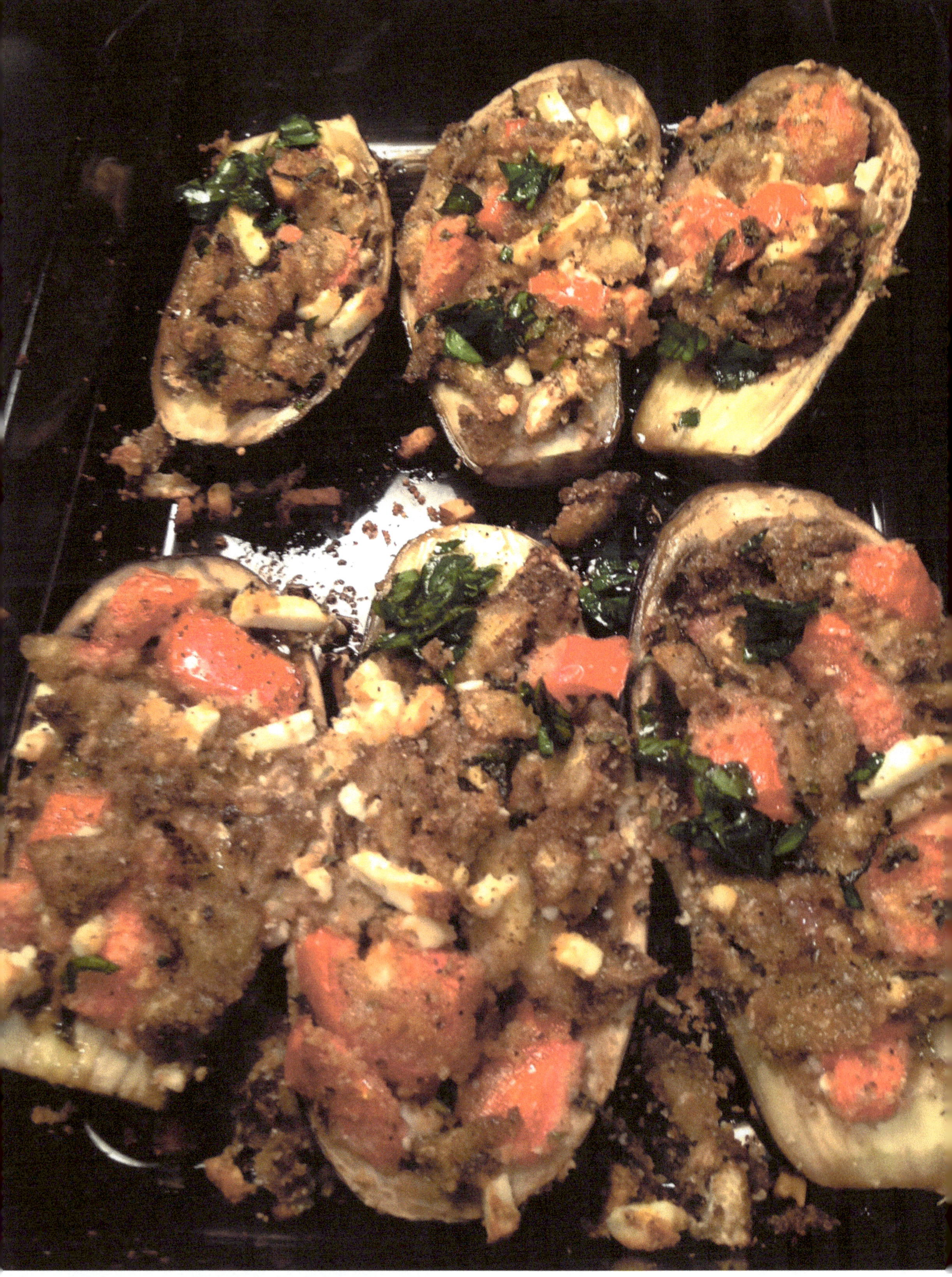

## *Baked Stuffed Eggplant*

1 eggplant
2 tomatoes, diced
1 cup bread crumbs
4 cloves garlic
Salt and pepper
6 basil leaves, chopped
1/2 cup parmesan cheese

1. Cut the eggplant in half and spoon out the pulp.
2. Dice the pulp and mix it together with all the other ingredients.
3. Place the stuffing back on the eggplant halves.
4. Drizzle with olive oil.
5. Bake at 350 degrees for 45 minutes.

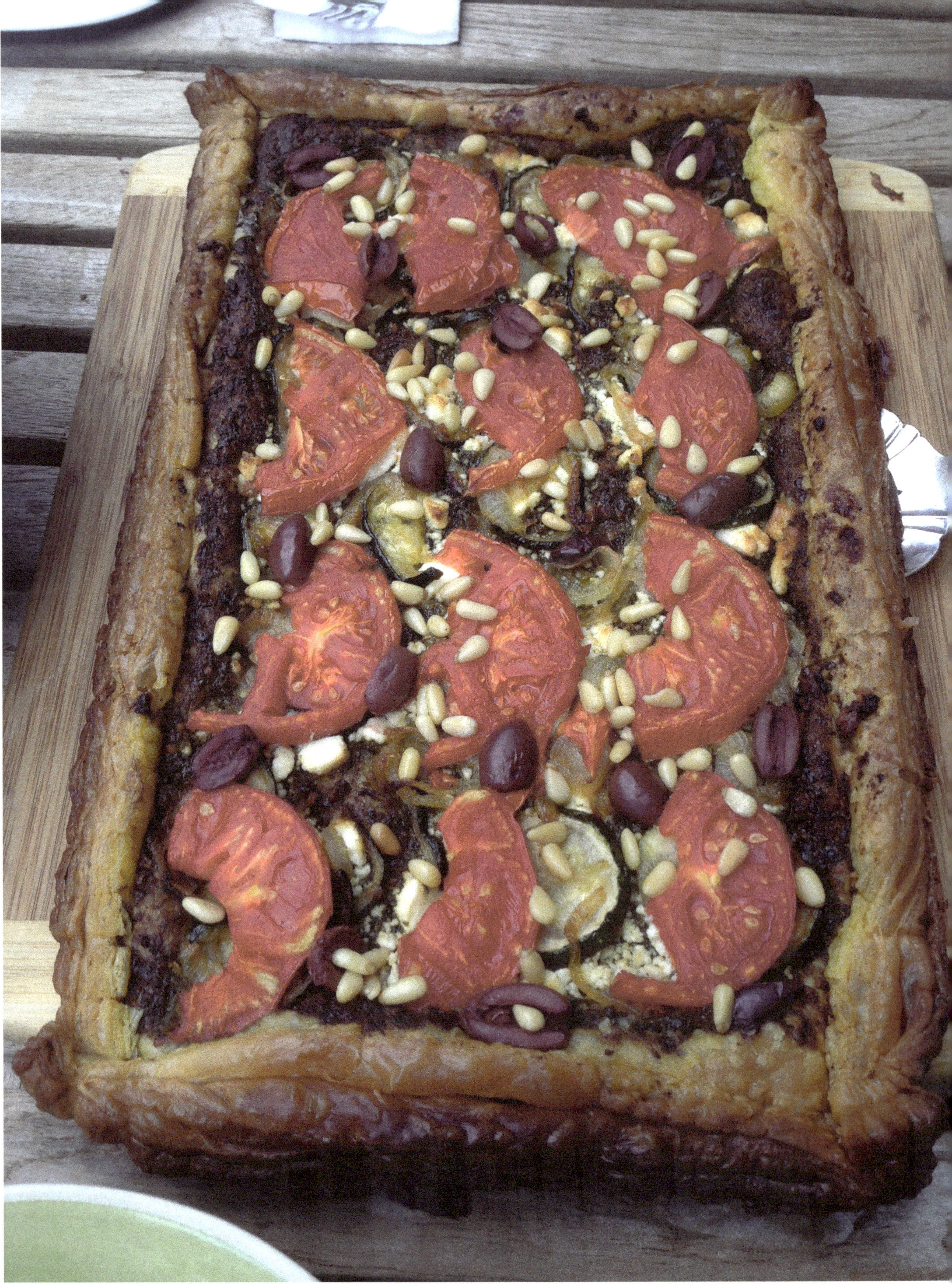

## *Tomato Zucchini Tort*

1 large phyllo dough
1/2 cup shallots
1 small zucchini, sliced
1/2 cup feta cheese
1 ripe tomato, sliced
1/2 cut pine nuts
Kalamata olives
1/2 teaspoon salt
1/2 teaspoon black pepper

1. Unroll phyllo dough onto cookie sheet.
2. Drizzle with olive oil.
3. Add chopped shallots, zucchini, feta cheese, pine nuts, olives, tomatoes, salt, and pepper.
4. Bake at 350 degrees until golden brown.

## *Steamed Spinach with Fresh Eggs*

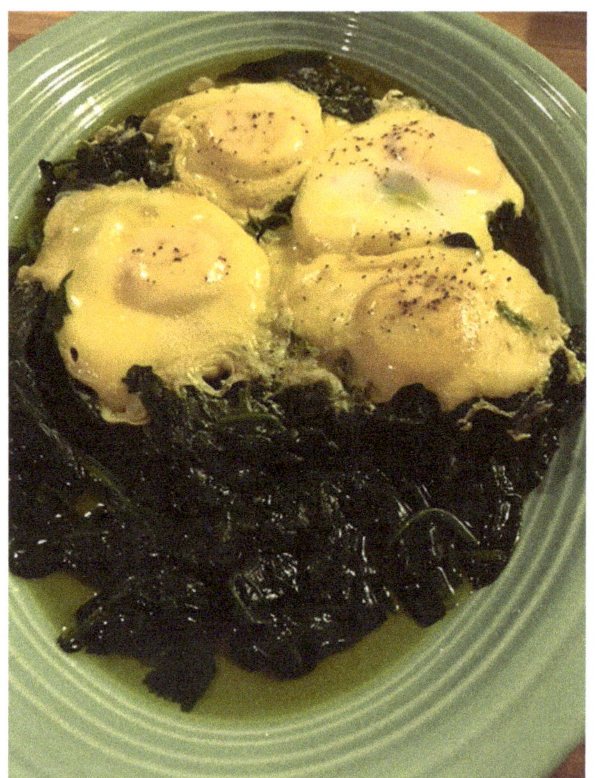

2 cloves garlic
4 tablespoons olive oil
2 cups chicken broth
3 bunches fresh spinach
3 eggs

1. Brown the garlic in the olive oil.
2. Add chicken broth and spinach.
3. Steam spinach in oil, broth, and garlic.
4. Make 4 depressions or nests in spinach.
5. Crack eggs into nests.
6. Reduce heat to medium.
7. Add salt and pepper to taste.
8. Cover until eggs are thoroughly cooked.
9. Serve with crusty bread.

*Fresh figs with Brie and comb honey on a date cracker are delicious.*

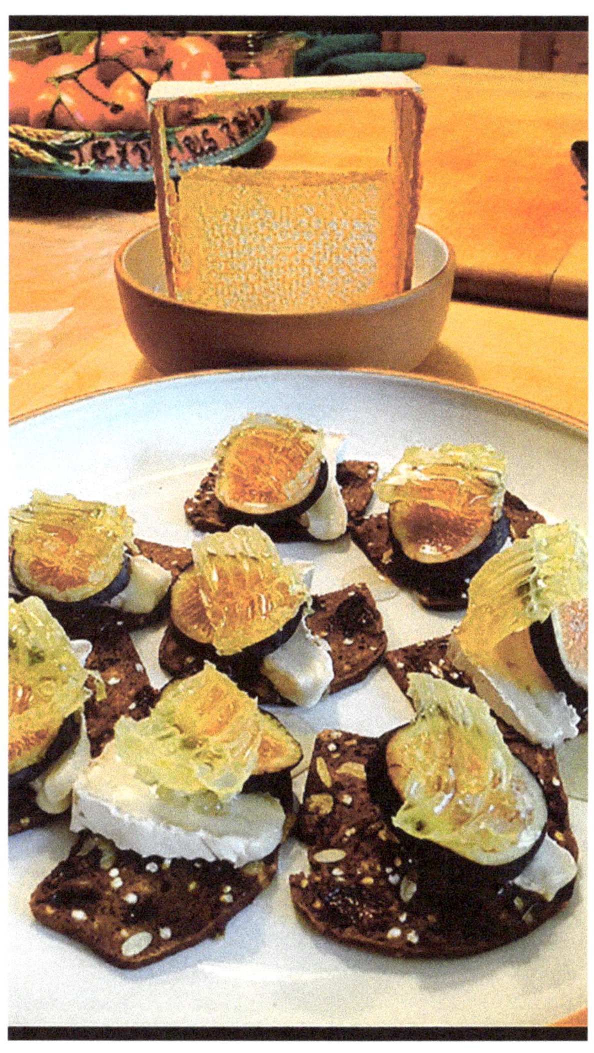

## *Lucy's Peanut Butter Honey Drops*

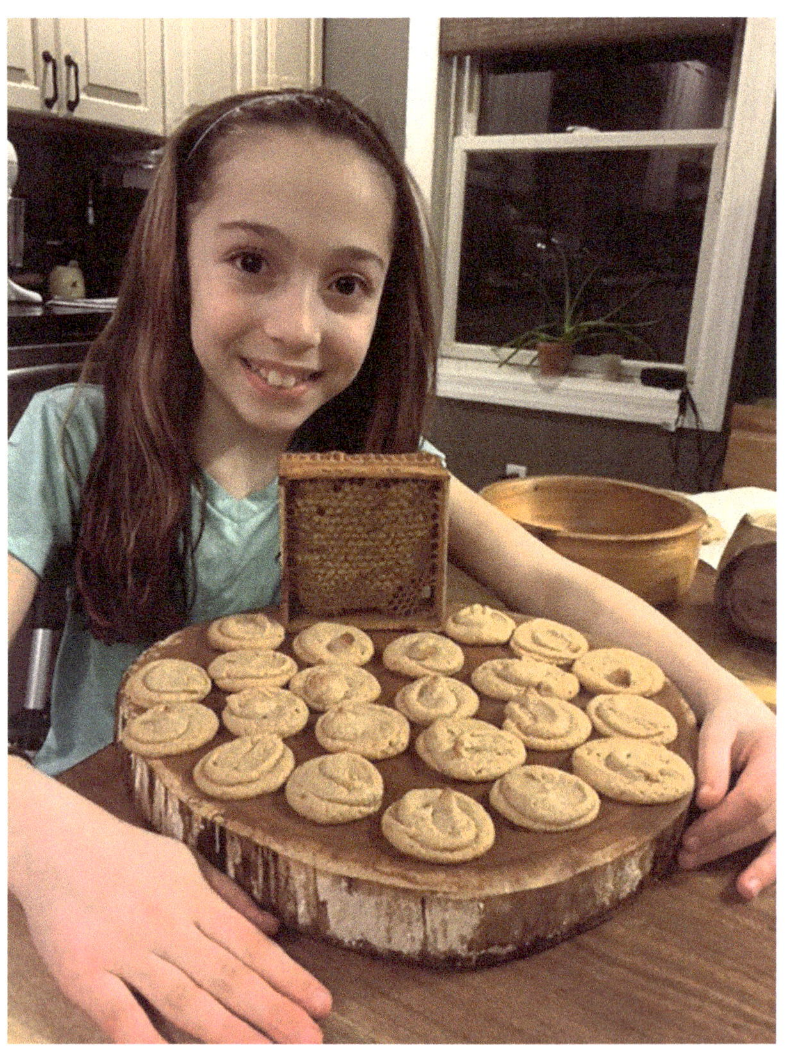

1 cup peanut butter
1 egg
1/2 cup sugar
1 teaspoon vanilla
3 tablespoons wildflower honey

1. Mix all ingredients together.
2. Place teaspoons of batter onto cookie sheet.
3. Bake at 350 degrees for 15 minutes until golden brown.

# Index

## B

### *Bees and Honey*

## C

### *Container Gardening*

# E

## *Eggs and Chickens*



# F

## *Fig Trees*

### Fishing



### Foraging



### Fruit Trees

## G

### *Gardening*

Lightning Source UK Ltd.
Milton Keynes UK
UKHW05f0523030818
326690UK00021B/715/P

9 781946 702029